DOGS IN SCHOOLS

Using a wealth of infographics and classroom examples, *Dogs in Schools* sets out the pedagogical principles that schools can employ to work with school dogs in a way that promotes the well-being of all participants and creates a safe environment for all.

This is the first book to combine theory and research with the views of experienced teachers and professionals working around the world, from the United Kingdom to India, from Australia to mainland Europe. Their perspectives illustrate the wide-ranging interest in school dogs but also highlight common concerns. For policymakers, this is a book not to ignore because it shows how dogs have the potential to make a significant contribution to children's well-being at a time of growing concern in this area. Simultaneously, the authors endorse the views of contributors who call for the introduction of humane regulations and fulsome guidance so that school dogs are viewed as sentient companions and not relegated to the latest educational fad.

This is a must-read book for all those who are serious about humane education and ensuring the well-being and happiness of both children and dogs.

Helen Lewis is an associate professor of education at Swansea University. Her research interests include animal-assisted interventions, the well-being of school dogs, and creative thinking.

Russell Grigg is Director of Initial Teacher Education at Swansea University. His research interests include teacher education and innovative pedagogy.

DOGS IN SCHOOLS

Pedagogy and Practice for Happy, Healthy, and Humane Interventions

Helen Lewis and Russell Grigg

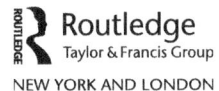
Routledge
Taylor & Francis Group

NEW YORK AND LONDON

Designed cover image: © Simon Dando

First published 2024
by Routledge
605 Third Avenue, New York, NY 10158

and by Routledge
4 Park Square, Milton Park, Abingdon, Oxon, OX14 4RN

Routledge is an imprint of the Taylor & Francis Group, an informa business

Library of Congress Cataloging-in-Publication Data
Names: Lewis, Helen (Helen E.), author. | Grigg, Russell, author.
Title: Dogs in schools : pedagogy and practice for happy, healthy, and humane interventions / Helen Lewis and Russell Grigg.
Description: New York, NY : Routledge, 2024. | Includes bibliographical references and index. |
Identifiers: LCCN 2023036307 (print) | LCCN 2023036308 (ebook) | ISBN 9781032189390 (hardback) | ISBN 9781032189383 (paperback) | ISBN 9781003257073 (ebook)
Subjects: LCSH: Animals in education. | Dogs–Therapeutic use. | Human-animal relationships.
Classification: LCC LB1044.9.A65 L49 2024 (print) | LCC LB1044.9.A65 (ebook) | DDC 371.33–dc23/eng/20230811
LC record available at https://lccn.loc.gov/2023036307
LC ebook record available at https://lccn.loc.gov/2023036308

ISBN: 9781032189390 (hbk)
ISBN: 9781032189383 (pbk)
ISBN: 9781003257073 (ebk)

DOI: 10.4324/9781003257073

For Grace and Sofie, and for Tom and Mia, with love.

CONTENTS

FOREWORD

Dogs in Schools: Pedagogy and Practice for Happy, Healthy, and Humane Interventions is a comprehensive textbook, drawing on careful examination of the evolutionary continuity of humane canine relationships, and the latest research and best practices.

School can be hard for many students. It can be difficult to navigate the academic and social expectations in such settings. This book illuminates the power of the human-canine connection, allowing us a compelling window into how our amazing canine colleagues can make a difference in the lives of children. This book moves our knowledge forward on many levels by offering numerous international and culturally responsive case examples to vividly explore the potential of canine supported education and clinical interventions.

This wonderful read offers the critical knowledge needed to incorporate dogs into educational environments and is packed with practical pedagogical frameworks and key ethical considerations for schools and educators who wish to introduce dogs into their classrooms. This useful compendium draws on carefully documented input from experts in the field, alongside years of practical experience from its authors. This results in a roadmap for schools to create successful, effective, safe, and ethically supported dog programmes.

This book in not only for educators and school administrators but also provides dog trainers, animal welfare advocates, and canine handlers interested in the well-being of dogs with the tools to ensure positive outcomes for their canine partners while optimising the impact of these interventions on children's academic and social-emotional development.

As the field of canine-assisted interventions has gained recognition and expanded to complex educational and clinical settings, fidelity to best practice guidelines is critical to ensure desired outcomes. This new offering is highly recommended as the go to source for educational settings that seek to establish healthy and humane environments for both students, teachers, staff, and dogs. By integrating these guidelines and recommendations, schools can demonstrate contemporary and innovative attention to evidence-supported practice centring both the student experience and canine well-being.

Incorporating dogs into the complexities of a school setting is also not without numerous challenges, and whether you are a teacher, educational counsellor, or school administrator, 'Dogs in Schools' offers in its carefully constructed chapters not only the foundational knowledge needed to understand the practical, operational considerations, but also to appreciate the species themselves and the historical significance of dogs in school settings.

Philip Tedeschi, LCSW
Clinical Professor
Institute for Human-Animal Connection *Affiliated Faculty & Director Emeritus*
Institute for Animal Sentience and Protection, *Co-Director*
Sturm College of Law – Animal Law Program, *Affiliated Faculty*
University of Denver, Graduate School of Social Work

ACKNOWLEDGEMENTS

We are grateful to **Dr. Janet Oostendorp-Godfrey** for her ongoing contribution to our projects on school dogs, to **Tom Bradraw**[1] for his wonderful sketches, to **Simon Dando** for capturing Barney the dog so beautifully as the cover image (in this case we hope people do judge our book by its cover!), and finally to our colleagues at Swansea University for their continued support.

We would like to thank the following undergraduate and postgraduate students from Swansea University, UK, for helping to enrich the content of this book, particularly Chapter 9. They provided valuable input, undertook research into aspects of AAE, showed genuine respect towards the dogs they encountered, and provided feedback on ideas and approaches.

Bethany Hill, Lydia Morgan, Marikris De-Leon, Shaun Witts, Anaya Rideout, Finn Reekie-Evans, Katarzyna Rees-Jauke, Sam Spurr, Amy Rattenbury, Alisha Gill, Lois Taylor, Lauren Reynolds, Danielle Willmott, Megan Driscoll, Abbie Johnson, Ella West, Natasha Thomas, Natalie Onwualu, Carys Ellis, and Carys Richards.

Thanks are also given to **Dr. Phillip Tedeschi, Jen Pearson, and the faculty and students** who were part of the 2022 Canine Assisted Intervention Specialist programme at University of Denver, Colorado. These sessions provided much food for thought when considering how to understand and respect the human-canine bond.

We would also like to give our thanks to **Dr. Risë VanFleet, Tracie Faa-Thompson and the wonderful community of the International Institute of Animal Assisted Play Therapy**®; not, their work on positive, playful interactions is always an inspiration.

We are grateful to the team at Routledge for their support, particularly Anna Moore, Alison MacFarlane, Georgina Clutterbuck and Sumati Agarwal.

And finally, our pages are full of stories and images of the wonderful dogs who enrich both our lives and those of our pupils. To **Carlo, Scarlet, Obie, Copper, Honey, Idun, Soef, Uni, Nemi, Šapa, Stella, Rollo, Barney, Tish, Toby, Dottie, Murren, Barnie, Bug, Java, Pearl, Murphy, Aled, Rafa and Flash, and all those school dogs who are not named individually but who play an important role**, we thank you for all you do, and the difference you make to so many people.

NOTE

1 https://scribeyak.com/sketchnotes

ABOUT THE CONTRIBUTORS

We are very grateful to the following contributors, who have shared their experiences with us. The examples that they provided have brought great depth to this book, particularly Part Two.

Dr. Sunday Agbonika is the founder of Dogalov Human Support Initiative, a Non-Profit Organization in Nigeria. He is a Veterinary Surgeon, with DVM degree from Ahmadu Bello University in Nigeria and holds a CHAIS (Certificate as a Human Animal Intervention Specialist) from Oakland University, in Michigan, the United States.

Nicky Barendrecht-Jenken is founder of Stichting AAI-maatje, a non-profit organisation based in Gouda (South Holland). Its goals are to promote responsible collaboration with dogs in educational settings and Dog Assisted Reading, as an affiliate group of Reading Education Assistance Dogs®, operated by the Intermountain Therapy Animals (ITA).

Vicki Cutting is a teacher who has worked in Special Educational Needs contexts for over 30 years. Her expertise lies in the areas of Emotional Health and Well-being. She is a qualified Children and Young People's 'Improved Access to Psychological Therapies' worker and part of an Additional Support Team (where referrals to work with the dog are triaged). She also has a Counselling Diploma and is an Advanced Drawing and Talking Practitioner. Vicki has qualifications in Animal Assisted Therapy qualifications from The Society for Companion Animal Studies and Animal Assisted Play Therapy (IIAAPT) and has completed the Autism Family Dog workshops from Dogs for Good. She currently works with her dog Wilf.

Geraldine Foley is headteacher of Marlborough Primary School in Cardiff, Wales. She has been a headteacher since 2004 and has been bringing her family dog, Rollo, into school since 2019.

Katie Howells and **Amber Roach** are dog trainers for Burns By Your Side, the reading with dogs scheme run by The John Burns Foundation in Kidwelly, South Wales. Working under the standards of Animal Assisted Intervention International, they use positive reinforcement methods, to train learning support dogs and their handlers to go into educational settings. The scheme, running since 2016, aims to build self-esteem and confidence in young learners, to help build a positive relationship with books. Burns By Your Side currently has 80 volunteer teams between South Wales and The Republic of Ireland, with 30 more expected to qualify by the end of 2023.

Sara Karlberg has been working with animal-assisted interventions in Sweden since 2008. She has worked both as a handler for social working dogs and trained pet teams within the field. She comes from a media background, but moved into dog training in 2007, and is undertaking a master's degree in environmental psychology with a focus on animal-assisted interventions. She is currently one of four partners in a research project with the Swedish University of Agriculture studying the health-economic benefits of school dogs working with children with problematic absence from school.

Poorvaja Kumar is based in New Delhi, India. She is an internationally certified Canine Trainer, Behaviourist, and Veterinary Assistant who works with therapy dogs (certified in Animal Assisted Therapy). Poorvaja has master's degrees in Social Psychology and Social work and is an experienced researcher. In 2016, she started 'Humans of Canines' dedicated to improving relationship between humans, pet-parents, and dogs. The services provided include canine assisted activities, canine therapy, and canine-led education.

Adele Lau is the founder of Animal-Assisted Interactions Singapore. Adele is a lawyer who has been working on animal welfare-related matters since called to the Singapore Bar in 2016. Realising that the law was a more reactive rather than a preventative tool to address animal welfare issues, she made the move to another department to work on animal welfare and management policies and legislation. Adele then took on the role of senior manager at the Centre of Animal Rehabilitation under the Animal & Veterinary Service at the National Parks Board of Singapore. During her time there, she continued to work on animal welfare policies, organised webinars, gave lectures on animal law, as well as designed and implemented animal-assisted programmes for youth from social service agencies. Since 2016, Adele has been pursuing further education in animal-assisted interventions. She currently sits on the board of the International Association for Human-Animal Interaction Organizations (IAHAIO). In 2022, Adele completed her Masters in Animal Law with the Centre of Animal Law Studies under the Animal Law Advocates Scholarship from the Lewis & Clark Law School.

Ceri Littlewood has been a headteacher at Oldcastle Primary school in Wales for 18 months following a varied teaching career of 23 years. Ceri was keen to put forward a proposal to school governors regarding a school well-being dog and has been delighted with the response that Barney has had with pupils, parents, and staff in Oldcastle Primary.

Katja Renaud Løvnes is a child and youth worker in Norway. She works with children with diverse needs such as Tourette's Syndrome, anxiety, and literacy challenges. Katja is passionate about working with children and animals and feels that the interaction between them provides magical moments in an otherwise demanding existence for many of the students. Besides her work at school, she also likes looking after the animals on the family farm, breeding copperdog puppies.

Roz Rimes is a passionate and experienced Canine-Assisted Educator with first-hand experience of the well-being benefits of Therapy Dog interactions with young people experiencing anxiety and at risk of self-harm. Roz has expertise across a diverse range of settings including working and volunteering with LGBTQIA+ and CALD communities, and in primary, secondary, and tertiary contexts. She has been enhancing student well-being with her highly trained and certified Therapy/Wellbeing Dogs since 2018 at the University of Melbourne. Roz holds a Master of Education Policy (International) and a Master of Applied Positive Psychology from the University of Melbourne, along with numerous advanced Animal-Assisted Therapy qualifications from Lead the Way Institute and La Trobe University.

Dr. Marieanna le Roux is a retired Research Psychologist from Stellenbosch University in South Africa. Her research interests include various aspects of human-animal interaction. Marieanna, a lifelong member of Pets as Therapy and ex-Chairperson, has been involved with PAT South Africa since 2006.

Dr. Sharyn Spicer is a lecturer in the Department of Sociology, at the University of the Western Cape (UWC). She is the undergraduate coordinator and launched a new inter-disciplinary post-graduate Human Animal Studies module in 2020 called Animals, Society & the Environment. Her latest research focuses on the relationships, interactions and entanglements between humans and other animal species. She runs TUFCAT, a UWC-based animal welfare project.

Mojca Trampuš is a highly experienced math teacher and home tutor at the Secondary School of Education, Gymnasium and Art Gymnasium, Ljubljana, Slovenia. She and her dogs work with students of different ages, including those training to be teachers. Mojca is also a member of the largest Slovenian volunteer association of therapeutic dogs, Tačke pomagačke.

Dr. Leigh Adams Tucker is a registered Clinical Psychologist and Senior Lecturer in the Department of Psychology at the University of the Western Cape in South Africa. Her research focuses on child development, youth mental health, and animal-assisted interventions in practice. She is the ex-Chairperson, and head of Research and Education for the non-profit organisation, Pets as Therapy (South Africa).

Jen VonLintel is a school counsellor at B.F. Kitchen Elementary in Loveland, Colorado. She has been implementing AAIs since 2011. During the summer, she works with older students as an adjunct instructor for the Institute for Human-Animal Connection at the University of Denver Graduate School of Social Work. She sits on the Board of Directors for the Association of Animal-Assisted Intervention Professionals (AAAIP) and is the administrator for the Facebook Group, School Therapy Dogs, which has 10,000 members world-wide.

Nurstasha Arifin Wong is a doctoral candidate of the Department of Anthropology at the University of Chicago. She studies the care and control of 'Singapore Specials,' local landrace stray dogs, across petrochemical industrial complexes and healthcare facilities in Singapore. Her research draws from feminist science and technology studies, medical anthropology, and multispecies ethnography. She is currently the Director of Animal-Assisted Interactions Singapore.

ABOUT THE AUTHORS

Dr. Helen Lewis is an associate professor of education at Swansea University. After studying animal and human behaviour at university, she became a primary school teacher and has worked in education for over 20 years. Part of her role in the university includes leading a module on animals in educational contexts, and she undertakes original research into practices relating to dogs in schools. She has written widely in this area, including co-authoring *Tails from the Classroom* (Crown House, 2021). She has a canine intervention specialist certificate from the University of Denver and a certificate in animal-assisted play therapy from the International Institute of Animal Assisted Play Therapy®. Her own three dogs support her and her students' well-being in playful ways. You can follow her on Twitter @HEL71_

Dr. Russell Grigg is Director of Initial Teacher Education at Swansea University and leads the Department of Education and Childhood Studies' Centre for Research into Practice. He has considerable experience as a teacher educator, education researcher, and school inspector. He has written extensively across a range of subjects, including pedagogy, creativity, school inspection, and the history of education. He is the author of the best-selling *Becoming an Outstanding Primary Teacher* (Routledge, 3rd edn, 2022) and co-author of *Tails from the Classroom* (Crown House, 2021). In his spare time, he collects old books and follows Swansea City FC. You can follow him on Twitter, @RussellGrigg.

LIST OF FIGURES

LIST OF PHOTOGRAPHS

LIST OF TABLES

INTRODUCTION

We started to write this book during the most significant challenge to global health in modern times. As the COVID-19 pandemic affected people's mental health, many people turned to their companion animals for comfort. Reports from around the world showed how dogs helped to take people's minds off negative thoughts, alleviated loneliness, and provided a sense of purpose (World Economic Forum, 2021). Following the easing of restrictions, schools and other educational settings increasingly focused on children and young people's well-being as a priority. Given the existing evidence, which suggests that dogs can make a positive contribution to this, it is not surprising to see the increasing interest in school dogs (Lewis et al., 2022). Recent studies have been reported in Australia (e.g., Henderson et al., 2020), Austria (e.g., Schretzmayer et al., 2017), Canada (e.g., Syrnyk et al., 2022), Finland (Meurer, 2019), Italy (e.g., Uccheddu et al., 2019), Portugal (e.g., Canelo, 2020), Slovenia (e.g., Torkar et al., 2020), South Africa (e.g., Le Roux et al., 2014), the United Kingdom (e.g., Steel, 2022; Steel et al., 2021), and the United States (e.g., Linder et al., 2018). In writing this book, we want to celebrate some of the innovative practices that are taking place around the world. However, one of our core messages is that bringing dogs into school is not a cure-all for children's poor well-being and there is a danger that the hype associated with school dogs overshadows what the most reliable research tells us. Above all, we want to emphasise that any intervention, particularly one that involves other-than-human animals, should try to ensure the happiness, health, and well-being of all participants.

We could have written this book to include many different species of animals which feature in educational settings. The choice of school dogs is partly personal. One of us (HL) has long been an avid dog lover and has for many years involved her own dogs in her work in varied educational settings. Another reason for choosing dogs is practical, because they are one of the most popular animals found in school and yet there is a lack of regulation and guidance for teachers. A third reason is more philosophical. We believe that there is a need to reframe the narrative around school dogs, reflected for example in the language that we use. We are mindful of not objectifying dogs (e.g., by referring to the dog as 'it') and we talk about 'involving' rather that 'using' them in our practice. Dogs are not tools or resources like pencils, software or reading schemes. They are individuals with thoughts, feelings, wants, needs, and desires. This means that we should not over-generalise when discussing dogs, just as we would not do so with children. In short, our book is a 'cautionary tail' which is a warning that while there is considerable appeal and joy in bringing dogs into school, there are also significant challenges which warrant very careful thought.

In broader society, there are regular reminders of how dogs are neglected, mistreated and abused. During 2022, record numbers of dogs were reportedly dumped at UK sanctuaries, greyhounds were forced to race during a deadly heatwave, and puppies stolen from breeding centres to be used for experiments in laboratories (Newkey-Burden, 2022). Kalof (2007) even coined the term 'misothery' (combining the Greek words for 'hatred' and 'animal') to describe the body of negative ideas

DOI: 10.4324/9781003257073-1

about animals and nature. While dogs are valued and loved in many households around the world, there are places where they are more welcome than others.

In 2022, one online insurance company composed a Dog Friendly Index comprising 51 countries, based on a range of metrics, including the number of dog-friendly hotels and vets, data from the Animal Protection Index rating (e.g., prohibition of animal suffering, and recognition of animal sentience) and animal rights legislation (Nash, 2022). The fact that a country has passed animal rights legislation is a step in the right direction but is, of course, no guarantee of consistent implementation of such laws. In 2008, the authorities in Switzerland introduced compulsory 4-hour practical training for dog owners with their pets after a young boy was killed by a group of Pitbull terriers near Zurich. However, this was controversially abandoned in 2016 when it was reported that there was no marked change in the behaviour of dog owners who had taken the course, many had missed the training altogether, and incidents of dog biting had not declined. Even within so-called dog-loving countries serious questions are asked around canine welfare.

The welfare and well-being of all participants should be the overriding consideration and we recognise the well-founded arguments against bringing dogs and other animals into schools. The success of any educational intervention is based on sound principles and shared values, which we discuss throughout the book. We argue that these include acknowledging the sentience of dogs, which means valuing their ability to experience emotions and recognising that they possess a degree of consciousness.

The language associated with the involvement of animals in education and other sectors can be confusing. One of us (HL) recently joined more than a hundred delegates to agree upon a shared understanding of key terms to describe animals working in support roles for people with support needs (Howell et al., 2022). We have opted for Canine Assisted Education (CAE) to describe interventions which feature dogs within educational settings for the purpose of achieving specific educational goals. This is very much an adaption of the American Veterinary Medical Association's definition of Animal-assisted education (AAE).[1] The important point to stress is that such interventions should have purpose and meaning. And our view is that the overarching purpose should be to foster happy, humane and healthy relationships between dogs and humans.

STRUCTURE OF THE BOOK

The book is divided into three parts: Part One (Chapters 1–3) focuses on context, research, and theory. The development of the human-dog attachment over the centuries is the subject of Chapter 1. Changes in animal-related attitudes are discussed including the rise in the practice of pet-keeping and, in modern times, the background to the growing interest in animal-assisted interventions. Chapter 2 reviews what research tells us about the benefits and challenges of bringing dogs into schools. It focuses on three areas which have most attracted scholarly interest: reading with dogs, the extent to which dogs support children with social and communication difficulties, and more broadly, how dogs enhance children's well-being. The chapter also highlights the limitations of research, notably the lack of rigour and the small-scale nature of most studies. Whether dogs should be brought into schools is discussed in Chapter 3. We support such practices provided certain preconditions are met relating to selection protocols: training, risk assessment, goal setting, monitoring, and evaluating. We also argue that if children are to benefit from the presence of dogs, educators need to follow a set of humane principles for effective pedagogy. First, they should respect everyone's feelings, spaces and thoughts, including the dogs. Second, they should build positive relationships. Third, they should create opportunities for playful interaction. And finally, they should ensure that the environment is safe for all.

Part Two (Chapters 4–7) explores the grounded experiences of contributors working in the field. Through personal networks and social media, we asked individuals in Spain, the Netherlands, Norway, Slovenia, Sweden, Wales, England, South Africa, Nigeria, Colorado (the United States), Singapore, Hong Kong, India, and Australia for their views on what is working well and the challenges they face in their respective contexts. We also wanted to know what impact the presence of dogs is having in their jurisdictions, and to celebrate their work in the field.

These stories are best regarded as snapshots of achievements and challenges rather than inclusive portraits. In conventional research methodology, they are more like field notes rather than case studies. We make no attempt to delve into the details of each case and the degree of contextual information varies considerably. Nonetheless, we value the individual contributions for providing authentic voices and perspectives on common issues. The contributors do not claim that what they report is representative of CAE within their respective countries.

Part Three (Chapters 8–10) provides guidance on planning, implementing and evaluating CAE. Chapter 8 focuses on the issue of selecting the right dog, matched to the needs of the children and the needs of the dog. It also compares models of practice (e.g., visiting dogs/permanent dogs) and draws on examples from schemes such as Burns By Your Side based in Wales. Chapter 9 discusses implementation, including providing practical guidance around risk assessment, animal welfare needs, and health and safety. How to understand canine communication, and plan for playful learning is considered. And finally, Chapter 10 details how to conduct research and evaluate dog assisted activities. It discusses key concepts, including a Theory of Change, causes and correlations, and research methods such as observations, interviews, surveys, randomised control trials, and quasi-experimental studies.

NOTE

1 'A planned and structured intervention directed and/or delivered by educational and related service professional with specific academic or educational goals.' https://www.avma.org/resources-tools/avma-policies/animal-assisted-interventions-definitions.

REFERENCE

Newkey-Burden, C. (2022). Britain's treatment of pets shows we're anything but a nation of dog lovers' *iNews*, 26 August, https://inews.co.uk/opinion/britain-treatment-pets-anything-but-dog-lovers-1815988

PART ONE
Background and Rationale

CHAPTER 1

THE HUMAN-DOG BOND IN HISTORICAL CONTEXT

When Frederick the Great, the eighteenth-century king of Prussia, lay on his death-bed, his final gesture was for a quilt to be placed over his favourite Italian greyhound who was shivering despite the warm night. While in better health, the king considered that in a selfish world, the only one that would not betray or deny him was his dog. As he lay dying, he asked to be comforted by the French philosopher and author Voltaire, although he was too ill to listen (Mitford & Williams, 2011). On the loyalty of dogs, Voltaire shared the sentiments of the dying king. They are rival claimants of the phrase 'a man's best friend is his dog'.[1] Frederick the Great's last will was to be buried alongside his Italian greyhounds 'without circumstance, without pomp, without splendour' (Timms, 2019).

Through history, dogs have shown their love, companionship, and protective inclination to people from all backgrounds and cultures in equal measure. This chapter traces the development of this special human-dog bond. It is divided into three parts: the first part comments on historical sources and challenges for a study of this relationship; the second part briefly discusses the specific roles that dogs have played in history; and the third part explains the background to the growing interest in bringing dogs into educational settings.

PART 1: SOURCES AND CHALLENGES

Historians depend on sources and their imagination to recreate and interpret the past. The earliest glimpse of the human-dog relationship can be found in ancient caves and other archaeological sites. These include a teenager's footprints and wolf-dog paw prints preserved in the soft clay floor of Chauvet cave (south-east France), formed around 30,000 years ago. These prints appeared alongside each other, which suggests the boy and dog were friends rather than foes. The discovery of 8,000-year-old rock carvings of dogs on leashes in north-western Saudi Arabia further illustrates the enduring, global nature of the human-dog relationship. Zooarchaeologists were so excited by the findings of the latter that they likened the experience to 'the closest thing you're going to get to a YouTube video' (Grimm, 2017). These motifs suggest that dogs and humans hunted together in a close-knit group (Andreae et al., 2021).

Archaeology has also revealed some poignant findings, notably the discovery in Israel of a 14,000-year-old human skeleton buried alongside a puppy with the hand resting on the dog's head, taken as a sign of affection. At another burial site in a Germany quarry, forensic analysis of prehistoric dog teeth revealed that a puppy had suffered from canine distemper 4–5 weeks before it died. During this time, archaeologists think that the dog had received intensive care from the two humans buried alongside (Janssens et al., 2018). Burials in Siberia around 8,000 years ago included

DOI: 10.4324/9781003257073-3

dogs wearing necklaces (Losey et al., 2011). Although such archaeological findings are scare, there is enough to show that the human-dog bond is both universal and very old.

While archaeology and DNA analysis of ancient bones provide tangible evidence of the human-dog relationship, it is more difficult to tease out the nature of their social bond from such material records. Hence, studies of preliterate societies often turn to myths, legends, and oral tradition, for example, one study of Tla'amin culture and society in northwest Columbia began with community memories of close relations between families and their hunting dogs. These were enriched by folklore (e.g., of women giving birth to dog children), oral tradition, ethnographic data from the 1930s, and interviews in the 1990s. These combined sources and methods highlighted how dogs have long been integrated into the daily lives and belief systems of the Tla'amin. In the words of one community member: '[Dogs] were so specialized in what they could do, they were actually a part of the people, the village, or the family' (Anza-Burgess et al., 2020, p. 434). Similarly, the Warlpiri people of northern Australia regard their dogs as family members (Musharbash, 2017). Their ancestors formed a special relationship with dingoes, the only animals that were given formal burials by Aboriginal people. Chambers et al. (2020) point out that although the Warlpiri do not regard dogs as people, they do hold them in higher regard than humans from outside the community. Such studies are important in counterbalancing traditional Eurocentric perspectives on the history of human-dog relationships (Taylor & Dalal, 2014; Walker, 2013).

Throughout history, dogs have been represented by humans in many ways including stories, poetry, tragedy, legal texts, historical accounts, proverbs, metaphors, comic jokes, mosaics, tombstone epithets, monuments, artefacts, pottery, tapestries, and paintings. For example, ancient Egyptian artists drew pictures of dogs wearing wide collars that announced their names, such as 'Town Dog' and made children's toys such as an ivory dog whose lower jaw could be moved by a lever (Kalof, 2007). Most of the written sources were either produced or commissioned by the literate, rich, and powerful. In medieval society, for example, descriptions of hunting dogs appear in courtly records and hunting manuals for wealthy landowners. In the seventeenth century, the individual traits of dogs started to appear in royal portraits of hunting parties (Sørensen, 2007). However, trying to retrace the everyday encounters between humans and dogs among the illiterate masses in premodern times is far more challenging.

Since the nineteenth century and the development of mass media, historians face a different challenge: an overabundance of material, with the advent of nineteenth-century dog shows and their records, care manuals, postcards, photography, newspapers, and popular magazines. In the twentieth century, dogs inspired television programmes, cartoons, films, a multi-billion-pound industry of paraphernalia, and social media followings. Rin Tin Tin, a German shepherd dog, became the first televised superstar of the modern age. Malamud (2007) relates how the original Rin Tin Tin was found in a bombed-out dog kennel in France at the end of World War I. He was named after a lucky charm that French children gave to American soldiers. Darryl F. Zanuck, a Hollywood film producer, saw the dog perform at a show and apparently leap 14 feet in the air, and imagined his screen potential. Hollywood legend has it that Rin Tin Tin won the nominations for Best Actor in the first-ever 1929 Academy Awards. However, his name was withdrawn, and the voting rerun because the organisers feared the event would not be taken seriously by the public. When Rin Tin Tin died in 1932, radio stations across the United States interrupted programmes to break the news and ran an hour-long tribute to the most famous dog in history (Orlean, 2012). The name passed to other German shepherds and spawned many films, radio broadcasts, and television series.

The modern-day Disneyfication of animals has seen dogs presented as loyal and courageous heroes while poor old rats have struggled to shake off their villainous stereotype (Stanton, 2021). Dogs such as Rin Tin Tin become famous because people make them so. Fame as a human construct is imposed on other animals, whether they like it or not. Acknowledging the individuality of animals is a rare occurrence because most are 'de-animalised'. Among the questions that occupy cultural histories (e.g., Kalof, 2007; Resl, 2007) in the field are the roles humans assigned to animals, their symbolism, representation in the arts, and entertainment. Dogs, for example, have acted as performers, media stars, and even astronauts. In 1957, Laika, a stray mongrel from Moscow, was the first dog sent into orbital space, where she died of overheating hours into the flight. She was a slave to the Space Race, despite her heroic status, memorialised across the Soviet Union. Her story is one of countless numbers illustrating how little animals really matter in the story of human progress (Malamud, 2007).

The notion that animals have a history, which warrants investigation, is a relatively new one. It began inauspiciously in the 1970s when it was suggested tongue-in-cheek that social historians might one day explore the history of pets, following on from such 'fads' as the histories of ethnic minorities, left-handed people, women, and homosexuality (Zelinger, 2021). Strangely prophetic, the 'animal turn' in historical writing over recent years has reflected serious scholarship and a desire to know more about the relationship between humans and other animals (Vandersommers, 2016). This is particularly true of the relationship between humans and dogs, the first animal to be domesticated.

One of the challenges in researching the history of the human-dog relationship relates to understanding conceptual changes. Fundamentally, the concept of what an animal is has changed over time.[2] In medieval texts, animal was often used in its strictest Latin sense (*animālis*) to describe all breathing, moving, living beings, thereby covering both humans and nonhuman animals. There was no single word that corresponded to the modern notion of animals referring to all nonhuman animals. Consequently, there is an anachronistic danger of modern scholars projecting modern-day concepts when they study the past (Resl, 2007).

On the matter of dogs (*Canis familiaris*), the word first seems to have appeared in the English language about 700 years ago to describe a particular breed, possibly a mastiff. Gradually, dog took over from *hund*, the old Anglo Saxon general term used to describe all domestic canines. It was rather like Hoover as a brand name overtaking vacuum cleaner. A few names for dog breeds are more easily traced. Spaniels were from Spain, collies derive their name from their black coats resembling coal, poodles were Germanic in origin, named after animals splashing in puddles, and terriers were named after the Latin *terra* ('earth').

The concept of personhood associated with dogs raises existential questions about how people were regarded as different to animals in the past. Here, philosophical, moral, and religious works are useful historical sources to consider. The Greek philosophical schools of the fourth and third centuries BCE provide the customary starting point for historians. Both Plato and his pupil Aristotle argued that humans were separated from animals by virtue of their ability to reason. Aristotle also claimed that only humans can contemplate the divine, have a language through which they can impart information and communicate ethical values to each other, and achieve true happiness based on mutual affection among their species (Newmyer, 2007). From the Renaissance (*c.* 1400–1600 AD) onwards, philosophical writings on the human-animal distinction are a rich source for philosophers and historians alike. For example, the sixteenth-century essayist Michel de Montaigne's mantra that 'Man is No Better Than the Animals' challenged the entrenched wisdom that humans were superior to animals. His work has been interpreted and re-interpreted with suggestions that it might be read as an early example of post humanist thinking: challenging the idea that humans are the only agents of the moral world (Wallen, 2015). Montaigne's famous utterance, 'When I am Playing with My Cat, How Do I Know She is Not Playing with Me?', raised questions around what it meant to be human and whether one could distinguish between 'human' (Homo Sapiens) and 'person' (any entity) (Frampton, 2011). Montaigne wanted people to see the world from the perspective of others. Such 'perspectivism' makes it more difficult to do harm, including torturing and abusing animals.

In such times, the debate over whether an animal had a soul really mattered because if they did, then they could gain salvation and deserved to be treated well. The seventeenth-century French philosopher René Descartes did not think animals had a soul – they were automata because they lacked language and general intelligence. In pursuit of his argument, Descartes had no qualms about dissecting animals, including chopping off the tail of his wife's dog, nailed to a board. Reacting to the challenge posed by the Cartesian 'animal machine', other Enlightenment thinkers such as Locke, Buffon, and Rousseau reappraised man's relationship to the animal world, acknowledging that animals had feelings and men had moral duties to consider these (Preece, 2002). John Stuart Mill's utilitarian philosophy carried with it the notion that in any given situation, the best course of action was to maximise pleasure and happiness of all interested parties. He considered any actions causing animals pain as ethically objectionable. As the founder of utilitarianism, Jeremy Bentham (1879, p. 309) asked in relation to animals: 'the question is not, Can they reason? nor, Can they talk? but, Can they suffer?'

Duncan (2006) traces the changing conception of animal sentience – the notion that they are capable of feelings such as pleasure, joy, pain, and distress that matter to them as individuals. Referencing the works of major behavioural scientists such as James, Watson, and Skinner, Duncan argues that their behaviourist theories eschewed the study of animal feelings for much of the twentieth century. It was the rise of the animal welfare movement that began to change the nature and direction of scientific research and the role of animals therein. In particular, the publication of *Animal Machines* (Harrison, 1964) raised public awareness around the sufferings of millions of animals subject to intensive farming and product testing. A UK government commissioned report (Brambell, 1965) on animal welfare followed and acknowledged animal sentience was key to their welfare, which had ethical implications for any future research. Nowadays, animal sentience is recognised by law in the United Kingdom, the European Union, New Zealand, and parts of Australia, while there are ongoing discussions in other countries (Browning & Veit, 2022).

The rise in environmental history in the late twentieth century has inevitably featured animals in discussions around the impact of changing landscapes and eco-systems. At the bequest of social historians, there have also been moves to broaden the narrative away from the deeds of 'great men' towards considering the historical agency of natural forces including animals. In psychological terms, agency describes the 'power to initiate action' (Bandura, 2001, p. 3). Conventionally, this has been only applied to humans. This matters because agency is a fundamental historical concept describing the ability of people to act intentionally to shape their worlds and convert their ideas into purposeful action. Social historians have shown how such agency has been exercised not only by powerful European elites but also by less privileged people, including those who were colonised, slaves, women, and children.

Nash (2005) argues that animals can exert their own agency if we rethink the concept as the outcomes of social milieus and interactions with nature rather than emanating from self-contained individuals confronting their worlds. She suggests: 'It is worth considering how our stories might be different if human beings appeared not as the motor of history but as partners in a conversation with a larger world, both animate and inanimate, about the possibilities of existence' (Nash, 2005, p. 69). Similarly, Shaw (2003) uses the term 'unities' to describe shared agency, as partners work together in the same direction, albeit not necessarily to achieve the same goal. He cites the example of militarised dogs and horses. Pearson (2013) illustrates this in his fascinating study of agency among army dogs during the World War I. He even cites one British dog handler as saying: 'It was my experience to find occasionally the canine 'conscientious objector' among the recruits'. Pearson points out that dogs differ in agency in comparison to other species, and even more importantly, within their species: 'Certain dogs, through their sense of smell, trainability, intelligence could also be said to possess more agency than other dogs, even those of the same breed' (Pearson, 2013, p. 135). The significance of conceptualising dogs as agentic is that they can then enter the historical record not as passive objects but as active beings in their relationship with humans. For historical studies, the evidential challenge remains in seeking to locate and analyse any remnants of animal agency in anthropocentric (human-centred) archives. This is likely to require creative research beyond texts to consider visual and oral sources.

PART 2: ROLES OF DOGS IN SOCIETY

The second part of this chapter discusses the varied roles played by dogs in their relationship with humans. Among academics, there is agreement that dogs descended from grey wolves (*Canis lupis*), whose nature and social organisation suited integration with human communities. The process may have begun around 30,000 years ago, although where and how long this took are points for debate (Shipman, 2021; Wang et al., 2016).

In prehistoric times, dogs' natural herding and hunting instincts were much valued by early peoples seeking food in tough climates (Fillios & Taçon, 2016; McIntosh, 2006). Across cultures, hunting dogs were highly valued for their loyalty, bravery, and tenacious spirit (Roberts, 2015), symbolising their owner's wealth and status (McIntosh, 2006). They are commemorated in mythology (e.g., the Greek Laelaps and the Irish Cú Chulainn) and considered the most noble of species. Hounds have been used to hunt slaves, for example, in the American South (Parry & Yingling, 2020), as well as animals. Huntsmen were expected to treat their hounds with considerable care. One medieval guide advised the nobility: 'herewith shall you rub every night the feet and folds between the clawes (sic) of your hands with a linen cloute'. As Bergman (2007, p. 65) observed, 'it is easy to see why noble hunters were accused of caring more for their dogs than their people'. Over the centuries, dogs have acted as guardians of other animals and protectors of households. Sheepdogs are mentioned in the records of the earliest civilisations including the Egyptians, Greeks, Babylonians, and Sumerians, credited with inventing the dog collar (Black et al., 2004). In largely rural Europe, the sheepdog became the archetypal working dog valued for its intelligence and initiative. It was not uncommon for sheepdogs to be left to care for flocks overnight.

Humans have long valued dogs as companions. One poignant example is of an ancient Roman tombstone showing the relief of a little girl sitting on a stool, reading an open scroll held in both hands (Photo 1.1). Behind her is a long-tailed, collared dog with lifted head and its right forepaw raised to touch the cushion on the stool, vainly hoping to gain her attention. The translated inscription reads that Avita died at the age of 10 years, 2 months (Toynbee, 1973); perhaps the first example of reading with (if not to) dogs.

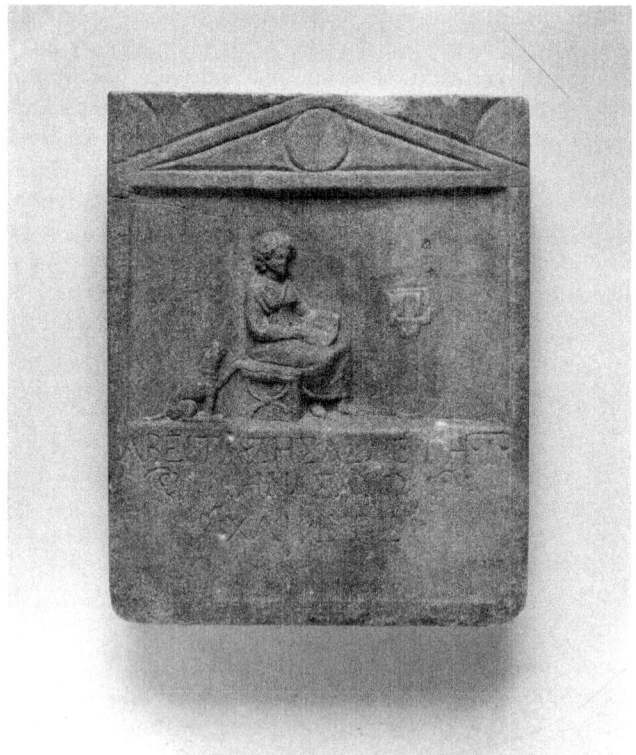

PHOTO 1.1 Reading with dogs in ancient Rome © The Trustees of the British Museum.
Source: https://www.britishmuseum.org/collection/object/G_1805-0703-187

In the Middle Ages, small dogs, cats, birds, and other species were pampered by the upper classes. In some cases, monks and nuns valued the companionship of dogs despite numerous injunctions that attempted to limit the practice. William Greenfield, Archbishop of York, complained in the early fourteenth century that bringing little dogs into the choir during divine services would 'impede the service and hinder the devotion of the nuns' (Walker-Meikle, 2013). It was not until the 1700s that owning a pet became more socially acceptable among the middle classes. Small dogs were not only good companions but they could also hunt rodents and warn of impending arrivals.

By the nineteenth century, Britain had established a reputation as a dog-loving nation. Much of this can be attributed to the personal interest shown by Queen Victoria and Prince Albert. Although King Charles I popularised through court portraits the spaniel named after him, Victoria and Albert's love of dogs took this to a new level. Sir Edwin Landseer was commissioned to paint Dash, Queen Victoria's spaniel since childhood while Albert's greyhound Eos accompanied him from Germany on his wedding day (and honeymoon). Victoria directed William Bambridge to systematically photograph the dogs in the royal kennels, established in the 1840s, where she banned the common practice of tail docking and ear cropping. Victoria took a keen interest in pedigrees, showing six of her Pomeranians at the first Crufts dog show in 1891. She became patron to both the Royal Society for the Protection of Cruelty to Animals (established in 1824) and Battersea Dogs Home (which opened in 1860). Undoubtedly, Victoria did much to popularise the notion of dogs as human's best friend.

PART 3: DOGS IN EDUCATIONAL SETTINGS

The story behind the involvement of dogs in schools and other educational settings can be traced to wide-ranging influences, from moral philosophy, experimental psychology and animal welfare reform to the rise of mass schooling, a growing market for children's books, educational psychology and interest in children's well-being.

In Britain, the seventeenth-century philosopher John Locke was among the first to suggest that children be given dogs and other animals to care for, to develop their empathy and responsibility. Such voices, however, had little impact beyond the home-educated children of the elite. With the nineteenth-century development of compulsory schooling for the poor came a recognition that teachers could use morality tales, stories, and 'object' lessons to transmit knowledge and instil values around caring for animals.

The English philanthropist Angela Burdett-Coutts was among those who campaigned for schools to teach children about the humane care of animals against a background of concern about their ill treatment in society. Given that teachers' salaries until the end of the century were tied in part to children's success in examinations in reading, writing, and arithmetic, the curriculum remained narrow and there was little appetite for innovation. Teachers mentioned dogs and other animals in the context of storytelling and instilling moral values, but it was not until the early twentieth century that the influence of progressive educationalists broadened the curricula and a few schools experimented with bringing animals on school grounds. Nature Study and local walks also gained popularity in the interwar years.

In the field of experimental psychology, the Russian neurologist Ivan Pavlov's systematic research highlighted that dogs could learn and unlearn things. But they were regarded as passive, experimental objects (Goldman, 2012; Todes, 2000). Pavlov said very little about the dogs' welfare and while he remains an icon in modern psychology textbooks, little was also said about the ethical side of his experiments, the conditions dogs experienced, or the details of the invasive procedures.

The notion of featuring dogs in therapeutic programmes can be traced to an accidental discovery. In 1953, Boris Levinson, a trained child psychiatrist working in America, noticed how the presence of his dog Jingles encouraged a withdrawn child to talk. Initially, Levinson did not pursue the idea and faced opposition in the scientific community, perhaps due to Levinson's strong spirituality. Nonetheless, by the 1960s he had published several papers advocating what he described as 'pet therapy' and the dog's potential as a 'co therapist' (Levinson, 1962; Levinson, 1964). His work gained credibility when biographers reported that Sigmund Freud, the founder of psychoanalysis, had noticed something similar in the 1930s when child and adult patients talked more openly to his own dog, Jofi.[3] Levinson's *Pet-Oriented Child Psychotherapy* appeared in 1969 and was the first to document the role of dogs in the psychological treatment of children (Mallon, 1994; Levinson & Mallon, 1997). As Fine (2017) notes, Levinson's contribution was to change perceptions on the human-animal bond.

Other researchers began to see the potential of pet-facilitated therapy in hospitals and nursing homes to improve communication and physical improvements among residential patients (Corson & Corson, 1978). In these early days, dogs were regarded very much as catalysts or 'social lubricants', a term coined by the Corsons, perceived as easing the communication between patient and staff. Such research inspired the mental health community to take animal-assisted interventions seriously.

In 1977, growing interest in the need for research in human-animal relationships led to the formation of the Delta Foundation in Oregon. This was renamed the Delta Society (1981) and its first President, the veterinarian Leo Bustad, is credited with introducing the term 'human–animal bond'. Among its achievements was the launch of *Anthrozoös* (1987), the leading peer-reviewed research journal in the field. In 2012, Delta Society was renamed Pet Partners to reflect its mission of promoting the health and well-being of both humans *and* animals, as partners. In terms of educational activity, Read With Me™ has proven one of its most successful programmes. Since its launch in 2016, thousands of volunteer animal therapy teams around the world are trained and assessed to work in schools and other settings. The academic argument draws on studies that suggest that children who read to dogs achieve higher end-of-year reading scores (Kirnan et al., 2016; Levinson et al., 2017). More recently, We Are All Ears is another Pet Partners initiative designed to make the most of pets' listening skills.

Over recent years, there has been a gradual shift from what was widely held as novel and unusual practices towards a drive for more rigorous interventions and evidence-based decisions. This is particularly important given the popularity of dogs in school promoted through social and print media soundbites and anecdotal evidence. Our scientific understanding of dogs has advanced considerably through genetics, anthrozoology, multi-species ethnography, and the emerging field of human-animal studies (HAS). Collectively, these studies have challenged the traditional people-focused humanities and social sciences, including psychology, by 'incorporating human relationships to nonhuman others and more-than-human worlds into theoretical frameworks and methodological approaches' (Adams, 2020, p. 121). The distinctive offer of HAS is to shift the focus to dogs and other nonhumans, moving 'beyond anthropocentric histories and social narratives by putting animal life in the spotlight' (Johnson, 2015, p. 299). The French anthropologist Claude Lévi-Strauss (1962, p. 89) asserted that animals are significant in human society not because they are 'good to eat' but because they are 'good to think'. He was discussing totemism, which describes beliefs about the relationship between humans and the natural world. The word 'totem' means 'a relative of mine' or 'one's brother-sister kin' in Ojibwe, an indigenous language of North America. Totemism suggests that the traditional relationship between humans and dogs needs to move beyond notions of human supremacy to appreciate the uniqueness and sentience of nonhuman animals.

Over recent decades, there have been moves towards understanding the human-dog relationship in the past from a variety of perspectives including art history, sociology, anthropology, literary criticism, philosophy, political science, and other social sciences (Pearson & Weismantel, 2010). For example, the multi-disciplinary field of HAS explores the experiences of nonhuman animals and how they figure in human lives. Since the 1980s and 1990s, journals such as *Anthrozoös*, the *Journal of Ethnobiology*, and *Society & Animals* have published inter- and multi-disciplinary academic works exploring the full range of human-animal relations, from their treatment in the humanities and arts, through to social, behavioural, biological, and health sciences. Comparative histories of human-dog relationships across cultures, drawing on anthropology, archaeology, and historical study, presents opportunities to tease out the narrative around the persistent reluctance in some quarters for humans to be conceptualised alongside animals. Anthropology can help historians recognise that the boundaries between humans and animals are more porous than Western assumptions often allow. Waldau (2013) argues that there is no reason why histories should be confined to human stories.

The new approach to thinking about the relationship between humans and animals is motivated by a desire to understand what it means to be human but always framed by consideration of the needs of other species in more-than-human worlds. It calls for a fresh look at seeing dogs not as passive objects for humans to act upon or 'use' as resources or tools (Mullin, 2010) but as species in their own rights. Through this lens, dogs are not viewed as laboratory animals subject to experimentation, but as sentient companions living in private homes and featuring in a range of contexts, including educational institutions, hospitals, prisons, and war zones. Researchers are no longer Pavlovian-style men in white coats but drawn from a range of experiences, including dog owners, who take the role of community scientists contributing 'to the systematic gathering of data from the comfort of their own homes' (Maclean et al., 2021, p. 2).

The reality is that our relationship with dogs is a multifaceted one reflecting a range of diverse beliefs, customs, and attitudes. History tells us that this relationship has endured for millennia but like all living relationships deserves to be fully understood, strengthened, nurtured, and respected. As other chapters in this book demonstrate, there is now a growing body of evidence which shows that dogs can bring wide-ranging social, emotional, physical, and psychological benefits to humans. Yet, we argue for greater humility in how we view such relationships.

Human exceptionalism assumes that we are superior in our complex thinking and feeling to other species. This can downplay nonhuman animals, including dogs, who experience a wide range of emotions such as grief when someone they care about dies (King, 2022). When we see ourselves as unique in value, it becomes easier to denigrate or harm nonhuman animals and to overlook their thoughts and feelings, especially when they do not match our own. The scientific evidence is clear about what dogs need, and these needs are not far removed from humans: love, attention, nutritious food, and regular exercise. The so-called 'new era of canine science' signals a reframing of the human-dog relationship by exploring what dogs can contribute to our understanding of ourselves, how we interact with other species, and the environmental challenges that we all face (Maclean et al., 2021).

The well-being of dogs and what benefits they derive from interacting with humans should always be a paramount concern, particularly in schools where children and young people should be educated to become well-rounded, caring citizens. There is a danger that bringing dogs into school is seized upon as the latest quick-fix initiative or driven by the particular interest of a dog-owning teacher. But unless animal-assisted interventions are carefully planned and implemented, then there are real possibilities of damaging the well-being of participants including dogs.

This chapter has highlighted the longevity in the human-dog relationship. It is almost impossible to disentangle the history of dogs from the history of humans. The story of dogs' domestication did not end with the Neolithic Revolution but continues in our day as humans find new ways to interact with dogs. Of all species, dogs have stood out for their attachment to humans. Writing in 1829 the first Scottish book about dogs, the naturalist Thomas Brown recognised that there was something very special about the human-dog relationship: 'while almost every other quadruped fears man as its formidable enemy, here is one which regards him as his companion, and follows him as his friend' (Brown, 1829, p. 26). Dogs are a permanent presence in the human psyche and culture. The relationship should not be romanticised because the responsibilities humans have in exercising power over dogs are not always upheld, resulting in unhappy, unhealthy, and inhumane relationships.

NOTES

1   Although recent ethnographic research (Chambers et al., 2020) suggests that women played a key role in the early domestication of dogs, forming a strong bond as they cared for puppies and small dogs unable to go hunting.

2   We adopt the shorthand convention of describing human animals as humans, and nonhuman animals as animals.

3   Freud claimed that he never needed to look at his watch during a session, as when the dog got up and yawned, it meant that the allotted hour was over (Freud, 1958, in Ruitenbeck, 1973, p. 379).

REFERENCES

Adams, M. (2020). The kingdom of dogs: Understanding Pavlov's experiments as human–animal relationships. *Theory & Psychology*, *30*(1), 121–141. https://doi.org/10.1177/0959354319895597

Andreae, M., Al-Amri, A., Hamad Al-Jibrin, F., & Alsharekh, A. (2021). Iconographic and archae-ometric studies on the rock art at Musayqira, Al-Quwaiyah Governorate, central Saudi Arabia. *Arabian Archaeology and Epigraphy, 32*(1), 153–182. https://doi.org/10.12759/hsr.40.2015.4.7-31

Anza-Burgess, K., Lepofsky, D., & Yang, D. (2020). "A part of the people": Human-dog relationships among the Northern Coast Salish of SW British Columbia. *Journal of Ethnobiology, 40*(4), 434–450. https://doi.org/10.2993/0278-0771-40.4.434

Bandura, A. (2001). Social cognitive theory: An agentic perspective. *Annual Review of Psychology, 52,* 1–26. https://doi.org/10.1146/annurev.psych.52.1.1

Bentham, J. (1879). *An introduction to the principles of morals and legislation.* T. Payne Son.

Bergman, C. (2007). A spectacle of beasts: Hunting rituals and animal rights in early modern England. In B. Boehrer (Eds.), *A cultural history of animals in the renaissance* (pp. 53–74). Blooms-bury Collections. https://doi.org/10.5040/9781350049550-ch-002

Black, J., Cunningham, G., Robson, E., & Zólyomi, G. (2004). *The literature of ancient Sumer.* Oxford University Press.

Brambell, F. W. (1965). *Report of the technical committee to inquire into the welfare of animals kept under intensive livestock husbandry.* HMSO.

Brown, T. (1829). *Biographical sketches and authentic anecdotes of dogs.* Oliver & Boyd.

Browning, H., & Veit, W. (2022). The sentience shift in animal research. *The New Bioethics, 28*(4), 299–314.

Chambers, J., Quinlan, M., Evans, A., & Quinlan, R. (2020). Dog-human coevolution: Cross-cultural analysis of multiple hypotheses. *Journal of Ethnobiology, 40*(4), 414–434. https://doi.org/10.2993/0278-0771-40.4.414

Corson, S. A., & Corson, E. O. (1978). Pets as mediators of therapy. *Current Psychiatric Therapies, 18,* 195–205.

Fillios, M. A., & Taçon, P. S. C. (2016). Who let the dogs in? A review of the recent genetic evidence for the introduction of the dingo to Australia and implications for the movement of people. *Journal of Archaeological Science: Reports, 7,* 782–792. https://doi.org/10.1016/J.JASREP.2016.03.001

Fine, A. H. (2017). Standing the test of time: Reflecting on the relevance today of Levinson's Pet-Oriented Child Psychotherapy. *Clinical Child Psychology Psychiatry, 22*(1), 9–15. https://doi.org/10.1177/1359104515589638

Frampton, S. (2011). *When I am playing with my cat, how do i know she is not playing with me? Montaigne and being in touch with life.* Faber and Faber.

Freud, M. (1958). Freud: My father. In H. M. Ruitenbeck (Ed.) (1973). *Freud as we knew him* (pp. 378–385). Wayne State University Press.

Goldman, J. G. (2012). *What is classical conditioning? (And why does it matter?).* 11 January, Scientific American. https://blogs.scientificamerican.com/thoughtful-animal/what-is-classical-conditioning-and-why-does-it-matter

Grimm, D. (2017). *These may be the world's first images of dogs—And they're wearing leashes.* 16 November, Science. https://www.science.org/content/article/these-may-be-world-s-first-images-dogs-and-they-re-wearing-leashes

Harrison, R. (1964). *Animal machines.* Vincent Stuart Publishers.

Janssens, L., Giemsch, L., Schmitz, R., Street, M., Van Dongen, S., & Crombré, P.. (2018). A new look at an old dog: Bonn-Oberkassel reconsidered. *Journal of Archaeological Science, 92,* 126–138. https://doi.org/10.1016/j.jas.2018.01.004

Johnson, E. R.. (2015). Of lobsters, laboratories, and war: Animal studies and the temporality of more-than-human encounters. *Environment and Planning D: Society and Space, 33*(2), 296–313. https://doi.org/10.1068/d23512

Kalof, L. (2007). *A cultural history of animals in antiquity* (Vol. 1). Berg.

King, B. (2022). Human exceptionalism imposes horrible costs on other animals. 1 November, *Psyche.* https://psyche.co/ideas/human-exceptionalism-imposes-horrible-costs-on-other-animals

Kirnan, J., Siminerio, S., & Wong, Z. (2016). The impact of a therapy dog on Children's reading skills and attitudes towards reading. *Early Childhood Education Journal, 44*(6), 637–651. https://doi.org/10.1007/s10643-015-0747-9

Levinson, B. (1964). Pets: A special technique in child psychotherapy. *Mental Hygiene, 48,* 243–248.

Levinson, B. M. (1962). The dog as a "co-therapist. *Mental Hygiene, 46,* 59–65.

Levinson, E. M., Vogt, M., Barker, W. F., Jalongo, M. R., & Van Zandt, P. (2017). Effects of reading with adult tutor/therapy dog teams on elementary students' reading achievement and attitudes. *Society & Animals, 25*(1), 38–56.

Lévi-Strauss, C. (1962). *Transl. the savage mind.* University of Chicago Press.

Losey, R., Vladimir, I., Bazaliiskii, S., Garvie-Lok, M., Germonpré, J., Leonard, A., Allen, M., Katzenberg, A., & Sablin, M. (2011). Canids as persons: Early Neolithic dog and wolf burials, Cis-Baikal, Siberia. *Journal of Anthropological Archaeology, 30*(2), 174–189. https://doi.org/10.1016/j.jaa.2011.01.001

Maclean, E., Fine, A., Herzog, H., Strauss, E., & Cobb, M. (2021). The new era of canine science: Reshaping our relationships with dogs. *Frontiers in Veterinary Science, 8.* https://doi.org/10.3389/fvets.2021.675782

Malamud, R. (Ed.) (2007). *A cultural history of animals in the modern age.* Berg. https://doi.org/10.5040/9781350049543

Mallon, G. P. (1994). A generous spirit: The work and life of Boris Levinson, *Anthrozoös, 7*(4), 224–231, https://doi.org/10.2752/089279394787001790

McIntosh, J. (2006). *Handbook to life in prehistoric Europe.* Oxford University Press.

Mitford, N., & Williams, K. (2011). *Frederick the great.* Vintage.

Mullin, M. (2010). Anthropology's animals. In M. DeMello (Ed.), *Teaching the animal: Human–animal studies across the disciplines* (pp. 145–201). Lantern Books.

Musharbash, Y. (2017). Telling Warlpiri dog stories. *Anthropological Forum, 27*(7), 95–113. https://doi.org/10.1080/00664677.2017.1303603

Nash, L. (2005). The agency of nature and the nature of agency? *Environmental History, 10*(1), 67–69.

Newmyer, S. T. (2007). Animals in ancient philosophy: Conceptions and misconceptions. In L. Kalof (Ed.). *A cultural history of animals in antiquity* (pp. 151–174). Berg. https://doi.org/10.5040/9781350049505-ch-006

Orlean, S. (2012). *Rin Tin Tin: The life and legend of the world's most famous dog: The life and legend of the world's most famous dog.* Atlantic Books.

Parry, T., & Yingling, C. (2020). Slave hounds and abolition in the Americas. *Past & Present, 246*(1), 69–108. https://doi.org/10.1093/pastj/gtz020

Pearson, C. (2013). Dogs, history and agency, *History & Theory, 52*(4), 128–145. https://doi.org/10.1111/hith.10683

Pearson, C., & Weismantel, M. (2010). A philosophical question: Does "The animal" exist. Without a trace; Or, are animals historical beings? In I. D. Brantz (Ed.), *Beastly natures. Animals, humans, and the study of history* (pp. 18–37). University of Virginia Press.

Resl, B. (Ed.) (2007). *A cultural history of animals in the medieval age.* Berg.

Roberts, A. (2015). *The celts.* Heron Books.

Shaw, D. G. (2003). The Torturer's horse. Agency and animals in history. *History and Theory, 52*(4), 146–167.

Stanton, R. (2021). *The Disneyfication of animals.* Palgrave Macmillan.

Taylor, C., & Dalal, N. (2014). *Asian Perspectives on animal ethics. Rethinking the nonhuman.* Routledge.

Timms, E. (2019, August 28). *A King's grave and his dogs.* Royal Central. https://royalcentral.co.uk/features/a-kings-grave-and-his-dogs-128646/

Todes, D. (2000). *Ivan Pavlov: Exploring the animal machine.* Oxford University Press.

Vandersommers, D. (2016, November 3). The "Animal Turn" in history. *Perspectives on History, 54*(8). https://www.historians.org/research-and-publications/perspectives-on-history/november-2016/the-animal-turn-in-history

Waldau, P. (2013). *Animal studies. An introduction.* Oxford University Press.

Walker, B. (2013). Animals and the intimacy of history. *History and Theory, 52*(4), 45–47.

Wang, G. D., Zhai, W., Yang, H. C., Wang, L., Zhong, L., Liu, Y. H., Fan, R. X., Yin, T. T., Zhu, C. L., Poyarkov, A. D., Irwin, D. M., Hytönen, M. K., Lohi, H., Wu, C. I., Savolainen, P., & Zhang, Y. P. (2016). Out of southern East Asia: The natural history of domestic dogs across the world. *Cell Research, 26*(1), 21–33. https://doi.org/10.1038/cr.2015.147

Zelinger, A. (2021). History of pets. In M. Roscher, A. Krebber, & B. Mizelle (Eds.), *Handbook of historical animal studies* (pp. 425–438). De Gruyter Oldenbourg.

CHAPTER 2

SCHOOL DOGS

What Does the Research Tell Us?

Over recent decades, the popularity of dogs featuring in schools and other educational programmes around the world has steadily increased (Lewis et al., 2022). Among the reasons cited are the relative convenience and low cost of such interventions along with the perceived gains in students' learning and well-being (Castellano, 2015; Friesen, 2010). The purpose of this chapter is to explore what systematic and rigorous research exists for the merits (or otherwise) of dogs' presence in educational settings. While 'research' can have a very broad application, we are using the term here to describe the process of investigation leading to new, publishable knowledge that stands up to academic review in reputable peer-reviewed journals.

The chapter highlights the main findings and evidential challenges in the three main areas that may be of particular interest to those working in schools, namely, reading with dogs, supporting children with difficulties in social interaction and communication, and the contribution dogs can make to children's well-being. While these are discussed separately for convenience, there is considerable overlap in outcomes for reading, social skills, and broader well-being. For instance, multiple studies (e.g., Connell et al., 2019; Crossman et al., 2020) show that children's interactions with dogs can foster positive reading dispositions, reduce anxiety, and boost feelings of self-confidence. The link is important because lower levels of stress are associated with clearer thinking (Scoffham & Barnes, 2011), better self-regulation (Gee et al., 2017), increased attentiveness and motivation (Borgi et al., 2016), and optimal engagement in reading (Ramirez et al., 2019). However, we recognise that much research in this area does not report on the impact interventions have on the dogs themselves.

READING WITH DOGS

The science behind reading suggests that it is not something that comes natural, unlike speaking and listening (Hanover Research, 2022; Stanovich, 1994). Reading is essentially a process of making sense of what is written, which requires the skills of decoding and comprehension. What makes this more challenging is the fact that words mean different things in different contexts. Even the word 'dog' can have several meanings, from a form of insult and unflattering description of a person to the act of following someone closely. Moreover, there is no consensus over how best to teach reading. In the 1990s, 'reading wars' surfaced with one side promoting whole-word meaning using look-and-say strategies and the other advocating the teaching of decoding skills, using phonics. For many, the choice should not be one or the other. Effective reading goes beyond mastering mechanical skills of decoding words

DOI: 10.4324/9781003257073-4

to include vocabulary acquisition, comprehension, and fluency, which means that teachers need to embrace a broad repertoire of strategies (Hanover Research, 2022). Advocates of balanced reading programmes recommend a mix of systematic phonics instruction, vocabulary development, fluency, guided oral reading, and whole-text comprehension (Pressley, 2006; Wyse & Bradbury, 2022).

Among the goals of teaching reading are for children to make sense of the text. Such comprehension operates at different levels. Initially, children acquire functional skills that enable them to decode what they can see and hear. This is sometimes referred to as 'on the page' or 'right there' comprehension. Beyond this surface level, children begin to make inferences and read between the lines. They draw on their prior knowledge of a topic and identify clues, such as words, images, or sounds, to make connections. Both surface and inferential comprehension can be achieved by young children (van den Broek et al., 2005). At the highest level of evaluative comprehension, good readers move beyond the text and link what they read to the wider context. They do not necessarily accept the text at face value and can challenge the viewpoints expressed. To fully understand what they read, children need a range of skills. They must learn to decode words, read at a pace, which allows them to maintain flow without missing the key points and apply general comprehension strategies such as predicting, self-correcting, and visualising. Thorndike (1917, p. 323) recognised that 'reading is a very elaborate procedure', where successful readers combine elements, make connections, and correctly weight each part in a sentence. Children also need background knowledge to connect the text to what they already know.

Based on a systematic review of the literature on the effective teaching of reading, Hattie and Donoghue (2016) suggest that instructional strategies should be organised along a continuum of skill, will, and thrill. The 'skill' describes children's prior or subsequent achievement, the 'will' refers to their various dispositions towards reading, and the 'thrill' is the motivation held by the children. 'Skill', 'will', and 'thrill' are considered both inputs and outcomes in the teaching of reading.

The roles of the teacher, student, and dog can be considered in relation to this skill, will, and thrill construct. The adult's main role is to teach the processing and comprehension skills that children need to acquire, with the most effective practices including direct instruction (Rosenshine, 1976, 2012) and modelling of how and when to use strategies (Dewitz et al., 2009). The former ('little di') describes a broad range of teaching behaviours, characterised by structured sessions in which teachers provide clear and concise instructions, and opportunities for children to learn new vocabulary and practise reading through guided and independent activities. Within the literature, this is not the same as Direct Instruction ('big DI'), which describes highly prescribed and sequenced curriculum programmes (e.g., *DISTAR*, *Reading Mastery*, *Connecting Math Concepts*, *Language for Learning*) characterised by step-by-step instructions, choral responding, and error correction (Engelmann & Carnine, 1992; Rolf & Slocum, 2021).

The nature of such explicit instruction with its teacher-led emphasis on correcting children's reading errors is at odds with the spirit of reading with dogs, which is often credited with providing children with a non-judgemental audience and minimal adult input. However, schools that deploy reading-with-dogs interventions do so as part of their broader provision, which means that during the dog sessions, the focus is very much on the interaction between the child and the dog. In these sessions, the teacher's role is primarily to create an environment that is conducive to reading. This means ensuring that the intervention occurs in a quiet, comfortable, well-lit space with few distractions, given that reading concentration suffers from noise, inappropriate temperature, and insufficient light (Chiang & Lai, 2008).

Dog-assisted reading programmes usually take two forms. In the first form, a child reads to a dog with the dog handler there to ensure the safety of all, without offering much guidance to the readers. In the second form, the educator provides reading instruction to a group of low-attaining readers in the presence of a trained dog. The children discuss their reading and practice strategies, while the dog acts as a comforting presence and perhaps carries out tasks such as distributing worksheets (Beetz & McCardle, 2017).

In practice, good readers make connections to what they already know when reading new material, predict, and set goals. While reading, they select strategies appropriate to the text, monitor their reading to check whether they understand, and demonstrate positive attitudes to reading (Brown & Briggs, 1989). They visualise scenes and infer meaning. At times, they skip forward on minor points and use context clues where they are uncertain. Through the reading process, they summarise and reflect on what the content means to them. Of course, children forget things and may not recall, ignore, or struggle to apply classroom strategies when faced with the excitement of a furry friend. The key message is for teachers to incorporate reading with dogs as part of their overall planning and preparation. While the teacher's focus is on skills, the dog's contribution lays in motivating young readers and providing 'a listening ear' – the will and thrill elements of the continuum. While children's attention naturally shifts towards the animal, it is important for children to understand what they need to do to improve their reading. These are sometimes referred to as reading behaviours (Figure 2.1).

Teachers also need to consider how to promote metacognition, namely, the skills of planning, monitoring, and evaluating their own reading. Metacognitive strategies

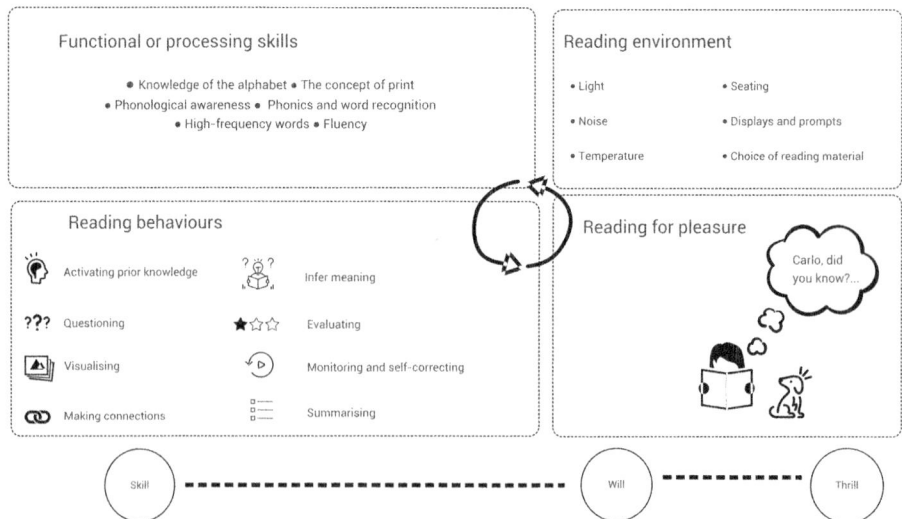

FIGURE 2.1 Reading skills and experiences with dogs.

and experience have long been recognised as significant in children's reading development (Jacobs & Paris, 1987; Paris & Oka, 1986; Williams & Atkins, 2009). Effective metacognitive strategies include goal setting, self-questioning, self-review, 'think-alouds', help-seeking, and deciding how much time to spend on an activity (Muijs & Bokhove, 2020). These low-cost strategies are designed to get children to think about their learning, although their impact depends very much on how well they are integrated with specific subject content (EEF, 2021). Moreover, high-quality talk is key to developing children's reading and so teachers need to pay close attention to what children say, rephrasing and validating as and when appropriate, modelling new language, asking a range of questions, and extending children's vocabulary at every opportunity (DfE, 2022).

Metacognitive strategies can be taught in the context of classroom topics and children then reminded before the reading-to-dog sessions to apply these. Occasional prompts might be appropriate, but overdoing these runs a high risk of children losing the joy of reading and interacting with the dog (Figure 2.2).

Metacognition and Reading to Dogs

1. Before

- Which book shall I read?
- What might interest Carlo?
- What do I think this book is about?
- What do I already know about this topic?

2. During

- This reminds me of...
- This is like...
- What do I feel about this?
- This makes me think...
- I'm not sure what this word means. I could skip this, or I could reread this bit.

3. After

- What have I learnt from this?
- Can I remember what this means?
- What could I read next?
- I found this bit hard because...
- Next time, I'm going to...
- I wonder whether Carlo liked this?

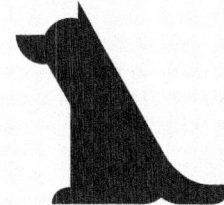

FIGURE 2.2 Promoting metacognition when reading with dogs.

Establishing effective sessions takes time and preparation. The presence of a dog in school inevitably creates excitement among children, particularly during the early visits. The primary literacy goal for reading with dogs sessions is children's enjoyment of books and the opportunity to talk about, practise and share their reading.

Motivation

Reading motivation has been defined as 'the individual's personal goals, values, and beliefs with regard to the topics, processes, and outcomes of reading' (Guthrie & Wigfield, 2000, p. 405). There is a well-established body of evidence, which highlights the strong links between children's attitudes to reading, their motivation, and their reading attainment (Medford & McGeown, 2011; Taboada et al., 2009; Wang & Guthrie, 2004). Motivation to read is a significant challenge for many children. In countries operating within the Organisation for Economic Co-operation and Development (OECD), it has been reported that around two-thirds of children say that they read for pleasure each day although this lessens as they get older (DfE, 2012; OECD, 2011). One recent UK survey reports that only one in four children (0–17) say they read for pleasure and one in five say they never do so (Farshore, 2022). Reading for pleasure matters because it feeds into the ability to read and write (literacy). If children find the experience of reading dull and uninspiring, then they are less motivated to read further. Children cannot take much pleasure from reading if they are finding words a struggle, which is one of the reasons for teaching phonics.

Readers can be motivated intrinsically, for example, through a desire to read about a topic, a belief in the value of reading, or satisfaction in reaching the end of a story; or they can be motivated extrinsically by the rewards on offer or environmental incentives. For some children and young people, the novelty of reading with dogs may act as an extrinsic motivation while for others the love of dogs forms an inner drive to reach out to them. In short, the presence of dogs can prove both an external and inner motivation. Moreover, when children have a choice over who they read to, as well as what they read, there is potential to increase their motivation. Experience of adverse criticism and setbacks in reading can lead readers to only read when they are expected to, which in turn reduces opportunities to practice and therefore succeed (Morgan & Fuchs, 2007).

Behaviourist learning theory suggests that positive external stimuli can act as rewards and reinforce desired behaviours. In the case of reading with dogs, children may receive immediate rewards in the form of the dog's positive body language, wagging tail, tilting head, or outstretched paw. Even when a dog has nodded off to sleep, a child may interpret this as positive feedback because the dog feels restful due to the reading (Pennac, 2009) although a counterview is that the child may perceive this as the dog being bored by the reading. It is certainly the case that dogs provide immediate feedback to children, which is widely recognised as helpful to children's development. Beetz (2017) suggests that dogs may have the power to reverse conditioned negative attitudes.

The conventional wisdom is that children are more likely to perform better in tests of their reading comprehension if they are intrinsically motivated than responding to external factors (Taboada et al., 2009; Wang & Guthrie, 2004; Wigfield & Guthrie, 1997a). One possible explanation is that extrinsically motivated readers focus too much on social rewards rather than comprehending the text. However, studies show that children can be well motivated to read by external factors. Much depends on the context. For example, one Japanese study found sustained benefits when teddy bears were used as a reading motivator during a children's sleepover at a library. The researchers reminded the children of the sleepover a month later, by hiding the stuffed animals and showing them the photographs again the next day. This led to a significant increase in the number of children reading to their stuffed animals (Yoshihiro et al., 2017). However, even Kirnan et al.'s (2016) longitudinal study of 169 children (kindergarten–grade 4) found that standardised reading test scores were only significantly different among the kindergarten class. Moreover, there is a danger of selection bias in overlooking those studies that show no significant difference in the reading behaviours of children in dog and non-dog groups (e.g., Booten, 2011).

Studies of children reading with dogs show that the experience can be highly motivating. Rousseau and Tardif-Williams (2019) found that when children were presented with a challenging text, they were significantly more interested and read for longer than when the dog was not present. Although this was a small-scale study (17 participants and their parents), the authors claim that this was the first within-in-study research in the field, which means that the same children experienced both conditions. Moreover, the reading passages were carefully selected for each child to ensure that they were suitably challenging.

Reading Attitudes and Dispositions

In psychological terms, attitudes have been described as 'evaluation of objects occurring in ongoing thoughts about the objects or stored in the memory' (Matsumoto, 2009, p. 59). Unlike feelings, attitudes involve cognitive evaluation. Dispositions are the 'recurrent intentions to think, feel, act or react in a particular way' (Matsumoto, 2009, p. 165). Attitudes and dispositions matter because they play an important role in children's developing reading proficiency (Clark, 2014; Clark & De Zoysa, 2011; Martinez et al., 2008; McKenna et al., 2012). Attitudes to reading are shaped by a wide range of factors including pupils' language and literacy skills, moods and beliefs, the influence of peers, teachers' interests and expertise, the nature of the reading material, role models at home, and the perceived usefulness and interest of the reading task. Hall et al. (2016) posit that children's moods are elevated when reading with dogs, which improves their attitudes to reading, their engagement, and skill. Studies of reading-with-dogs programmes show that they can inspire children to read and persist in their reading (Friesen, 2013; Uccheddu et al., 2019). For example, a small-scale study (based on 18 participants) reported that preschool children in contact with their pet dogs at home were more likely to show initiative in communication than those without pet dogs (Filiatre et al., 1986).

Reading for Pleasure

For children to see themselves as effective readers in a range of contexts, they must see reading as valuable and enjoyable (Geist, 2011; Parshall, 2003). Enjoyment of reading is among the attitudes that the OECD (2021b) identifies as key to lifelong learning and educational success. The concept of reading for pleasure is often used synonymously with reading for enjoyment, recreational reading (Ross et al., 2006), and independent self-selected reading (Martin, 2003). International evidence suggests that it is more important for children's academic success than their family's socio-economic status (Clark & Rumbold, 2006; OECD, 2002). Many studies point out that reading for pleasure is associated with increases in reading attainment, as well as gains in other language skills, general knowledge, and cultural awareness (Clark & Rumbold, 2006; Howard, 2011; Wigfield & Guthrie, 1997b). There is strong evidence highlighting the positive relationship between reading frequency, reading enjoyment, and attainment (Clark & De Zoysa, 2011; Clark & Douglas, 2011). Children who hold negative attitudes towards reading are less likely to choose to read, and read less often, than those who take pleasure from reading (McKenna et al., 1995; Sainsbury & Schagen, 2004).

The pleasure children derive from reading with dogs is cited as among the greatest benefits of such interventions (Hall et al., 2016; Henderson et al., 2020; Linder et al., 2018; Noble & Holt, 2018). It seems that most children find reading with dogs an exciting and enjoyable experience (Lane & Zavada, 2013). Such pleasure can take different forms. Children may enjoy experimenting with tone and using different 'voices', in the safe knowledge that the dog might respond positively, building confidence and fluency. Children can also take pleasure from choosing what material they think the dog might like to hear – choice can empower and engage children, although such choices should be informed by specific elements such as the text difficulty, genre, and desired reading experience (Clark & Phythian-Sence, 2008). Children who believe that their reading brings joy to the dog may also receive a confidence boost, a sense of pride and achievement, which reinforce positive attitudes to reading. Affective factors such as self-concept (Katzir et al., 2009), engagement, (De Naeghel et al., 2012), and literacy interest (Hume et al., 2015) all play a role in children's attainment in reading. Maintaining children's interest is key to their continuous engagement with reading (Guthrie et al., 2006).

Although there is an emerging consensus that dog-assisted reading programmes foster children's positive attitudes to reading (Henderson et al., 2020), it is less conclusive whether children's reading skills and attainment improve through such experiences. This is largely because there are questions over the methodological rigour of research, the small sample size, and absence of control groups (Brelsford et al., 2017) while it has also been suggested that different dogs may have different effects (Kropp, 2017). Matching the individual dog to the individual children and the activity is discussed in Chapter 3.

Hall et al. (2016) conducted one of the few systematic literature reviews that focused specifically on the perceived benefits to children of reading with dogs. Although they adopted broad inclusion criteria, given the relative newness of the field, they could identify less than 50 relevant academic papers. Of these, only a handful met the higher levels of quality set out by the Oxford Centre for Evidence-Based Medicine. The authors concluded that reading to a dog could benefit behavioural processes, which contribute to a positive effect on the environment in which reading is practiced, leading to improved reading performance. Their tentative conclusions denote a need for more robust research, which builds in appropriate controls so researchers can draw causal inferences on whether or how reading with dogs may benefit children's reading practices.

It is less common to find studies that report of children who respond adversely when reading with dogs. This reflects a general bias in the field. It is logical to assume that some children's experiences of reading with dogs will not be a pleasurable one, or at least to posit that children may be distracted by the dog's presence, which impacts their learning. Gee et al. (2017) acknowledge that children who dislike and fear dogs are unlikely to make much progress in their, if a dog is present.

There are a few studies that suggest a positive correlation between reading with dogs and children's reading proficiency. Levinson et al. (2017) found that reading with a dog tended to increase children's (grades 2–5) scores on a test of oral reading fluency much more than reading aloud to peers. Although the sample size was small, it seems that elementary school children benefit more than older ones as the effect sizes get smaller the older the children become. This has implications when considering at what age this intervention would be most effective. Another study randomly allocated children (aged 7–13 years) to three experimental groups and one control group. Twenty-seven children read to a dog in the presence of a Pets as Therapy volunteers, 24 children read directly to an adult, while 26 children read to a teddy bear in the presence of an adult suggests that the animal-assisted reading programme did impact positively on the reading skills of the students who read to a dog (le Roux et al., 2014). Such studies are promising but are still few.

Moreover, it does not necessarily follow that reading to a dog builds children's confidence and where it does so, this does not always extend to improved reading skills. For example, Uccheddu et al. (2019) found that children (6–11-year-olds) with autism who read to a dog had better attendance and were better motivated than those who did not, but there were no significant differences in cognitive and reading tests between the two groups. We do not know why there is a disparity in these cases between reading motivation and skill. It may be due to the short duration of most reading-to-dog programmes.

CHILDREN WITH SOCIAL AND COMMUNICATION DIFFICULTIES

Children are social beings, naturally predisposed to interact with other humans, non-human animals, and living things. The term 'natural childhood' describes children's primal urge to connect with the natural world around them (Fromm, 1964), which is seen as part of their biological and evolutionary heritage. As Chapter 1 noted, dogs have long played an important role as a companion to humans. Wilson's (1984) theory of biophilia posits that children are genetically driven to connect with animals and nature, although this does not necessarily mean that this is a positive connection. The relationship can become 'unlikable and unfriendly, if not threatening and harmful' (Kahn, 1997, p. 2). Yet, social commentators have argued that children's opportunities to interact with nature and the animal world in general has declined in modern times for a range of reasons, including sedentary lifestyles, over-protective parents, the rise of a risk-adverse culture, a lack of green play spaces, and the obsession with technologies (Louv, 2005; Palmer, 2007; Postman, 1982). Not only are children allegedly missing out on nature, but concerns have also been raised that the social skills of the present generation are not as well developed as previous generations. In fact, setting aside the COVID-19 pandemic, and the associated social distance restrictions, the evidence suggests that social skills are not in decline (Downey & Gibbs, 2020). Rather, children are increasingly interacting in different, nonlinear ways. The Internet, for example, may hinder social skills in some ways but promote them in others. There are pet dogs with millions of followers on Instagram. And increasingly, schools are tapping into social media to publicise their therapy dogs and engage parents and the wider community.[1]

Over recent decades, therapy dogs have featured in educational settings for the purpose of supporting children with a range of social and communication difficulties. Most notably, studies (e.g., Kern et al., 2011; Redefer & Goodman, 1989; Sams et al., 2006) have focused on the impact of dogs on children with Attention-deficit/hyperactivity disorder (ADHD), medical conditions (Barker et al., 2015), emotional and behavioural difficulties (Barker & Dawson 1998; Nagengast et al., 1997), and physical conditions (Hooker et al., 2002).

The general picture is a positive one. Dogs are reported to be a source of non-verbal, non-judgemental companionship, enabling children to rehearse social skills without the stressful presence of adults (Grigore & Rusu, 2014; Solomon, 2010). Reading with a dog can reduce the amount of stress experienced compared to reading to a friend or adult (Jalongo et al., 2004). Meintz et al. (2022) show that dog-assisted interventions can reduce stress levels in school children with effects lasting over the school term. Even the presence of a guinea pig improved social behaviours in children with autism spectrum disorders (O'Haire, 2013). Pets are considered a source of support (Van Houtte & Jarvis, 1995), providing children with qualities that people cannot (Bueche, 2003). Dogs are perceived to promote acceptance and trust (Anderson & Olson, 2006; Thigpen et al., 2005).

There is a growing body of research exploring the impact of dogs in supporting children with disabilities. Autism is a developmental disability that affects how people communicate and interact with others. Children with autism, which is derived from the Greek word *autos* ('self'), are often self-absorbed in their own private worlds in which they struggle in different ways to communicate with others. Hence, a spectrum is used to capture the wide range of social, communication, and behavioural challenges. Children with autism struggle to understand the nuances of communication and complexities of social relationships because of their tendency to think in concrete and literal terms. They may have problems understanding the actions, intentions, and emotions of others, and have difficulties with organising, planning, and managing (executive functioning) themselves. The unpredictable nature of school environments can prove unsettling and heighten anxiety. Hence, educators often use visual timetables, calendars, timers, checklists, simple sequenced instructions (e.g., 'Now, Next, Then'), and carefully labelled items, to reinforce familiar routines. They also break activities into small chunks with calming moments in between so that children with autism have time to regulate their feelings (Watson, 2022).

In caring for dogs and taking responsibility for their training, children enhance their perspective-taking skills as they respond to the animal's feedback. O'Haire and Gabriels (2017, p. 90) identify the following eight evidence-based benefits of animals for children with autism (Figure 2.3).

The authors also acknowledge that dogs and other animals pose additional potential risks for children with autism; for example, distraction from their work, fear or dislike of animals, allergic reactions, and harm for the animals. However, each of these can be ameliorated through careful planning and preparation. Picture

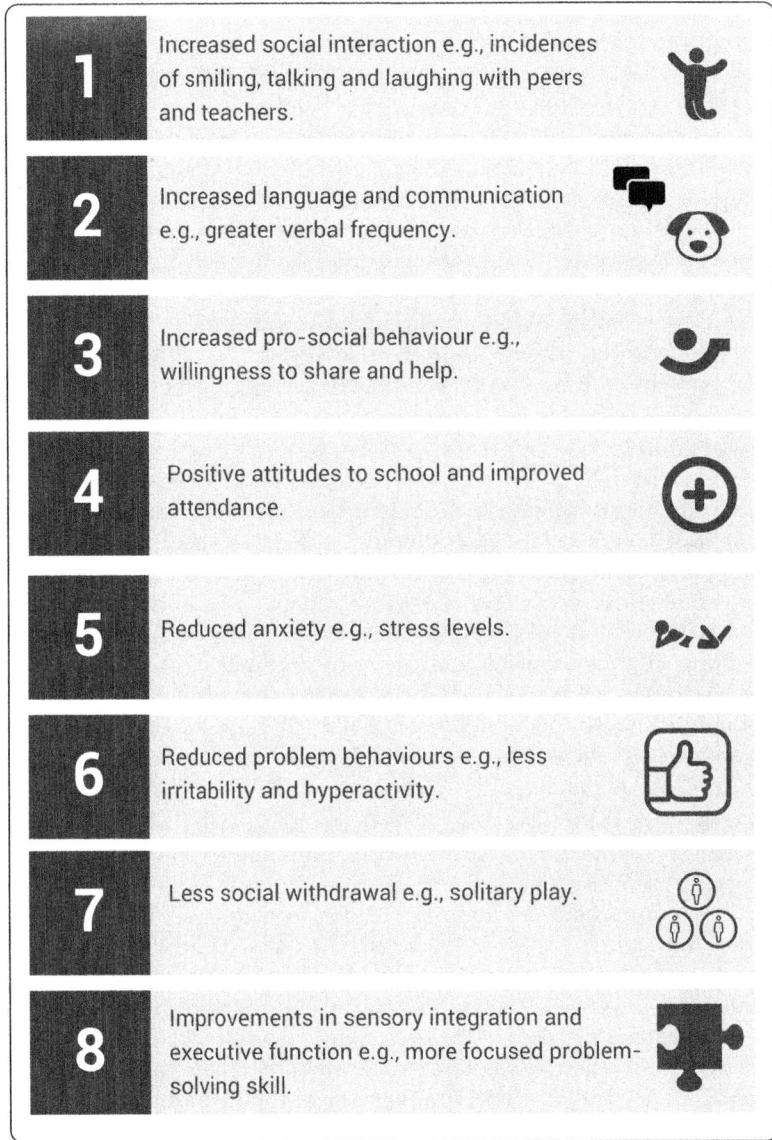

FIGURE 2.3 Benefits of animals for children with autism.

schedules can help children understand routines of feeding, grooming and exercising dogs, while symbols can be devised to remind children of the rules when interacting with dogs, such as using a quiet voice and gentle touch. Selecting a quiet, clean space for the intervention to take place, with reminders that dogs also dislike chaotic, noisy environments, can provide further reassurance for children who prefer routine. Children with autism spectrum disorder (ASD) may demonstrate more prosocial behaviours in the company of a dog, including talking, looking at faces, and touching (Harris & Sholtis, 2016). Children's social interaction with dogs may also see a reduction in the frequency of prompting from an adult (Fung, 2017). In the words of one 11-year-old diagnosed with Asperger's syndrome, interviewed for CBS News, 'Anyone who has autism, anybody in the world would just benefit from this. She's just like a healing dog' (Solomon, 2010, p. 143).

A growing number of UK charities are specialising in providing trained dogs to work with autistic children and adults. Examples include Helpful Hounds Assistance Dogs, Dogs for Autism, Dogs for Good, Autism Dogs Charity, and Support Dogs. The developing evidence (e.g., Leung et al., 2022) suggests that such assistance dogs are effective in promoting the quality of social interaction and communication skills of individuals with ASD. Parents perceive the benefits to include the emotional comfort and sense of freedom afforded to their children (Burgoyne et al., 2014), and their increased participation in daily routines (Hellings et al., 2022), although canine assistance alone by itself is not seen as sufficient therapy (Hill et al., 2020).

Supporters of animal-based humane education, with its emphasis on displaying compassion, empathy, and respect for all living beings, argue that their programmes promote the social skills children need. This seems to be particularly so for children with autism, the most common neurobehavioural childhood disorder. By adopting the role of dog trainers and mentors, children with ADHD have shown respect, kindness, compassion, and other prosocial behaviours (Chadwick et al., 2022; Plumer & Stoner, 2005). In Project Positive Assertive Cooperative Kids (P.A.C.K.), 24 children with ADHD and their parents participated in a randomised clinical trial (see Chapter 10) using a canine-assisted intervention over a 12-week period. The control group received cognitive-behavioural therapy. Across both treatment groups, parents reported improvements in children's social skills and a reduction in the severity of ADHD symptoms. However, the greatest reductions were experienced by children within the dog-assisted intervention (Schuck et al., 2015).

While there is a shortage of rigorous scientific research on how dogs impact children with social and communication difficulties, there is plenty of anecdotal evidence worth considering. One school librarian in Yorkshire relates the story of a girl with selective mutism who according to her mother had never read to anyone other than close family at home. When she was first introduced to the idea of reading to a dog, the girl settled down next to the dog and started whispering to him as she read: 'The longer she stroked him the more relaxed she became and by the end of the book, she was reading aloud' (Local Government Association, 2022). In summarising anecdotal reports on the impact of animal-assisted interventions (AAIs) on children with ADHD, Schuck and Fine (2017, p. 17) convey the following messages: children are less worried and stressed when animals are around; they seem less active but better at academic tasks in the presence of an animal; taking care of animals makes them more responsible; and animals improve the social milieu of group activities like peer to peer mentoring. The authors argue that children's social competence improves through peer mentoring programmes involving therapy dogs and that the prosocial skills benefit the whole school community.

Steel (2022) reports a case study in which the *most vulnerable* children in a Scottish primary school made the greatest gains in well-being and engagement in reading with dogs. However, a cautionary note is needed. The novelty of a dog can distract children from their learning and in some cases add anxiety (Steel, 2022; Steel et al., 2021). One study reports children performed better without a dog present, albeit in only one out of ten physical tasks (Gee et al., 2007).

CHILDREN'S WELL-BEING

Much of the literature on dogs in educational settings focuses on their contribution to promoting children and young people's well-being, described by the Council of Europe (n.d.) simply as 'the experience of health and happiness'. A more detailed definition is offered by the UK's National Institute for Health and Care Excellence (2018, p. 3): 'happiness, confidence and not feeling depressed, resilience to cope with difficulties, ability to have good relationships with others, think clearly, participate in decision making, and have optimism, sense of control and self-efficacy'. While definitions of well-being vary, reflecting different disciplinary and cultural perspectives, educators and policymakers recognise the need to approach well-being holistically (OECD, 2021b).

Common themes in the well-being literature revolve around satisfaction with life, emotional self-regulation, a sense of optimism, and possessing the personal resources to cope with challenges (Oberle, 2018; Statham & Chase, 2010). Prominent theoretical perspectives include the notion of 'havings' (natural and social goods e.g., intelligence, health, and income) that individuals need for the good life (Rawls, 1971); and the extent to which people have the freedom of opportunity to achieve outcomes that they value and have reason to value (Sen, 1999). Other theorists contend that relationships matter above all else and well-being emerges from these rather than what people have: 'it inheres in the dance; it is not the property of individual dancers' (White, 2015, p. 11).

There is a strong relationship between children's well-being and their learning. Clearly, children who feel good about themselves and receive appropriate emotional support when needed are more likely to be in the right frame of mind to explore new ideas and ways of thinking, which are key to academic achievement. Physical activity is associated with improved learning and the ability to concentrate. Strong, supportive relationships help children to develop self-confidence and belief to step out of their intellectual 'comfort zone'. Hence, there is an emerging consensus, which endorses a multidimensional view of well-being, which goes beyond single metrics, to embrace emotional, social, physical, psychological, and economic domains (Ruggeri et al., 2020). Both objective data and subjective views are now seen as important sources in understanding well-being although the latter has gained in status over recent years. This is largely due to the rise in the children's rights movement and an emphasis on their agency in framing what well-being means to them.

EMOTIONAL WELL-BEING

Companion animals can offer something that humans often struggle with – unconditional love and emotional support (Jalongo et al., 2004). Emotional well-being describes how well children and young people perceive the emotional quality of their everyday experiences. Psychologists have conceptualised emotions in different ways, from Ekman's (1999) list of eight basic emotions (anger, fear, sadness, disgust, surprise, anticipation, trust, and joy) shared around the world, to a far more nuanced set of 27 inter-related gradients of emotions (Cowen & Keltner, 2017). Plutchik (1980) proposed a Wheel of Emotions as a means of understanding how primary emotions combine to trigger behavioural patterns, while Goleman (1995) popularised the importance of emotional intelligence or quotient (EQ) in building strong relationships, succeeding at school, and achieving goals. Dog-assisted interventions have the potential to boost each component of a child's EQ: self-awareness, self-management, social awareness, and social skills. Through interactions with therapy dogs, children can build their sense of optimism, confidence, and self-efficacy, learning to cope with life's challenges (Oberle, 2018).

The importance of learning to effectively regulate emotions in self and others has been advocated for many years (Mayer et al., 2011; Salovey & Mayer, 1990). This has led to a range of school-based programmes aiming to promote social and emotional learning (e.g., DfE, 2010). However, success in terms of both emotional and academic outcomes hinges on how well interventions are embedded into routine school practices and the degree and quality of professional development and training for staff (EEF, 2019). It is also important to ensure that materials are accessible for students and teachers receive appropriate guidance. Chapter 4 discusses SponsorDogs, a Swedish programme, which aims to develop empathy and other aspects of children's emotional and social well-being. Children participate in games, and learn basic greetings and how to act respectfully around the dog. Afterwards, they complete colouring sheets to record their actions while teachers receive curriculum guidance and a storybook, which highlights the importance of pro-social behaviour when interacting with dogs (Figure 2.4).

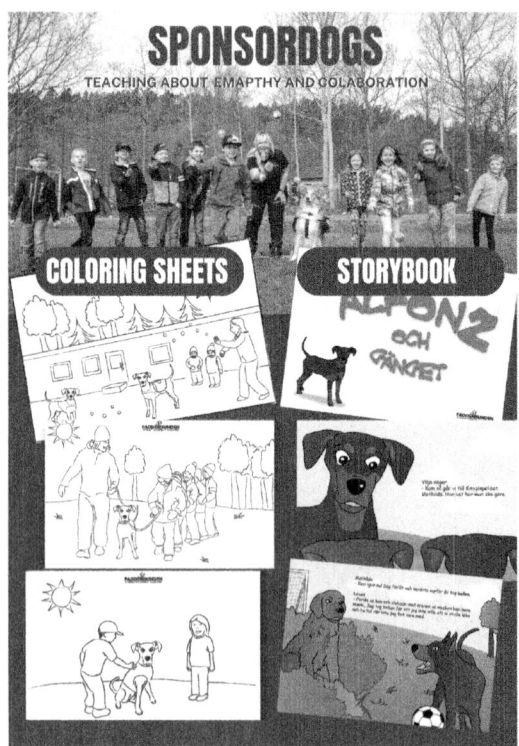

FIGURE 2.4 SponsorDogs. Teaching about empathy and collaboration.

The literature suggests that children who are emotionally secure are likely to make most progress in primary school, are more engaged in secondary school, and achieve higher academic grades (Gutman & Vorgaus, 2012). In terms of AAIs, Fredrickson (2004) posits that as children experience enhanced moods when reading with dogs, these contribute to more enduring cognitive and social reserves. For example, they acquire new knowledge and understanding, increase self-esteem and develop the skills necessary to interact successfully with others. Further, Fredrickson (2001) speculates that such positive emotions undo the negative ones that children may bring to reading tasks. This effect could explain why some children say they enjoy reading even when they are not capable readers (Reading Agency, 2015).

SOCIAL WELL-BEING

Social well-being involves the development of meaningful, positive relationships. The extent to which we connect with others and feel a sense of belonging is closely associated with our emotional well-being and mental health. In the absence of significant, sustained, and loving relationships, the likelihood of experiencing loneliness, negative emotions and more serious depression, and suicidal thoughts increases (Baumeister & Leary, 1995). Various theories have been put forward to explain how these develop. Most notably, Bowlby's (1969) theory of attachment suggests that young children develop a psychosocial bond with a specific person, which shapes the extent to which the child sees the world as a safe, trustworthy place. Interestingly, studies show that individuals with an insecure attachment style form a particularly strong emotional attachment to their companion animals (Lass-Hennemann et al., 2022). Touch, proximity, and mind-body interaction with animals contribute to stress reduction and trauma recovery (Yorke, 2010).

There are several theoretical models that seek to explain the nature of the human-animal bond. For example, Gee et al. (2021) refer to a biopsychosocial model. From this perspective, the dynamic nature of the human-canine relationship may differentially interact with each of the three influencers of human health and well-being. Biological influencers include physiological changes such as heart rate, psychological influencers include emotions, and social influencers include relationships with peers. These influencers are not fixed but rather interact with each other over time.

In terms of forming relationships and attachments, it seems that children aged between 6 and 10 years of age prefer dogs and cats over other species (Hirschenhauser et al., 2017). It is difficult to cuddle a fish or tortoise, while dog behaviour particularly supports anthropomorphic play. Companion animals positively influence children's social development and play a valuable role in therapy (Endenburg & van Lith, 2011).

The theory of social support suggests that AAIs are effective because animals provide comfort, reassurance, and a sense of belongness and promote confidence and self-esteem (McNicholas & Collis, 2006). In some aspects of social support, animals excel in providing non-judgemental companionship and consistent availability. Unlike humans, dogs do not lie, retaliate, or betray trust (Serpell, 2002). And the basis of good social relationships is trust. Studies suggest that when children develop positive relationships with animals, this might mitigate negative feelings towards

humans by building trust (Beetz et al., 2012; Julius et al., 2013). There is some biological evidence to support this view with reported reductions in salivary cortisol and
skin conductance responses following participation in AAIs (e.g., Meints et al., 2022;
O'Haire et al., 2014). Shy children and those who have experienced rejection by
their peers say that they feel more confident as a result of regular interactions with a
dog (Lane & Zavada, 2013).

In one study of the personality of dogs and their German and Austrian owners,
Haubenhofer (2009) found that a 'typical' dog owner involved in AAIs was active,
assertive, considerate, committed, and self-confident. When asked to describe the
qualities of their dogs, most chose the same qualities: sociable, calm, well balanced,
fond-of-children, clever, and obedient. However, it is important to note that within
the same breeds, dogs have different temperaments and personalities. A dog's breed
is reported to explain only 9% of behavioural variation among different dogs (Morrill
et al., 2022). Even behavioural traits that appear to be breed-specific, such as bidda-
bility (how readily a dog responded to commands), have been found to vary significantly among individual animals within the same breed. In short, a dog's breed is not
always a good predictor of its behaviour, which is an important consideration for
schools choosing their dogs. This is explored in more detail in Chapter 8.

Most children and young people who have participated in AAIs are reported
to have gained in terms of their social and emotional well-being. Studies point
to improved relationships, greater responsibility, and the exercising of empathy
and care (Gee et al., 2017). The dog's presence is said to act as a 'social lubricant'
(Wells, 2019, p. 527), creating a calm ambience in which children feel at ease in
sharing their thoughts and feelings, while also fostering closeness, cooperation,
and other prosocial behaviours. Research by Beetz (2013) found that children
who had a school dog-teacher team in the classroom through the course of a year
held more positive attitudes to school and prosocial behaviours than the control
group.

What makes dogs different to us is that they represent 'what you see is what you
get' (Walsh, 2009, p. 471) without the more complex aspects of human behaviour
and friendship. For children who have experienced adverse childhoods, such as
experiences of domestic violence or abuse, dogs project a safe and accepting zone to
express (or not express) feelings, thus fulfilling children's social, emotional, and psychological need for companionship without fear. This is also the case for those children who have experienced rejection or stigma, which is why AAIs feature strongly in
special schools and units. We also know that the presence of a therapy dog can promote social inclusion. In one study, children without disabilities were ten times more
likely to interact with peers who had disabilities when such children were accompanied by a dog (Katcher, 1997).

One of the most important aspects of social well-being is the feeling of being
listened to. Children can be reassured through their interactions with dogs that
they will receive the attention they need because dogs are commonly perceived as
'good listeners' who do not interrupt or hurry children, giving them the space and
time to express themselves (Klotz, 2014). In contrast, the typical classroom power
dynamics and logistics of 30 or so competing voices means that there are individuals
whose voices remain relatively unheard. In some cases, the experience of reading
with dogs improves children's oracy skills more so than their reading (Levinson
et al., 2017).

Social well-being is not only about children's experiences now, but also their well-becoming. In other words, thinking forwards to the quality of life that children should experience and how this can be achieved. Since the late 1980s, the growing emphasis on children's rights, particularly their right to be heard alongside the development of more learner-centred curricula, has presented opportunities to capitalise on children's interests. Given the universal popularity of dogs, schools are increasingly seeing their potential to break down barriers to children's learning and well-being. These include a lack of motivation and reported widespread boredom with traditional teaching practices.

Nowadays, the principles of effective pedagogy, such as giving serious attention to learner voice, building on their prior experience, and meeting their diverse needs (Husbands & Pearce, 2012), align well with incorporating animals into approaches to well-being, teaching plans, and practices. Instructional quality is complex, and there is no single route to successful learning outcomes with both child-centred learning and direct instruction having merit (OECD, 2012). A capability approach (CA) focuses on how children can exercise more informed choices over how they learn, take increasing responsibilities for their learning, and pursue goals that they value and have reason to do so (Biggeri & Santi, 2012).

PHYSICAL WELL-BEING

Children's physical well-being has been defined as 'the ability to perform physical activities and carry out social roles that are not hindered by physical limitations and experiences of bodily pain, and biological health indicators' (Capio et al., 2014, p. 4805). Animals have long been utilised in educational settings to help develop children's motor and physical skill development (Chandler, 2001). Children with moderate physical impairments may be capable of dropping or throwing a ball to a dog, brushing it, or pouring water into a bowl. Most older children can take a dog for a walk in the school grounds or join in more active games such as running or orientation exercises. Such physical exertions can develop both fine and gross motor movements (Siegel, 2004).

Given the widely reported physical and cognitive benefits of walking, there is surprisingly few studies that have focused on the impact of dog-facilitated physical activity for children. A recent Australian study of 150 dog-owning parents and children reported a range of benefits as children played with the family dog, including overall physical activity, socio-emotional development, self-regulation, self-esteem, empathy, and level of attachment to their dog (Ng et al., 2021). However, there are potentially detrimental outcomes with children being the most at-risk population regarding minor dog bites, serious injuries, and fatalities (Giraudet et al., 2022), so interventions need careful planning and management.

MENTAL HEALTH AND PSYCHOLOGICAL WELL-BEING

The World Health Organisation (WHO, 2022) defines mental health as 'a state of well-being in which an individual realises his or her own abilities, can cope with the normal stresses of life, can work productively and fruitfully, and is able to make a contribution to his or her community'. Alongside this positive view is the notion of mental disorders and symptoms of mental illness, such as excessive anxiety, extreme mood changes, and social isolation. The WHO (2021) estimates that 13% of children and adolescents (10–19) experience mental health issues. Psychological well-being covers a wider range of cognitive aspects of mental health than affect and life satisfaction such as mastery and a sense of control, having a purpose in life, a sense of belonging, and positive relationships with others.

Dog-assisted programmes have been reported to benefit children and young people's mental health across a range of settings. Grajfoner et al. (2017) found a significant reduction in anxiety levels among university students when the dogs were present, compared to those interacting solely with the handler while the difference between the two conditions in which the dogs were present was not significant. The findings reinforced those from previous studies (e.g., Lannon & Harrison, 2015), which report improvements in well-being among college students attending therapy dog sessions. Guzmán et al. (2022) report reductions in emotional and behavioural outbursts of 23 child outpatients in a Barcelona hospital, compared to the days that the dog-assisted therapy interventions were not carried out. These children, suffering from severe mental disorders, improved their attendance, emotional self-regulation, and social skills through participating in therapy sessions with dogs through the course of a year. However, based on parental feedback, it seems that these gains were not demonstrated outside of the hospital setting. The authors speculate that this was possible because the changes were easier to observe in a controlled environment.

Across the United Kingdom, the rise in mental health problems among children and young people over recent decades, exacerbated by the pandemic, has led to government strategies to improve mental health support and services (Grimm et al., 2022). Despite the growing body of evidence to show that AAIs can have a positive impact on mental health, they rarely feature in official policy discourse and tend to rely on charities such as Pets as Therapy to support their implementation. In reviewing the growing presence of therapy dogs in further education, Mersinoglu (2019) cites the former education secretary Damian Hinds admitting that he 'had not realised the incidence of well-being dogs in education providers until he visited classrooms'. But he added that 'it was a great thing for learners and can be really uplifting'.

LIMITATIONS OF RESEARCH

It would be a one-sided chapter if we did not note the limitations of existing research and the potential drawbacks of bringing dogs into school. One of the most enduring criticisms of AAIs is the need for more rigorous scientific research to improve the methodological quality in the field. Stern and Chur-Hansen (2013, p. 127) point out that there are too many anecdotal accounts and 'experimental studies undertaken are often flawed in aspects of design, conduct and reporting'. The authors provide a detailed review of the limitations associated with research in the field. These include inconsistent terminology, small sample sizes (average between 30 and 40), a lack of consensus over how interventions are administered, variation in the duration of sessions (from 3 to 90 minutes), and in the nature of the intervention, which makes it difficult to prove causation. They point out that in some research projects dogs are held on a lead while in others they are left unleashed to interact with participants, while conducting a session with an individual in a private room may be a very difference experience to a group scenario. Although the authors were reviewing literature relating to canine-assisted interventions for older people residing in long-term care, many of these limitations apply to school settings.

While there are many studies that report the positive effects of dog-assisted interventions in educational settings, selection bias needs to be considered. Such studies usually include participants that choose to select dogs. More generally, it is also worth noting that interactions with dogs have negative consequences in terms of financial cost, while children's anxieties around dogs may well be underreported. The size and universality of these effects are unclear. Krouzecky et al. (2019) highlight that media reports of dogs relieving human stress are exaggerated. More generally, the media is quick to vaunt the amazing capabilities of dogs, but there is something to be said for moving the narrative on from magic to science.

One area that has received less attention is the dog's specific characteristics: for example, its breed, size, and age. Children may prefer one breed over another, larger or smaller dogs and respond better to puppies over adult dogs, although this then raises questions over the dogs' welfare. Hirschenhauser et al. (2017) found that younger children's (6–10-year-olds) relationships co-varied with taxonomic order of their pets. In contrast, 11- to 14-year-old children reported similarly high scores of attachment with their mouse or iguana as with their dog or cat, and the relationship patterns did not co-vary with taxonomic order.

Many papers are unclear in describing who was present during the intervention and their exact roles. The basic assumption in the AAI literature is that it is the dog (or other animal) that makes the difference in the intervention. Even when this seems to be the case, however, it is less clear which specific attributes of the animal contribute to the reported effects. For safety reasons, it is almost always the case in school settings that the dog is accompanied by either the teacher or a trained handler or both. At times, this makes it difficult to ascertain what role the dog plays in the intervention and the extent to which they act autonomously. Hall and Malpus (2000) argue that the critical interaction in an intervention may be between the subject and the handler and not the animal.

A further limitation is that if research reports on a dog-assisted intervention over a short duration, it is possible that any gains may be due to the novelty factor of having a dog in school rather than the intervention itself. There is also the possibility that any positive effects from touching or interacting with a dog may be short-lived, lasting during and shortly after the interaction. This does not make the experience of less significance for the participants, but clearly educators are looking for interventions to produce lasting impact.

Despite these limitations, Wagner et al. (2022) identified 176 studies that fulfilled their inclusion criteria of investigating an AAI, having control conditions for comparison, and were published in English or German. Their systematic review included studies of animals other than dogs, such as dolphins, mice, and horses, in a range of settings other than schools. They also avoided publication bias by including non-peer-reviewed manuscripts, although they acknowledge that this meant the study quality was sometimes low. Their stark conclusion is a reminder that there is still a long way to go in the field: 'research still cannot answer the question of how and why

AAIs work'. (Wagner et al., 2022, p. 1). The authors recommend making greater use of placebo research, which deliberately includes fake or no-effect treatments, to tease out participants' perceptions of the intervention such as information and expectations about the treatment' (Wagner et al., 2022, p. 23). Here they are referring to AAIs in hospital settings, but they also suggest the use of robotic dogs to confound the novelty aspect of AAIs. This might have potential with schools using educational programmes or apps featuring virtual pet dogs compared to living creatures. The authors also advocate the use of component studies which look more closely at the contribution of individual components of an intervention independently or in some combination to determine the contribution of each.

Gee et al. (2017) highlight the danger of publication bias, where studies report only significant treatment effects than null findings. They point out that reporting disappointing results is important to help inform the selection of interventions to support students. In areas such as well-being, which at times is loosely defined, it can be challenging for researchers to identify exactly which areas AAIs target. Making comparisons of well-being in different social and cultural contexts is also difficult because factors such as language, religions, gender, age, social expectations can all shape what well-being means to an individual. With an increase in the popularity and prevalence of Reading to Dogs (RTD) interventions designed to support children's literacy, mental health and well-being (Brelsford et al., 2017; Hall et al., 2016; Reilly et al., 2020), there is a need for more research to understand and examine the experiences and impact of including dogs in educational settings (Lewis & Grigg, 2021). In the future, there is also a need for more systematic cross-cultural research and longitudinal studies to better understand the impact of child-dog interactions.

Finally, but importantly, while this chapter has focused on how dogs contribute to children's well-being, the potential 'will and thrill' for dogs in such interactions needs to be more closely examined. There is also a danger of dogs being unintentionally viewed as a resource or pedagogical tool. This awareness of the needs and desires of the dog as an active partner in any interaction will form part of the recommendations for pedagogy discussed in the next chapter.

NOTE

1 https://www.thetelegraphandargus.co.uk/news/19912006.harden-primary-school-dog-archie-instagram-tiktok-hit/; https://www.countesswear.devon.sch.uk/percy-our-school-dog

REFERENCES

Anderson, K. L., & Olson, M. R. (2006). The value of a dog in a classroom of children with severe emotional disorders. *Anthrozoös: A Multidisciplinary Journal of the Interactions of People & Animals, 19*, 35–49. https://doi.org/10.2752/089279306785593919

Barker, S. B., & Dawson, K. S. (1998). The effects of animal-assisted therapy on anxiety ratings of hospitalized psychiatric patients. *Psychiatric Services, 49*(6), 797–801.

Barker, S. B., Knisely, J. S., Schubert, C. M., Green, J. D., & Ameringer, S. (2015). The effect of an animal-assisted intervention on anxiety and pain in hospitalized children. *Anthrozoös: A Multidisciplinary Journal of the Interactions of People & Animals, 28*(1), 101–112.

Baumeister, R. F., & Leary, M. R. (1995). The need to belong: Desire for interpersonal attachments as a fundamental human motivation. *Psychological Bulletin, 117*(3), 497–529.

Beetz, A. (2013). Socio-emotional correlates of a schooldog-teacher-team in the classroom. *Frontiers in Psychology,* 886. https://www.frontiersin.org/articles/10.3389/fpsyg.2013.00886/full

Beetz, A., & McCardle, P. (2017). Does reading to a dog affect reading skills? In N. Gee, A. Fine, & R. McCardle (Eds.), *How animals help students learn* (pp. 111–123). Routledge.

Beetz, A., Uvnäs-Moberg, K., Julius, H., & Kotrschal, K. (2012). Psychosocial and psychophysiological effects of human-animal interactions: The possible role of oxytocin. *Frontiers in Psychology, 3,* Article 234. https://doi.org/10.3389/fpsyg.2012.00234

Beetz, A. M. (2017). Theories and possible processes of action in animal assisted interventions. *Applied Developmental Science, 21*(2), 139–149.

Biggeri, M., & Santi, M. (2012). The missing dimensions of children's well-being and well-becoming in education systems: Capabilities and philosophy for children. *Journal of Human Development and Capabilities, 13*(3), 373–395. https://doi.org/10.1080/19452829.2012.694858

Booten, A. E. (2011). Effects of animal-assisted therapy on behavior and reading in the classroom [Doctoral Dissertation, Marshall University]. https://mds.marshall.edu/etd/22

Borgi, M., Loliva, D., Cerino, S., Chiarotti, F., Venerosi, A., Bramini, M., & Cirulli, F. (2016). Effectiveness of a standardized equine-assisted therapy program for children with autism spectrum disorder. *Journal of Autism and Developmental Disorders, 46*(1), 1–9. https://doi.org/10.1007/s10803-015-2530-6

Bowlby, J. (1969). *Attachment and loss: Vol. 1. Attachment.* Basic Books.

Brelsford, V. L., Meints, K., Gee, N. R., & Pfeffer, K. (2017). Animal-assisted interventions in the classroom—A systematic review. *International Journal of Environmental Research and Public Health, 14*(7), 669. https://doi.org/10.3390/ijerph14070669

Bueche, S. (2003). Going to the dogs: Therapy dogs promote reading. *Reading Today, 20,* 46.

Burgoyne, L., Dowling, L., Fitzgerald, A., Connolly, M., Browne, J. P., & Perry, I. J. (2014). Parents' perspectives on the value of assistance dogs for children with autism spectrum disorder: A cross-sectional study. *BMJ Open, 4*(6), e004786. https://doi.org/10.1136/bmjopen-2014-004786

Capio, C. M., Sit, C. H. P., & Abernethy, B. (2014). Physical well-being. In A. C. Michalos (Ed.), *Encyclopedia of quality of life and well-being research* (pp. 4805–4807). Springer.

Castellano, J. (2015). Pet therapy is a nearly cost-free anxiety reducer on college campuses. https://www.forbes.com/sites/jillcastellano/2015/07/06/pet-therapy-is-a-nearly-cost-free-anxiety-reducer-on-college-campuses/#131248e17c59

Chadwick, Z., Edmondson, A., & MacDonald, S. (2022). Engaging with animal-assisted interventions (AAIs): Exploring the experiences of young people with ASD/ADHD diagnoses. *Support for Learning, 37*(1), 44–61.

Chandler, C. K. (2001). *Animal-assisted therapy in counseling and school settings.* ERIC Clearinghouse on Counseling and Student Services.

Chiang, C., & Lai, C. (2008). Acoustical environment valuation of joint classrooms for primary schools in Taiwan. *Building and Environment, 43*(4), 1619–1632.

Clark, C. (2014). *The reading lives of 8 to 11-year-olds 2005–2013. An evidence paper for the read on get on coalition.* National Literacy Trust.

Clark, C., & De Zoysa, S. (2011). *Mapping the interrelationships of reading enjoyment, attitudes, behaviour and attainment.* National Literacy Trust.

Clark, C., & Douglas, J. (2011). Young people's reading and writing. In C. Clark, & C. Phythian-Sence (Eds.), *Interesting choice: The (relative) importance of choice and interest in reader engagement.* National Literacy Trust.

Clark, C., & Rumbold, K. (2006). *Reading for pleasure: A research overview.* National Literacy Trust.

Connell, C. G., Tepper, D. L., Landry, O., & Bennett, P. C. (2019). Dogs in schools: The impact of specific human–dog interactions on reading ability in children aged 6 to 8 years. *Anthrozoös, 32*(3), 347–360. https://doi.org/10.1080/08927936.2019.1598654

Cowen, A. S., & Keltner, D. (2017). Self-report captures 27 distinct categories of emotion bridged by continuous gradients. *Proceedings of the National Academy of Sciences, 114*(38), E7900–E7909.

Crossman, M. K., Kazdin, A. E., Matijczak, A., Kitt, E. R., & Santos, L. R. (2020). The influence of interactions with dogs on affect, anxiety, and arousal in children. *Journal of Clinical Child & Adolescent Psychology, 49*(4), 535–548. https://doi.org/10.1080/15374416.2018.1520119

De Naeghel, J., Van Keer, H., Vansteenkiste, M., & Rosseel, Y. (2012). Relation between elementary students' recreational and academic reading motivation, reading frequency, engagement, and comprehension: A self-determination theory perspective. *Journal of Educational Psychology, 104*, 1006–1021.

Department for Education (DfE). (2010). *Social and emotional aspects of learning (SEAL) programme in secondary schools: National evaluation.* DfE.

DfE. (2012). *Research evidence on reading for pleasure education standards research team.* DfE.

DfE. (2022). *The reading framework. Teaching the foundations of literacy.* DfE.

Dewitz, P., Jones, J., & Leahy, S. (2009). Comprehension strategy instruction in core reading programs. *Reading Research Quarterly, 44*(2), 102–126.

Downey, D. B., & Gibbs, B. G. (2020). Kids these days: Are face-to-face social skills among American children declining? *American Journal of Sociology, 125*(4), 1030–1083.

Education Endowment Foundation (EEF). (2021). *Metacognition and self-regulated learning guidance report.* EEF.

EEF. (2019). *Improving social and emotional learning in primary schools: Guidance report.* EEF.

Ekman, P. (1999). Basic emotions. In T. Dalgleish, & M. J. Power (Eds.), *Handbook of cognition and emotion* (pp. 45–60). John Wiley & Sons Ltd.

Endenburg, N. & van Lith, H. (2011). The influence of animals on the development of children. *The Veterinary Journal, 190*(2), 208–214.

Engelmann, S., & Carnine, D. (1992). *Theory of instructional design: Principles and applications.* Irvington Press.

Farshore. (2022). Reading for Pleasure and Purpose. https://s28434.pcdn.co/wp-content/uploads/sites/46/2022/03/Reading-for-Pleasure-and-Purpose-Report-Farshore.pdf.

Filiâtre, J. C., Millot, J. L., & Montagner, H. New data on communication behaviour between the young child and his pet dog. *Behavioural Processes, 12*(1):33–44.

Fredrickson, B. L. (2001). The role of positive emotions in positive psychology. The broaden-and-build theory of positive emotions. *American Psychologist, 56*(3), 218–226. https://doi.org/10.1037//0003-066x.56.3.218

Fredrickson, B. L. (2004). The broaden-and-build theory of positive emotions. *Philosophical Transactions of the Royal Society: Biological Sciences, 359*, 1367–1377.

Friesen, L. (2010). Exploring animal-assisted programs with children in school and therapeutic contexts. *Early Childhood Education Journal, 37*(4), 261–267.

Friesen, L. (2013). Establishing a climate of care and safety: Considerations for volunteers' entry and sustained involvement in animal-assisted literacy programs in elementary classrooms. In M. Jalongo (Ed.), *Educating the young child: Advances in theory and research, implications for practice* in the volume *teaching compassion: Humane education in early childhood* (pp. 149–160). Springer.

Fromm, E. (1964). *The heart of man.* Harper and Row.

Fung, S. C. (2017). An observational study on canine-assisted play therapy for children with autism: Move towards the phrase of manualization and protocol development. *Global Journal of Health Science, 9*(7), 67–86. https://doi.org/10.5539/gjhs.v9n7p67

Gee, N., Fine, A., & McCardle, R. (Eds.) (2017). *How animals help students learn.* Routledge.

Gee, N. R., Harris, S. L., & Johnson, K. L. (2007). The role of therapy dogs in speed and accuracy to complete motor skills tasks for preschool children. *Anthrozoös, 20*(4), 375–386.

Gee, N. R., Rodriguez, K., Fine, A. K., & Trammell, J. P. (2021). Dogs supporting human health and well-being: a biopsychosocial approach. *Frontiers in Veterinary Science, 8.* https://www.frontiersin.org/articles/10.3389/fvets.2021.630465/full

Geist, T. S. (2011). Conceptual framework for animal assisted therapy. *Child and Adolescent Social Work Journal, 28*(3), 243–256.

Giraudet, C., Liu, K., McElligott, A., & Cobb, M. (2022). Are children and dogs best friends? A scoping review to explore the positive and negative effects of child-dog interactions. *PeerJ*, e14532. https://doi.org/10.7717/peerj.14532

Goleman, D. (1995). *Emotional intelligence*. Bantam Books.

Grajfoner, D., Harte, E., Potter, L. M., & McGuigan, N. (2017). The effect of dog-assisted intervention on student well-being, mood, and anxiety. *International Journal of Environmental Research and Public Health*, 14(5), 483. https://doi.org/10.3390/ijerph14050483

Grigore, A. A., & Rusu, A. S. (2014). Interaction with a therapy dog enhances the effects of social story method in autistic children. *Society and Animals*, 22(3), 241–261.

Grimm, F., Alcock, B., Butler, J. E., Crespo, R. F., Davies, A., Peytrignet, S., Piroddi, R., Thorlby, R., & Tallack, C. (2022). *Improving children and young people's mental health services*. The Health Foundation.

Gutman, L., & Vorgaus, J. (2012). *The impact of pupil behaviour and wellbeing on educational outcomes*. Institute of Education, University of London Childhood Wellbeing Research Centre.

Guthrie, J. T., & Wigfield, A. (2000). Engagement and motivation in reading. In M. L. Kamil, P. B. Mosenthal, P. D. Pearson, & R. Barr (Eds.), *Handbook of reading research* (Vol. 3, pp. 403–422). Lawrence Erlbaum Associates Publishers.

Guthrie, J. T., Wigfield, A., Humenick, N. M., Perencevich, K. C., Taboada, A., & Barbosa, P. (2006). Influences of stimulating tasks on reading motivation and comprehension. *Journal of Educational Research*, 99, 232–245.

Guzmán E. G., Rodríguez L. S., Santamarina-Perez, P., Hermida Barros, L., Giralt M. R., Elizalde, E. D., Ubach, F. R., Gonzalez, M. R., Pastor Yuste, Y. P., Téllez C. D., Cela, S. R., Gisbert, L. R., Medina, S. M, Ballesteros-Urpi, A., & Liñan, A. M. (2022). The benefits of dog-assisted therapy as complementary treatment in a children's mental health day hospital. *Animals (Basel)*, 12(20), 2841. https://doi.org/10.3390/ani12202841

Hall, S., Gee, N. R., & Mills, D. S. (2016). Children reading to dogs: A systematic review of the literature. *Public Library of Science ONE*, 11(2). https://doi.org/10.1371/journal.pone.0149759

Hall, P. I., & Malpus, Z. (2000). Pets as therapy: Effects on social interaction in long-stay psychiatry. *British Journal of Nursing*, 9, 2220–2225.

Hanover Research. (2022). *The science of reading*. https://portal.ct.gov/-/media/SDE/Academic-Office/Reading-Leadership-Implementation-Council/The-Science-of-Reading–A-Literature-Review-April-2022-Update.pdf

Harris, K., & Sholtis, S. (2016). Companion angels on a leash: Welcoming service dogs into classroom communities for children with autism. *Childhood Education*, 92(4), 263–275. https://doi.org/10.1080/00094056.2016.1208003

Hattie, J., & Donoghue, G. (2016). Learning strategies: A synthesis and conceptual framework. *Science of Learning*, 1, 16013. https://doi.org/10.1038/npjscilearn.2016.13

Haubenhofer, D. (2009). *The other Side of the effect: Analysis of personality, self-perception and physiological arousal of owner-dog teams working in animal-assisted interventions*. Südwestdeutscher Verlag für Hochschulschriften.

Hellings, D., Joosten, A., Hatfield, M., & Netto, J. (2022). Benefits and challenges of assistance dogs for families of children on the autism spectrum: Mothers' perspectives. *Qualitative Health Research*, 32(11), 1648–1656.

Henderson, L., Grové, C., Lee, F., Trainer, L., Schena, H., & Prentice, M. (2020). An evaluation of a dog-assisted reading program to support student wellbeing in primary school. *Children and Youth Services Review*, 118. https://doi.org/10.1016/j.childyouth.2020.105449

Hill, J., Ziviani, J., Driscoll, C., Teoh, A. L., Chua, J. M., & Cawdell-Smith, J. (2020). Canine assisted occupational therapy for children on the autism spectrum: A pilot randomised control trial. *Journal of Autism and Developmental Disorders*, 50(11), 4106–4120.

Hirschenhauser, K., Meichel, Y., Schmalzer, S., & Beetz, A. M. (2017). children love their pets: Do relationships between children and pets co-vary with taxonomic order, gender, and age? *Anthrozoös*, 30(3), 441–456. https://doi.org/10.1080/08927936.2017.1357882

Hooker, S. D., Freeman, L. H., & Stewart, P. (2002). Pet therapy research: A historical review. *Holistic Nursing Practice, 17*, 17–23.

Howard, V. (2011). The importance of pleasure reading in the lives of young teens: Self-identification, self-construction and self-awareness. *Journal of Librarianship and Information Science, 43*(1), 46–55.

Hume, L. E., Lonigan, C. J., & McQueen, J. D. (2015). Children's literacy interest and its relation to parents' literacy-promoting practices. *Journal of Research in Reading, 38*, 172–193.

Husbands, C., & Pearce, J. (2012). *What makes great pedagogy? Nine claims from research.* National College for School Leadership.

Jacobs, J., & Paris, S. (1987). Children's metacognition about reading: Issues in definition, measurement, and instruction. *Educational Psychologist, 22*(3–4), 255–278. https://doi.org/10.1080/0046 1520.1987.9653052

Jalongo, M. R., Astorino, T., & Bomboy, N. (2004). Canine visitors: The influence of 29 therapy dogs on young children's learning and well-being in classrooms and hospitals. *Early Childhood Education Journal, 32*(1), 9–16.

Julius, H., Beetz, A., Kotrschal, K., Turner, D., & Uvnäs-Moberg, K. (2013). *Attachment to pets.* Hogrefe.

Kahn, P. (1997). Developmental psychology and the biophilia hypothesis: Children's affiliation with nature. *Developmental Review, 17*, 1–61.

Katcher, A. H. (1997). New roles for companion animals mean new roles for veterinarians. *The Newsmagazine of Veterinary Medicine, 29*(6), 12–16.

Katzir, T., Lesaux, N. K., & Kim, Y. S. (2009). The role of reading self-concept and home literacy practices in fourth grade reading comprehension. *Reading and Writing, 22*, 261–276. https://doi.org/10.1007/s11145-007-9112-8

Kern, J. K., Fletcher, C. L., Garver, C. R., Mehta, J. A., Grannemann, B. D., Knox, K. R., Richardson, T. A., & Trivedi, H. (2011). Prospective trial of equine-assisted activities in autism spectrum disorder. *Alternative Therapies in Health and Medicine, 17*(3), 14–20.

Kirnan, J., Siminerio, S., & Wong, Z. (2016). The impact of a therapy dog on children's reading skills and attitudes towards reading. *Early Childhood Education Journal, 44*(6), 637–651. https://doi.org/10.1007/s10643-015-0747-9

Klotz, K. (2014). Promoting humane education through intermountain therapy animals' R.E.A.D. program. In M. R. Jalongo (Ed.), *Teaching compassion: Humane education in early childhood* (pp. 175–195). Springer.

Kropp, J. J. (2017). Review of the research: Are therapy dogs in classrooms beneficial? *Forum on Public Policy.* https://files.eric.ed.gov/fulltext/EJ1173578.pdf

Krouzecky, C., Emmett, L., Klaps, A., Aden, J., Bunina, A., & Stetina, B. U. (2019). And in the middle of my chaos there was you? Dog companionship and its impact on the assessment of stressful situations. *International Journal of Environmental Research and Public Health, 16*, 3664. https://doi.org/10.3390/ijerph16193664

Lane, H. B., & Zavada, S. D. (2013). When reading gets ruff: Canine-assisted reading programs. *Reading Teacher, 67*(2), 87–95.

Lannon, A., & Harrison, P. (2015). Take a paws: Fostering student wellness with a therapy dog program at your university library. *Public Services Quarterly, 11*, 13–22. https://doi.org/10.1080/15228959.2014.984264

Lass-Hennemann, J., Schäfer, S. K., Sopp, M. R., & Michael, T. (2022). The relationship between attachment to pets and mental health: The shared link via attachment to humans. *BMC Psychiatry, 22*, 586. https://doi.org/10.1186/s12888-022-04199-1

Leung, J. Y., Mackenzie, L., & Dickson, C. (2022). Outcomes of assistance dog placement in the home for individuals with autism spectrum disorder and their families: A pilot study. *Australian Journal of Occupational Therapy, 69*(1), 50–63. https://doi.org/10.1111/1440-1630.12768

le Roux, M. C., Swartz, L., & Swart, E. (2014). The effect of an animal-assisted reading program on the reading rate, accuracy and comprehension of grade 3 students: A randomized control study. *Child & Youth Care Forum, 43*(6), 655–673. https://doi.org/10.1007/s10566-014-9262-1

Levinson, E. M., Vogt, M., Barker, W. F., Jalongo, M. R., & Van Zandt, P. (2017). Effects of reading with adult tutor/therapy dog teams on elementary students' reading achievement and attitudes. *Society & Animals*, 25(1), 38–56.

Lewis, H., & Grigg, R. (2021). *Tails from the classroom. Learning and teaching through animal-assisted interventions.* Crown House.

Lewis, H., Grigg, R., & Knight, C. (2022). An international survey of animals in schools: Exploring what sorts of schools involve what sorts of animals, and educators' rationales for these practices. *People and Animals: The International Journal of Research and Practice*, 5(1), Article 15. https://docs. lib.purdue.edu/paij/vol5/iss1/15

Linder, D. E., Mueller, M. K., Gibbs, D. M., Alper, J. A., & Freeman, L. M. (2018). Effects of an animal-assisted intervention on reading skills and attitudes in second grade students. *Early Childhood Education Journal*, 46(3), 323–329.

Local Government Association. (2022). Read2Dogs. 9 May, https://www.local.gov.uk/case-studies/ read2dogs.

Louv, R. (2005). *Last child in the woods.* Algonquin Books.

Martin, T. (2003). Minimum and maximum entitlements: Literature at key stage 2. *Reading Literacy and Language*, 37(1), 14–17.

Martinez, R. S., Aricak, O. T., & Jewell, J. (2008). Influence of reading attitude on reading achievement: A test of temporal-interaction model. *Psychology in the Schools*, 45, 1010–1023.

Matsumoto, D. (Ed.). (2009). *The Cambridge dictionary of psychology.* Cambridge University Press.

Mayer, J. D., Salovey, P., Caruso, D. R., & Cherkasskiy, L. (2011). Emotional intelligence. In R. J. Sternberg & S. B. Kaufman (Eds.), *The Cambridge handbook of intelligence* (pp. 528–549). Cambridge University Press. https://doi.org/10.1017/CBO9780511977244.027

McKenna, M., Kear, D., & Ellsworth, R. (1995). Children's attitudes toward reading: A national survey. *Reading Research Quarterly*, 30(4), 934–956.

McKenna, M. C., Conradi, K., Lawrence, C., Jang, B. G., & Meyer, J. P. (2012). Reading attitudes of middle school students: Results of a U.S. Survey. *Reading Research Quarterly*, 47, 283–306.

McNicholas, J., & Collis, G. (2006). Animals as social supports: Insights for understanding animal-assisted therapy. In A. H. Fine (Ed.), *Handbook on animal-assisted therapy: Theoretical foundations and guidelines for practice* (pp. 49–71). Academic Press.

Medford, E., & McGeown, S. (2011) Cognitive and motivational factors for reading in J. Franco and A.Svensgaard (Eds.) *Psychology of motivation: New research.* Nova Science Publications.

Meintz, K., Brelsford, V., Dimolareva, M., Maréchal, L., Pennington, K., Rowan, E., & Gee, N. (2022). Can dogs reduce stress levels in school children? Effects of dog-assisted interventions on salivary cortisol in children with and without special educational needs using randomized controlled trials. *PLOS ONE*. https://doi.org/10.1371/journal.pone.0269333

Mersinoglu, Y. (2019) Ofsted praise college therapy dogs as popularity on the rise. 29 November, *FE Weekly*. https://feweek.co.uk/ofsted-praise-college-therapy-dogs-as-popularity-on-the-rise/

Morgan, P. L., & Fuchs, D. (2007). Is there a bidirectional relationship between children's reading skills and reading motivation? *Exceptional Children*, 73(2), 165–183.

Morrill, K., Hekman, J., Li, X., McClure, J., & Karlsson, E. (2022). Ancestry-inclusive dog genomics challenges popular breed stereotypes. *Science*, 376, 6592. https://doi.org/10.1126/science. abk0639

Muijs, D., & Bokhove, C. (2020). *Metacognition and self-regulation: Evidence review.* Education Endowment Foundation.

Nagengast, S. L., Baun, M. M., Megel, M., & Leibowitz, J. M. (1997). The effects of the presence of a companion animal on physiological arousal and behavioral distress in children during a physical examination. *Journal of Pediatric Nursing*, 12(6), 323–330.

National Institute for Health and Care Excellence. (2018). *Health and social care directorate. Quality standards and indicators.* Briefing Paper. https://www.nice.org.uk/guidance/gid-qs10070/ documents/briefing-paper

Ng, M., Wenden, E., Lester, L., Westgarth, C., & Christian, H. (2021). A study protocol for a randomised controlled trial to evaluate the effectiveness of a dog-facilitated physical activity minimal intervention on young children's physical activity, health and development: The PLAYCE PAWS trial. *BMC Public Health, 21*(1), 51. https://doi.org/10.1186/s12889-020-10034-7

Noble, O., & Holt, N. (2018). A study into the impact of the reading education assistance dogs scheme on reading engagement and motivation to read among early years foundation-stage children. *Education 3-13, 46*(3), 277–290.

Oberle, E. (2018). Early adolescents' emotional well-being in the classroom: The role of personal and contextual assets. *Journal of School Health, 88*(2), 101–111. https://doi.org/10.1111/josh.12585

O'Haire, M. E. (2013). Animal-assisted intervention for autism spectrum disorder: A systematic literature review. *Journal of Autism and Developmental Disorders, 43*, 1606–1622.

O'Haire, M., & Gabriels, R. (2017). The impact of animals in classrooms assisting students with autism and other developmental disorders. In N. Gee, A. H. Fine, & R. R. McCardle (Eds.), *How animals help students learn* (pp. 83–97). Routledge.

O'Haire, M. E., McKenzie, S. J., McCune, S., & Slaughter, V. (2014). Effects of classroom animal-assisted activities on social functioning in children with autism spectrum disorder. *The Journal of Alternative and Complementary Medicine, 20*(3), 162–168.

Organisation for Economic co-operation and Development (OECD). (2002). *Reading for change: Performance and engagement across countries: Results from PISA 2002.* OECD.

OECD. (2012). *Teaching practices and pedagogical innovation.* OECD.

OECD. (2021b). *Measuring what matters for child well-being and policies.* OECD.

Palmer, S. (2007). *Toxic childhood. How the modern world is damaging our children and what we can do about it.* Orion Books.

Paris, S., & Oka, E. (1986). Children's reading strategies, metacognition, and motivation. *Developmental Reading, 6*(1), 25–56.

Parshall, D. P. (2003). Research and reflection: Animal-assisted therapy in mental. *Counseling and Values, 48*(1), 47–56.

Pennac, D. (2009). *Dog. In search of a well-trained owner.* Walker Books.

Plumer, P., & Stoner, G. (2005). The relative effects of classwide peer tutoring and peer coaching on the positive social behaviors of children with ADHD. *Journal of Attention Disorders, 9*(1), 290–300.

Plutchik, R. (1980). *Theories of emotion.* Academic Press.

Postman, N. (1982). *The end of education.* Vintage Books.

Pressley. (2006). *Reading Instruction that works: The case for balanced teaching.* Guilford Press.

Ramirez, G., Fries, L., Gunderson, E., Schaeffer, M. W., Maloney, E. A., Beilock, S. L., & Levine, S. C. (2019). Reading anxiety: An early affective impediment to children's success. *Reading, Journal of Cognition and Development, 20*(1), 15–34. https://doi.org/10.1080/15248372.2018.1526175

Rawls, J. (1971). *A theory of justice.* Harvard University Press.

Reading Agency. (2015). *Literature review: The impact of reading for pleasure and empowerment.* BOP Consulting.

Redefer, L. A., & Goodman, J. F. (1989) Brief report: Pet-facilitated therapy with autistic children. *Journal of Autism and Developmental Disorders, 19*, 461–467. https://doi.org/10.1007/BF02212943.

Reilly, K. M., Adesope, O. O., & Erdman, P. (2020). The effects of dogs on learning: A meta-analysis. *Anthrozoös, 33*(3), 339–360. https://doi.org/10.1080/08927936.2020.1746523

Rolf, K. R., & Slocum, T. (2021). Features of direct instruction: Interactive lessons. *Behavior Analysis in Practice, 4*(3), 793–801.

Ross, C. S., McKechnie, L., & Rothbauer, P. M. (2006). *Reading matters: What research reveals about reading, libraries and community.* Libraries Unlimited.

Rosenshine, B. (1976). Recent research on teaching behaviors and student achievement. *Journal of Teacher Education, 27*(1), 61–64.

Rousseau, C., & Tardif-Williams, C. (2019). Turning the page for spot: The potential of therapy dogs to support reading motivation among young children. *Anthrozoös, 3*(25), 665–677. https://doi.org/10.1080/08927936.2019.1645511

Ruggeri, K., Garcia-Garzon, E., Maguire, Á, Matz, S., & Huppert, F. A. (2020). Well-being is more than happiness and life satisfaction: A multidimensional analysis of 21 countries. *Health Qual Life Outcomes, 18*(192). https://doi.org/10.1186/s12955-020-01423-y

Sainsbury, M., & Schagen, I. (2004). Attitudes to reading at ages nine and eleven. *Journal of Research in Reading, 7*(4), 373–386.

Salovey, P., & Mayer, J. D. (1990). Emotional intelligence. *Imagination, Cognition, and Personality, 9,* 185–211.

Sams, M., Fortney, E., & Willenbring, S. (2006). Occupational therapy incorporating animals for children with autism: A pilot investigation. *American Journal of Occupational Therapy, 60*(3), 268–274.

Schuck, S. E., Emmerson, N. A., Fine, A. H., & Lakes, K. D. (2015). Canine-assisted therapy for children with ADHD: Preliminary findings from the positive assertive cooperative kids study. *Journal of Attention Disorders, 19*(2), 125–137. https://doi.org/10.1177/1087054713502080

Sen, A. K. (1999). *Development as freedom.* Oxford University Press.

Scoffham, S., & Barnes, J. (2011). Happiness matters: Towards pedagogy of happiness and wellbeing. *Curriculum Journal, 22*(4), 535–548.

Serpell, J. (2002). Anthropomorphism and anthropomorphic selection—Beyond the "Cute response". *Society & Animals, 10*(4), 437–454.

Siegel, W. L. (2004). The role of animals in education. *Revision, 27*(2), 17–26.

Solomon, O. (2010). What a dog can do: Children with autism and therapy dogs in social interaction. *Journal of the Society for Psychological Anthropology, 38*(1), 143–166.

Stanovich, K. (1994). Romance and reality. *The Reading Teacher, 47,* 280–291.

Statham, J., & Chase, E. (2010). *Childhood wellbeing: A brief overview.* Childhood Wellbeing Research Centre. https://assets.publishing.service.gov.uk/government/uploads/system/uploads/attachment_data/file/183197/Child-Wellbeing-Brief.pdf

Steel, J. (2022). Children's wellbeing and reading engagement: The impact of reading to dogs in a Scottish primary 1 classroom. *Education 3-13.* https://doi.org/10.1080/03004279.2022.2100442

Steel, J., Williams, J. M., & McGeown, S. (2021). Reading to dogs in schools: An exploratory study of teacher perspectives. *Educational Research, 63*(3), 279–301, https://doi.org/10.1080/00131881.2021.1956989

Stern, C., & Chur-Hansen, A. (2013). Methodological considerations in designing and evaluating animal-assisted interventions. *Animals, 3,* 127–141.

Taboada, A., Tonks, S., Wigfield, A., & Guthrie, J. (2009). Effects of motivational and cognitive variables on reading comprehension. *Reading and Writing, 22,* 85–106.

Thigpen, S., Ellis, S., & Smith, R. (2005). Special education in juvenile residential facilities: Can animals help? *Essays in Education, 14,* 1–15.

Thorndike, E. L. (1917). Reading as reasoning: A study of mistakes in paragraph reading. *Journal of Educational Psychology, 8*(6), 323–332. https://doi.org/10.1037/h0075325.

Uccheddu, S., Albertini, M., Pierantoni, L., Fantino, S., & Pirrone, F. (2019). The impacts of a reading-to-dog programme on attending and reading of nine children with autism spectrum disorders. *Animals, 9*(8), 491. https://doi.org/10.3390/ani9080491

van den Broek, P., Kindeou, P., Kremer, K., Lynch, J., Butler, J., White, M. J., & Pugzles Lorch, E. (2005). Assessment of comprehension abilities in young children. In Scott. G. Paris and Steven. A. Stahl (Eds.), *Children's reading: Comprehension and assessment.* Mahwah, Lawrence Erlbaum Associates.

Van Houtte, B. A., & Jarvis, P. A. (1995). The role of pets in preadolescent psychosocial development. *Journal of Applied Developmental Psychology, 16*(3), 463–479. https://doi.org/10.1016/0193-3973(95)90030-6

Wagner, C., Grob, C., & Herdiger, K. (2022). Specific and non-specific factors of animal-assisted interventions considered in research: A systematic review. *Frontiers in Psychology, 13.* https://doi.org/10.3389/fpsyg.2022.931347

Walsh, F. (2009). Human-animal bonds I: The relational significance of companion animals. *Family Process, 48*(4), 462–480. https://doi.org/10.1111/j.1545-5300.2009.01296.x

Wang, J. H., & Guthrie, J. T. (2004). Modeling the effects of intrinsic motivation, extrinsic motivation, amount of reading, and past reading achievement on text comprehension between U.S. and Chinese students. *Reading Research Quarterly, 39*(2), 162–186.

Watson, K. (2022). *Good autism practice for teachers.* Critical Publishing.

Wells, D. (2019). The state of research on human–animal relations: Implications for human health. *Anthrozoös, 32*(2), 169–181. https://doi.org/10.1080/08927936.2019.1569902

Wigfield, A., & Guthrie, J. T. (1997a). Relations of children's motivation for reading to the amount and breadth of their reading. *Journal of Educational Psychology, 89,* 420–432.

Wigfield A., & Guthrie J. T. (1997b). Motivation for reading: individual, home, textual, and classroom perspective. *Educational Psychology, 32,* 57–135.

Williams, J. P., & Atkins, J. G. (2009). The role of metacognition in teaching reading comprehension to primary students. In A. Graesser., D. Hacker, & J. Dunlosky (Eds.) *Handbook of metacognition in education.* Routledge.

Wilson, E. (1984). *Biophilia.* Harvard University Press.

White, S. C. (2015). *Relational wellbeing: A theoretical and operational approach.* University of Bath.

World Health Organization (WHO). (2022). *Mental health: Strengthening our response.* www.who.int/en/news-room/fact-sheets/detail/mental-health-strengthening-our-response.

WHO. (2021). *Mental health of adolescents,* 17 November, https://www.who.int/news-room/fact-sheets/detail/adolescent-mental-health

Wyse, D., & Bradbury, A. (2022). Reading wars or reading reconciliation? A critical examination of robust research evidence, curriculum policy and teachers' practices for teaching phonics and reading. *Review of Education, 10,* e3314. https://doi.org/10.1002/rev3.3314

Yorke, J. P. (2010). The significance of human–animal relationships as modulators of trauma effects in children: A developmental neurobiological perspective. *Early Child Development and Care, 180,* 559–570.

Yoshihiro, S. O., Atsushi, A., Kentaro, I., & Yuki, Y. (2017). The stuffed animal sleepover: Enhancement of reading and the duration of the effect. *Heliyon, 3*(2), e00252. https://doi.org/10.1016/j.heliyon.2017.e00252

CHAPTER 3

TOWARDS A PEDAGOGY FOR EFFECTIVE PRACTICE

One of the long running debates in education policymaking is the extent to which schools should be afforded autonomy from centralised authorities in making decisions in the key areas of the curriculum, instruction, assessment, finance, and resources. The degree of autonomy varies from one country to the next and in many cases is exercised within multiple levels of governance. On average, schools operating within OECD are fully responsible for nearly one in three decisions (OECD, 2018). Therefore, it becomes incumbent on schoolteachers and leaders to be clear on the desired outcomes of any new programmes, including AAIs. This is particularly so in a climate of tightening education budgets and the need to exercise value for money.

In recent years, interest in bringing dogs into school appears to have grown significantly. Ofsted, the school inspectorate in England, has reported positively on the presence of dogs in school as the following media extracts reveal:

Monkseaton Middle School celebrates Good Ofsted report – with the help of Berta the Bloodhound – North Tynside Council, 7 March 2022.

Derby's school's therapy dog helps get it a 'good' Ofsted report
Derby Telegraph, 22 November 2021 (Kingsmead special school, Alvaston).

Puppy love for school from Ofsted after even its pet dog praised
Chester and Cheshire News, 5 July 2019 (Broken Cross Primary, Macclesfield).

How Betty is top dog with Ofsted school inspectors
East Anglia Daily Times, 16 February 2020 (Woodhall Primary School, Sudbury).

Ofsted gives pat on head for school dog Bramble
Wigan Today, 26 October 2019 (Hindley All Saints CE Primary School, Wigan).

Between 2016 and 2019, the publication *Schools Week* found that 12 Ofsted reports had praised the presence of school dogs. Woodland Academy Trust bought dogs for each of its four primary schools in London. Julie Carson, its director of education, explained that she wanted to lower the 'high number of children coming into schools with anxiety and mental health difficulties' and was encouraged by research in the United States (Carr, 2019). Testimonies from teachers suggest that school dogs make an important contribution to children who have suffered trauma. Matthew Fuller, the headteacher of Woodhall Primary School in Sudbury, explained the value of Betty the school labradoodle: 'She is great for children who are going through difficult times, such as family bereavement or break-up. One of our children would only talk to an adult through her'. Children's personal development was ranked outstanding by school inspectors (Langford, 2020).

DOI: 10.4324/9781003257073-5

The growing interest in school dogs also follows on from greater coverage in academic literature. Although there are no reliable statistics on the number of schools involving dogs, the impression from both print and social media is that the trend is a fast-growing one. Databases such as PubMed (maintained by the United States National Library of Medicine and National Institutes of Health) show a significance rise (roughly threefold) in the number of articles relating to AAIs over the last decade or so, a high proportion of which feature dogs.

Given the global interest in bringing dogs into school, however, there is a surprising lack of guidance on the pedagogical implications which this chapter seeks to address. It begins by exploring relevant perspectives on pedagogy before proposing a set of principles to guide teachers and school leaders and explores two possible models of practice – a visiting dog or a permanent school dog.

DEFINING PEDAGOGY

The term 'pedagogy' derives from the ancient Greek notion of a male attendant (*paidagōgos*) leading a boy to school. Both the gendered nature and the association with the process of upbringing have since been replaced with an emphasis on the 'science of teaching' and professional practice (Hayes, 2010; Wallace, 2015). Other definitions include the artistry of teachers who make the most of unexpected moments (Marzano & Brown, 2009). Less tangible elements include the teacher's personality (Kim et al., 2019), humour (Şahin, 2021), and tacit knowledge (Elliott et al., 2011). Some commentators stress the broader links between pedagogy, the curriculum, and assessment, as educators combine these to create purposeful learning experiences (Leach & Moon, 2008).

There are more precise definitions of pedagogy. For example, Alexander (2004, p. 11) sees pedagogy as 'what one needs to know, and the skills one needs to command, in order to make and justify the many different kinds of decisions, of which teaching is constituted'. Such decisions are shaped by beliefs about learning, the wider social context and norms. Watkins and Mortimore (1999) are eager to define pedagogy in a way which goes beyond the role of the teacher and teaching (didactics) to take the learner into account. Hence their definition of pedagogy is 'any conscious activity by one person designed to enhance learning in another' (Watkins & Mortimore, 1999, p. 3). Whilst there is some debate over whether dogs are 'persons' (see Herzog, 2013), this broad definition is in keeping with this book.

Pedagogy is a widely used term across mainland European countries although less so in the United Kingdom, reflecting different traditions (Hamilton, 1999). For some UK critics (e.g., Didau, 2015), pedagogy has become little more than a pretentious, vacuous term used by 'experts' who look down upon 'just teaching'. However, Shulman's (1987) work has highlighted important subtleties, for example, relating to pedagogical content knowledge, which describes how teachers convey topics in ways that learners can understand. It is the difference between knowing something, and knowing how to help others understand it, for example through explanations, illustrations and models. Shulman has also drawn attention to 'signature pedagogies' which stand out in different professions, such as the bedside teaching of doctors, dialogic methods in law school or fieldwork amongst geographers (Shulman, 2005; Thomson et al., 2012).

In the academic community, there is a readiness to adopt pedagogy for a range of purposes. Pedagogical 'encounters' present fresh ways of thinking about 'self' and 'other' and new possibilities for teaching about difference (Inayatullah, 2022; Nayak & Jaramillo, 2020). There is scope here to use such thinking to reframe how the interactions between dogs and children are perceived, with a stronger emphasis on the agency of non-human animals. Rather than seeing dog-human interactions in bilateral terms, these can be reimagined and reworked to afford a more balanced relationship which goes beyond meeting the basic welfare needs of the dog to aspiring to provide enriching experiences for all.

Critical pedagogy is based on the belief that educators should challenge existing inequalities and empower students with the competences to critique these (Freire, 1970; Giroux, 1997). There is a strong association with historical, social, and cultural analysis in areas such as 'equity-oriented pedagogy' (Phuong et al., 2017), which is committed to finding fairer ways to improve learning for all. Such a critical perspective could be extended to the way in which dogs are treated. Informed by social and philosophical commentators, there are arguments for humans to demonstrate a more empathetic understanding of how non-human animals think and feel (Derrida, 2008; Kahn, 2009; Pedersen, 2004). According to Pedersen (2004, p. 2), within the world of scientific research, non-human animals are only valued for instrumental uses rather than as 'beings living for their own sake and with their own purposes'. The suffering of non-human animals is often legitimatized in the name of scientific advancement within university research laboratories. Many years ago, Russell and Burch (1959) advocated three Rs in the hope of transforming how animals were used in scientific research through 'alternative methods':

- replacing the use of nonhuman animals with alternatives;
- reducing the numbers of nonhuman animals used; and
- refining procedures to keep nonhuman animal suffering to a minimum where it is 'unavoidable'.

These sentiments were expressed more than 50 years ago and were directed at animal experimentation in scientific research. However, it would be wrong to dismiss such thinking as outdated and irrelevant to dogs who may be perceived as being out of harm's way in school. There are organisations that strongly maintain that dogs should not feature in schools and be replaced by alternatives. The People for the Ethical Treatment of Animals (PETA), the largest animal rights organization in the world, concludes: 'A classroom is an unhappy 'home' for animals'.[1]

Whilst schools may seem less likely contexts within which non-human animals are exposed to suffering, at the very least there is a danger that they are objectified. Moreover, there is a danger that the sufferings of dogs could go undetected or unreported especially amongst those who are not under the care of trained and experienced handlers. Too often, glib headlines appear in the media extolling the virtues of bringing dogs into school and the presumed benefits for children: 'Why every school should bring dogs into the classroom' (Weller, 2015); 'Every School Should Have A Therapy Dog' and 'Every school 'needs dog as stress-buster' (Coughlan, 2019). These examples illustrate why schools may perceive that they are doing the right thing by bringing in a dog. We would argue that before making such a big decision, school leaders (and indeed the school as a community) need to give serious thought to developing a robust pedagogy which considers both their learners and the dogs.

Traditionally, pedagogy has been tied closely to the education of young children. In the context of early years' practice, Siraj-Blatchford et al. (2002) regards effective pedagogy as high-quality interactions between a learning environment's components. If a school dog initiative is to be effective, the interactions between humans, canines, and the environment must be of high quality. The concept of pedagogy, however, is no longer limited to young children or schooling. It extends into the community and informal contexts (Sandlin et al., 2010). Here, the work of Lave and Wenger (1991) has relevance to Canine Assisted Education (CAE). Their notion of communities of practice describes groups of people who share a concern or passion for something they do and learn how to do it better as they interact (Farnsworth et al., 2016; Lave & Wenger, 1991).

In the United Arab Emirates, for example, Reading Dogs UAE comprises a group of animal professionals, dog handlers, dog trainers, animal owners, and volunteers who share a passion for dogs and children's reading. Like many such groups, they actively engage in social media sharing news stories, photographs, feedback from schools, and invitations to events. The team continually reflect on how to celebrate achievements and address the challenges they face, such as misconceptions around Islamic attitudes towards dogs and the inclination amongst a few schools to involve dogs that are not trained, to save costs. Reading Dogs UAE are amongst those organisations that treat the welfare of its dogs seriously.

The first pedagogical decisions school leaders need to make is whether dogs should be brought into educational settings and, if so, why. This is discussed in detail in Chapter 9. Few would doubt that dogs can have a powerful impact in people's lives. For example, Shaun, a university student in Wales, explains the difference his dog, Harley, has made to the quality of his life:

> I was diagnosed with Cerebral Palsy as a baby and with autism when I was 10 years old. I was born 15 weeks prematurely, weighing 1lb 11oz. During the birth, I suffered a massive intraventricular haemorrhage, and my parents were told that I would never walk or talk and would be blind and deaf. When I was 18 days old, I caught pneumonia and needed an emergency baptism. I had another brain hemorrhage and died that night. Miraculously, I was resuscitated but, even more miraculously, a brain scan revealed that the second hemorrhage had dispersed the first so, even though I still have considerable brain damage, the damage is not all condensed in one area, so my prognosis improved. I spent 4 months in a Special Care Baby Unit before being released home on oxygen and 23 drugs a day.
>
> Throughout my life, I have had physiotherapy, hydrotherapy, occupational therapy and speech therapy, but the therapy that helped me most started in November 2011 – Harley therapy! Harley is a Sprocker Spaniel that my parents bought after hearing how getting a dog had helped other autistic children. Before we got Harley, I hardly spoke, and I did not enjoy doing my physiotherapy or walking; this all changed when I had a puppy! I love taking him out for walks, my physiotherapy exercises are fun with him "helping" and we swim together all the time on holiday. As well as physically helping me, Harley has helped with my confidence and my communication skills; from being almost mute, I started to feel comfortable talking to other dog walkers about the dogs and having Harley has given me something to talk about even if he is not there. Harley also helps me study; he sits with me through every online lecture and being able to stroke him and seeing him looking at me with his big, brown eyes makes me feel happy and less stressed.

It is clear from this testimony that Harley has made a big difference to Shaun's life, and this is echoed in the relationships many people, over many generations, have had with dogs. It is hardly surprising then that the perceived benefits of bringing dogs into school are often seen to outweigh the practical challenges, risks, and disadvantages.

Nonetheless, there are potential challenges at a strategic and operational level. Strategically there needs to be a clear rationale for such activity, with an evaluation plan in place. At an operational level, the demands on a teacher when an additional responsibility is placed on them can be considerable, and measuring how effective these interventions are can be challenging, for example, making decisions about well-being can be subjective (e.g., Ng in Tedeschi & Jenkins, 2019). It is essential that teachers and children are aware of how to engage positively and humanely with their dogs, and how to develop meaningful, enriching activities for all concerned.

PRECONDITIONS

On balance, our view is that suitable dogs, accompanied by their handlers, should be invited into school on four preconditions (Figure 3.1).

The first precondition is that children and their teachers receive appropriate training on how best to interact with dogs. By bringing a dog into a setting, children can be taught how to observe the dog's natural behaviour, 'read' their signs, and respond in the right way. This can be done virtually or in real life. Children can be shown clips on social media to illustrate dogs' body language, as well as their social and emotional intelligence (which can prompt discussion about how to be a good friend or about what it means to learn). Alternatively, games can be played using pictures and photographs of dogs to build children's knowledge and empathy.

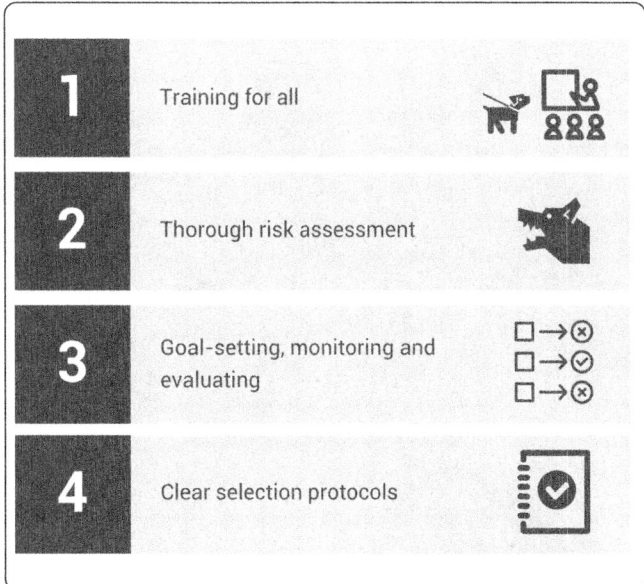

1 Training for all

2 Thorough risk assessment

3 Goal-setting, monitoring and evaluating

4 Clear selection protocols

FIGURE 3.1 Four preconditions for bringing dogs into school.

Children can practise how to meet and greet a dog, how to stroke a dog carefully (e.g., on the chest not on the head), and how to stand near a dog (e.g., not looming over or crowding around the dog) initially using large stuffed toys. The dog also needs appropriate, positive training so that the interactions that are planned can be as safe as possible. These ideas are explored in more depth in Chapter 9.

Second, that risk assessment is robust enough to ensure that the health and safety of all participants are given due consideration at all times. Given the popularity of dogs as pets, learning how to be safe around them is a life skill. In the United Kingdom alone, dog bites account for nearly 70% of all hospital admissions for mammalian bites and cost the NHS an estimated £10 million per year (NHS, 2015). The research has identified two age groups of children that are bitten most often, those under the age of 2 years, and those aged 9–12 (Fein et al., 2019). Jakeman et al. (2020) suggest certain patterns in terms of who is most at risk of a bite:

- children under 5 years are more likely to be bitten in the head or neck;
- boys are more likely to be bitten;
- children are most often bitten in the home;
- the dog is owned by the family in most cases;
- paediatric dog bites tend to occur in the early evening or on the weekend and are more common in the summer months.

Social media is awash with images of dogs and people interacting, but frequently these interactions place dogs in difficult situations – such as being hugged, kissed, or jumped upon. For example, Figure 3.2 is adapted from a photograph on social

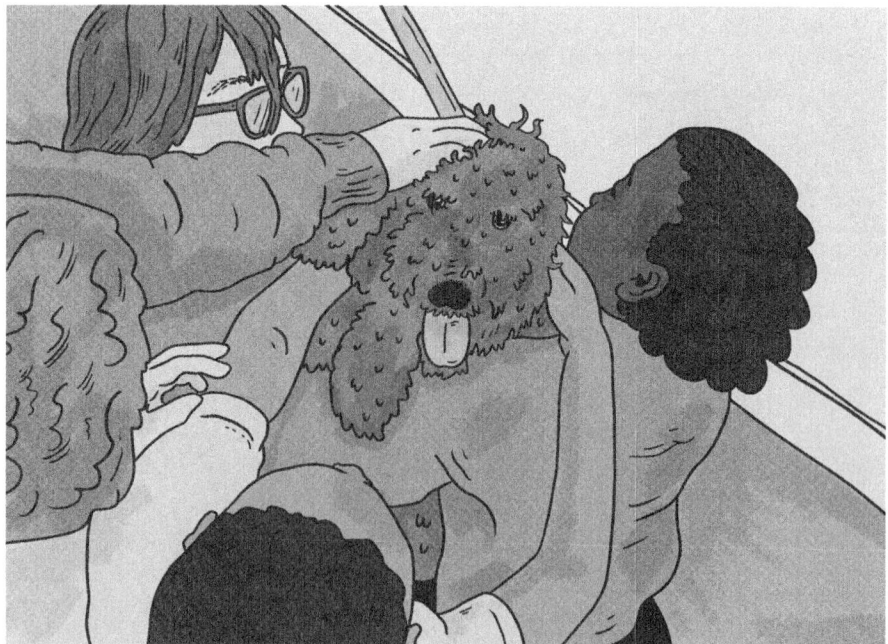

FIGURE 3.2 Hugging the dog: picture adapted from social media.

media. Without knowing the individual dog, it is impossible to know whether this was a comfortable interaction for her. However, there are some potential concerns that the image raises. Firstly, it shows a dog being hugged by several children, who are all gathered closely around her, and some of whom are stroking her on her head. Many dogs would find this overwhelming. The dog has been lifted, which may remove her feeling of a sense of control over the situation, and she has no easy escape route. She has her tongue out, which may be a sign that she is feeling hot, stressed, or anxious. The children are all in very close proximity to her, and this may lead her to feeling crowded. Whilst this individual dog may manage the situation well, in terms of risk, there are several ways the interaction should be improved. Children should neither pick up the dog nor stroke her on the head. The number of children involved in an interaction should be carefully managed, and the dog should be able to leave an activity at any point.

Therefore, to establish routines that will allow the dog to also feel happy in any interactions, she should be brought into school and introduced in a carefully prepared and managed manner. This ensures there is opportunity not only to plan specific activities around individual needs but also to educate children, teachers, and the wider community about safe and healthy interactions with dogs. Certainly, school dogs need to be 'well-mannered, but they don't have to suffer calmly through a frightening or traumatic situation' (Howie, 2015, p. 3).

The third precondition for successful CAE is for school leaders to treat the intervention as a serious attempt to improve aspects of children's learning or well-being. This requires a commitment to appropriate educational goals and then monitoring and evaluating progress towards achieving these (see Chapter 10). From an educational viewpoint, there should always be sound pedagogical reasons for bringing dogs into school. Unless teachers and school leaders are clear about the rationale for any intervention, especially those involving live animals, then they simply cannot say with authority whether these have been worthwhile. Having a clear rationale also helps select the individual dog best suited to the activities that are going to take place, which will help to ensure that they are happy to participate as well. This links to the fourth precondition.

Finally, there is a need to establish clear selection protocols for children, dogs, and handlers. Selection of the dog-handler team may be managed by an outside agency or by the school itself. Regardless of which approach is used, it is essential to recognise that there needs to be a match between the right dog for the right child and in the right environment if the intervention is to succeed. This is an ongoing process, which recognises that all participants are individuals, with the right to make choices about when and with whom they interact. This is explored in more depth in Chapters 8 and 9.

Having met these preconditions, we suggest that the actions of teachers, leaders, and other members of the school community should be governed by a set of principles or moral precepts to guide the teaching and learning experiences.

PEDAGOGICAL PRINCIPLES

It is widely agreed that effective educators work according to pedagogical principles, which are the fundamental truths that should underpin their teaching practices. Amongst the more common principles is a recognition that teachers should provide

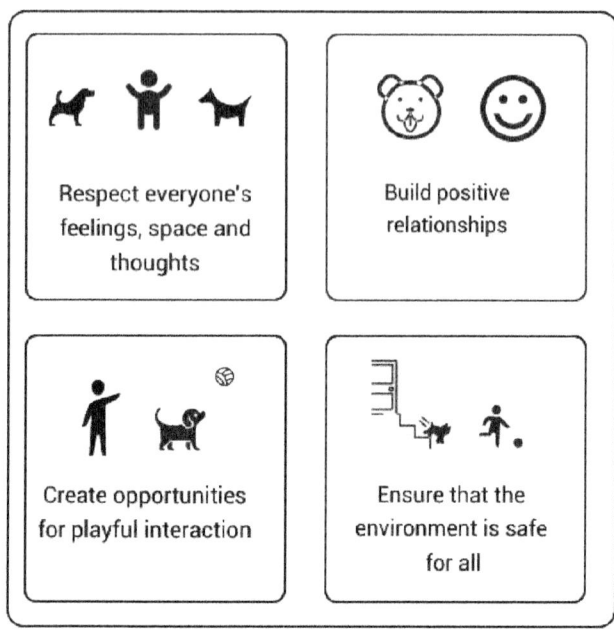

FIGURE 3.3 Pedagogical principles for AAIs (Lewis & Grigg, 2021).

real-world or authentic contexts for learning, build on prior knowledge, aim to challenge and motivate learners, and support their learning through immediate feedback (Grigg, 2022; Husbands & Pearce, 2012; James & Pollard, 2011; Rosenshine, 2012). Elsewhere, we have proposed four pedagogical principles (Figure 3.3) suitable for AAIs when working with children in school contexts (Lewis & Grigg, 2021). Whilst such principles are aligned specifically to the rationale behind England's Early Years Foundation Stage, they have broader appeal in underpinning healthy, happy, and humane interactions for children of all ages and the dogs they develop relationships with. In the next section, we expand upon these principles.

RESPECT EVERYONE'S FEELINGS, SPACES AND THOUGHTS

It is important for all children to learn that animals have their own feelings and thoughts that deserve respect and protection. Respect means allowing dogs to be themselves rather than seeing them as tools or resources. However, this brings challenges. For example, children will need to be taught when it is and is not appropriate to approach a dog. Dogs do not have a choice in whether they are present in a school environment, but it is important that educators recognise their sentience, and that a dog can indicate their consent to interact in several non-verbal ways. This means getting to know the dog as an individual, observing their behaviour throughout the interaction, and having a plan in place if the dog indicates that they do not want to join in with a planned activity, for example, by having a stuffed toy dog on standby.

From a young age, children should be helped to learn to read and respect a dog's body language. Any signal must always be interpreted in the specific context because similar signs have different meanings in different situations. For example, a dog yawning might mean that she is tired, but it could also mean she is nervous. And when a dog licks their lips, this may be to convey stress not necessarily hunger. A head cocked to the side and a lifted paw can be signs of curiosity and anticipation or an appeasement signal when the dog feels anxious. This is discussed further in Chapter 9.

In our own experiences, before taking a dog into a setting, we visit the setting and work with the children in preparatory activities such as:

- talking about whether any children have dogs at home or know of any dogs in the wider family or community;
- drawing pictures of dogs;
- sorting pictures of dogs into 'happy' and 'sad' categories and discussing what they thought dogs in different postures were trying to say;
- asking children to think about what they might do to help a dog who was looking sad or scared;
- playing with stuffed toy dogs to practise standing still like a statue and using their 'quiet voices' ready to meet the dog;
- talking about how to approach a dog safely after asking the owner 'please' ('Pat, Pet, Pause').

These activities prepare children for safe real-time interactions and support wider conversations about feelings and emotions. It is essential to avoid a situation where a dog is forced to interact, and it is tolerating (because it is well-trained and eager to please) the situation rather than enjoying it. We also need to ensure that the handler understands what a respectful relationship is and strives to keep this at the forefront of their pedagogy. For example, in Figure 3.4, the needs of Polo the dog must be paramount. The post suggests that she is no longer comfortable with some of the activities taking place when she is in school. As the reply comments indicate, respecting Polo's boundaries, and what she is trying to communicate is essential.

BUILD POSITIVE RELATIONSHIPS

The success of dog-assisted interventions rests on the quality of relationships between children, adults, and animals. Successful relationships are based on values such as care, kindness, and connection. Dogs can act as a non-judgmental friends. Kurdek (2008) suggests that children respond positively to the security and proximity of dogs. In one pre-school setting, young children enjoyed exploring whether Honey the golden retriever preferred sausages or dog biscuits as her treat (she chose sausages!). This led to lots of conversation about favourite things and opportunities to compare each other's ideas of a perfect treat. Children explored the concept of healthy snacks and began to think about the needs of themselves compared to the needs of Honey. For example, Honey brought her washbag to each session, which prompted the children to discuss and agree upon a rota for brushing Honey's coat.

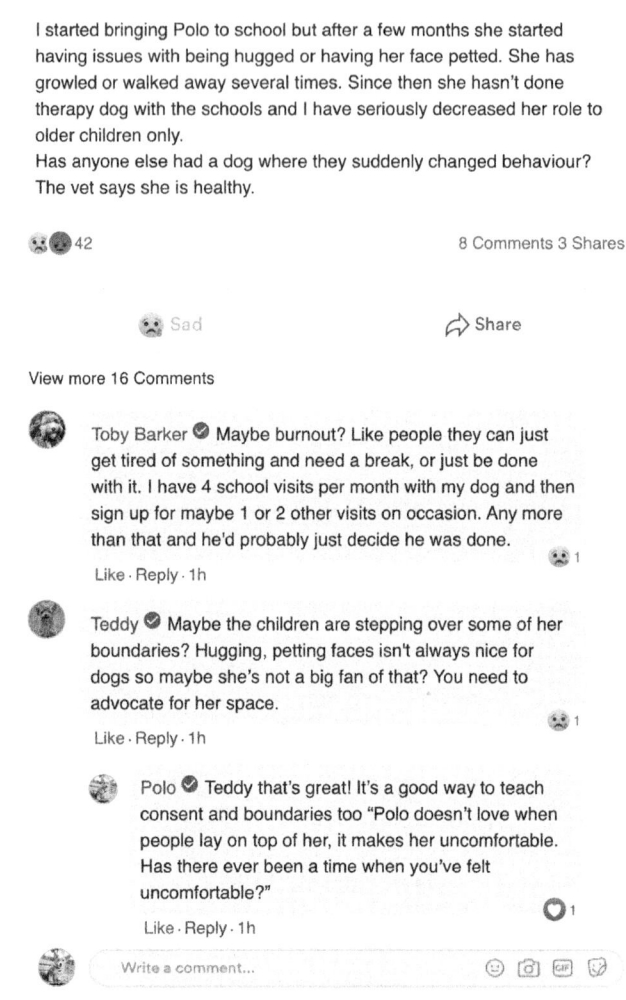

Polo the school dog Midwestern school
Yesterday at 10am ·

I started bringing Polo to school but after a few months she started having issues with being hugged or having her face petted. She has growled or walked away several times. Since then she hasn't done therapy dog with the schools and I have seriously decreased her role to older children only.
Has anyone else had a dog where they suddenly changed behaviour? The vet says she is healthy.

42   8 Comments 3 Shares

              Sad   Share

View more 16 Comments

Toby Barker ✅ Maybe burnout? Like people they can just get tired of something and need a break, or just be done with it. I have 4 school visits per month with my dog and then sign up for maybe 1 or 2 other visits on occasion. Any more than that and he'd probably just decide he was done.

Like · Reply · 1h

Teddy ✅ Maybe the children are stepping over some of her boundaries? Hugging, petting faces isn't always nice for dogs so maybe she's not a big fan of that? You need to advocate for her space.

Like · Reply · 1h

Polo ✅ Teddy that's great! It's a good way to teach consent and boundaries too "Polo doesn't love when people lay on top of her, it makes her uncomfortable. Has there ever been a time when you've felt uncomfortable?"

Like · Reply · 1h

Write a comment...

FIGURE 3.4 Social media post: dog boundaries.

They talked about why she had a toothbrush and a flannel, making connections to their own personal hygiene, and developing fine and gross motor skills and coordination as they gently groomed her, clipped on her lead, and walked her around the playground. This also led to opportunities for authentic conversations with her owner about things the children wanted to know more about Honey with her owner (Lewis, 2017).

However, we also need to accept that just like people dogs will have preferred friends, and may be less willing to interact with some people. Berkoff (2018) reminds us that, just like people, dogs do not love unconditionally. Several factors may influence this, from a person's appearance or behaviour, to how they smell. Dogs may also pick up on social and emotional cues. For example, one study by Albuquerque et al. (2022) found that that dogs actively acquire information from affective cues produced by people and make functional use of this to solve problems. This may impact on who a dog may wish to spend time with. This needs to be carefully managed as it may have the opposite impact to the intended one. For instance, if a dog chooses not to interact with a particular child, they may feel bitterly disappointed, and this may have detrimental effects on their well-being.

Furthermore, as Van Fleet and Faa-Thompson (2017) point out, relationship building cannot be rushed. In our own work, we have seen children and dogs become better at interacting with each other over time. In one primary school, it took more than four visits before Omar the child and Roxy the dog interacted positively. In the first session, Omar was reluctant to look at or touch Roxy, and Roxy was not interested in Omar at all, preferring to sit close to her handler. The school was unsure whether to continue the programme for Omar, but his parents were keen, and Roxy's handler felt confident that Roxy was enjoying visiting the school. Over time, and in a series of very small steps (e.g., Week 2, Omar looks at Roxy three times; Week 3, Omar threw a treat on the floor for Roxy; Week 4 Roxy accepted a treat from Omar's hand), the relationship steadily blossomed. After ten sessions, the relationship was still in its early stages, but Omar would talk to Roxy and sit close to her, occasionally stroking her. He was more excited to see her and talked about her after the session. Roxy would approach Omar confidently and often chose to interact with him. If we accept the notion of dog sentience, we need to acknowledge that relationships take time and effort to grow.

CREATE OPPORTUNITIES FOR PLAYFUL INTERACTION

Dogs are social beings, just like children and adults. They enjoy playing and having fun, and for children and dogs, play promotes learning and builds rapport. Working with Honey the retriever in one pre-school setting, several boys who were reluctant to speak were able to use gestures to encourage her to interact with them, patting their knees to call her over for a game of ball. They were able to recognise how much Honey enjoyed this game, and that she kept returning for 'more'. They also began to interact with each other more frequently, even on the days that Honey was not there. In time they began to talk to Honey, and about Honey. This included talking at home about their experiences, which was a useful way to increase parental engagement with learning. The parents of children in the setting were often as keen as their children to hear about Honey's day.

It is important that the interactions between children, adults, and dogs are based on playful learning. This does not mean that dogs should be regarded as playthings. Rather, it suggests that children can learn with, from and about the dog, whilst recognising that dogs need attention, love, and active play to stay healthy. Playful learning also benefits dogs because it helps their mental health and enables strong bonds to form (Van Fleet & Faa-Thompson, 2017). Scarlet, a cockerpoo, visited a reception class to work with two children identified as having some difficulties making friends with other children. Opportunities to play games with Scarlet helped develop their self-confidence. The children were motivated to interact with each other and decided to take it in turns to hide a treat for Scarlet and then ask her to 'find it'. They were amazed by her ability to sniff out treats that were hidden from view, and she delighted in the game as well. Undergraduate students in Swansea University enjoyed sessions with Carlo the Spinone. His love of his stuffed squirrel toy meant that he was keen to play games such as 'Find It', and the excitement was shared by the group. The students felt that playing with him was 'a great chance to stop worrying about assignment deadlines' and to 'laugh and have fun with one another'.

Dogs learn through association (ideally positive) and classical conditioning, and, more so than humans, rely heavily on scent and visual cues (Kokocińska-Kusiak et al., 2021). They often pick up the meaning of gestures a lot quicker than spoken commands. This can be beneficial for children who lack confidence in speaking aloud and can also help children see cause and effect in action. For instance, when Sally the dog visited an autistic unit in a primary school setting, several children were able to benefit from successfully teaching her simple tricks, using short verbal phrases or gestures. These active sessions were also enjoyable for Sally, who also benefited from engaging with some enriching experiences.

ENSURE THAT THE ENVIRONMENT IS SAFE FOR ALL

Clearly, any educational intervention requires careful planning to ensure the environment is safe for all, but this is particularly so when other living beings are involved. Both children and practitioners need to recognise and respect the uniqueness of each animal. Within dog breeds, there are individual dogs who are calm and others more boisterous, and all will have different preferences, just like children. Careful thought needs to be given to selecting the right dog for any intervention and expert advice should always be sought. We also need to recognise the unique factors of any environment. These will be very different to the dog's home environment, and care must be taken not to overwhelm them with new sights, sounds, and smells. Not all settings, not all children, and not all dogs are suitable for face-to-face interactions with one another.

There may be phobias or anxieties amongst some children, or cultural reasons why a dog may not be suitable. There is no such thing as a completely hypoallergenic dog (although some breeds may not moult many people with allergies are allergic to dander rather than fur itself), so health issues may be a problem. Clear communication with parents, staff, and children is essential, as is careful risk assessment. Any animal and any child can be unpredictable. We have found that practitioners need to prepare for the unexpected – even the best trained and mild-mannered dog can bark, toilet, or jump up whilst in school. It is vital that we know and understand the dog as fully as we can so that we can predict the things that they will delight in and anticipate the things that may worry them. Many organisations working with dogs in schools recommend that the dog is at least 18 months old before they begin interacting with children in an educational setting, and many also expect the dog to have lived with their handler for at least a year. Conducting a detailed risk assessment and having a first aid kit on hand for the dog as well as for children are also important.

An enabling environment applied to CAE means not only ensuring appropriate health and safety measures are in place to minimise harm to all participants but also that the environment enriches the experiences of all participants. Organisations involved in AAIs will have their own risk-assessment policies, and these typically cover identifying hazards (e.g., lack of supervision, injury to children, damage caused to school property, dog fouling), degree of potential injury, controls to eliminate or reduce such risks (e.g., adult supervision, training children), and the probability of an accident happening. And equally importantly, any AAI should be planned to be exciting and enjoyable for children, adults, and the animals themselves. But we need to go beyond this and understand what motivates, engages, and interests both children and dogs so that we can provide an environment that enriches their experiences.

There also need to be clear guidelines regarding the dog's right to space in the school environment. All school dogs need a quiet space to retreat to, where they can rest and relax. Figure 3.5, adapted from a social media post, shows an interaction that could be described as unsafe. The dog appeared to be trying to rest, and the child approached and started to touch the dog on his head. Whilst this individual dog may welcome the child stroking them whilst they are in bed, typically this is not an interaction to be encouraged. It is essential that children and adults respect this and allow the dog the opportunity to make choices of when to enter this space. Establishing clear boundaries is important. These matters are considered in more detail in Chapters 8 and 9.

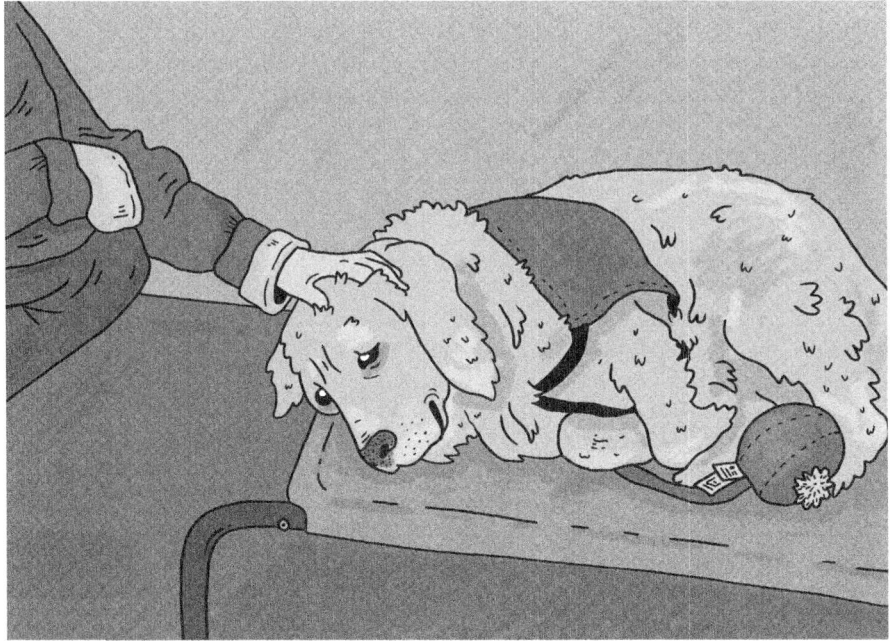

FIGURE 3.5 The dog's personal space: image adapted from social media.

Reprinted with permission from tom Bradshaw.

THE ROLE OF THE HANDLER

In establishing these principles in practice, the role of the handler is key. Glenk and Foltin (2021, p. 226) remind us that:

adding a sentient being to a therapeutic setting, therefore, creates a triangular relationship rather than a bidirectional one. Having an additional sentient partner requires the adept skills of the AAI handler in order to split attention, maintain desired outcomes, and respond quickly and appropriately to all participants throughout a session.

Howie (2015, p. 15) talks about therapy dogs and their handlers being a team. She argues that a handler must be fully present, close to their dog, carefully observing them, touching them and speaking to them throughout an activity or visit. This means that emotional and physical support is in place for the dog, which helps them also benefit from the interactions. These principles form the basis of Howie's 'STEPs' approach to guide interactions:

S – speak conversationally to your dog;
T – stay in touch with your dog;
E – keep your eyes on your dog;
P – maintain close proximity to your dog.

We must also consider the role we have in how our dogs behave. As mentioned previously, dogs are highly attuned to reading human body language and verbal cues (Albuquerque et al., 2022; Bekoff, 2019). Dogs perceive minute changes in our body language, and seemingly tiny movements can have great impact on how the dog responds (McConnell, 2002). I am (HL) always amazed how my dogs can tell when I come downstairs in the morning whether I am heading to work or if we are heading out for a walk. Something in the way I move and the gestures I make must allow them insight into the activity that is to come. They react accordingly by either remaining in their beds or rushing excitedly to the door.

However, these sensitivities can also prove challenging – for there is the possibility that dogs may experience 'emotional contagion' when working with children who are experiencing negative emotions themselves (Huber et al., in Tedeschi & Jenkins, 2019, p. 312).

Partnerships between handler and dogs require both parties to have confidence in each other. Fredrickson-MacNamara and Butler (2010, p. 137) note that both come to an interaction with different levels of confidence in one another, alongside different levels of skill, experience, talent, and comfort in each situation. These factors highlight the complex nature of any interaction, and the influence all parties have on one another. A well-trained dog may not have the talent to interact with several unfamiliar people even if they are willing to tolerate this. A confident dog handler may not have the talent to speak to children with specific needs, even if they wish to support them. Alongside the dog and the handler, the environment also has an important role with factors such as the nature of physical space, population, staff, other animals, and the types of other activities taking place all having potential impact on how an interaction takes place. Fredrickson-MacNamara and Butler (2010) indicate that in the most successful interactions, handler, dog, and environmental factors need to balance (Figure 3.6).

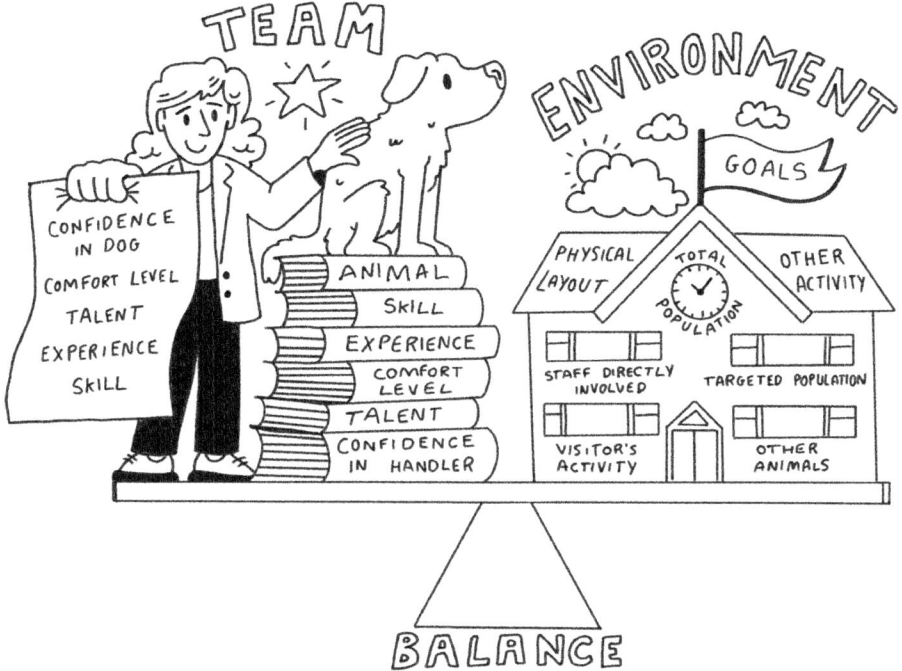

FIGURE 3.6 Balancing various needs in successful CAE.
Reprinted with the permission of Tom Bradshaw.

The Animal Assisted Intervention International Standards and Competencies (2019) emphasise that the dog needs to be able to rely on their human partner to provide a safe base to obtain their needs and to explore their external environment. In CAE experiences, dogs may experience frequently changing environments such as classrooms, playgrounds and offices; different people, and a wide range of sensory information (e.g., Lewis et al., 2022). As a practical recommendation, Glenk and Foltin (2021) recommend that handlers offer exploration opportunities to their dog each time they enter a setting, allowing the dogs time to explore this setting in their own time. Handlers should not guide them or intervene in their movements or choices, the dogs should be able to explore unrestrictedly and freely.

PART 2: MODELS OF PRACTICE

Some of these factors may look different depending on the approach or model of pedagogy adopted by a school. In Part 2, we explore two common models of practice. One is to have a visiting dog, brought in by an external agency, such as the internationally recognized R.E.A.D., or Burns By Your Side (based in South Wales and Ireland). The dog is brought in on a regular basis by their handler, who is typically their owner. The other approach is to have a permanent school dog (or dogs) who belongs to a member of staff, or to the school. Both models of practice are illustrated in the international case studies in Part 2 of this book, and both models have strengths and limitations. Both need careful planning, preparation, and ongoing evaluation.

BENEFITS AND CHALLENGES OF A VISITING DOG APPROACH

Visiting dog schemes are well-established internationally. There are many benefits of having a visiting dog team come into school. Typically, administrative and financial implications are relatively small – these programmes usually rely on volunteers from an external agency, and many of these provide free or low-cost visits. The school does not need to find a suitable dog as the assessment, training, insurance, and selection of a visiting dog team are typically arranged by this organisation. For example, Burns By Your Side includes 16 weeks of training for dog and handler, plus additional taught sessions for the handler about the underpinning reasons for bringing a dog into school. Initial temperament assessments are followed by in-school observations and a yearly re-assessment. There is on-going support available, regular events, and a social media group for volunteers.

A visiting dog approach means timetabling the sessions with the dog can be made simple, as usually the visiting dog will come on the same day and at the same time every week or fortnight. This helps planning to manage risk, for example, in the case of children with fears of allergies challenges can be reduced as the team will typically be on-site for a limited number of hours and on specific days. Fewer demands are placed on school staff because the dog is the responsibility of the volunteer throughout the visit, and the volunteer will know their dog very well. This also means that this approach is relatively low risk to the dog. Providing the volunteer has depth of knowledge regarding canine communication, and understands their dog well, they will be able to identify if the dog is enjoying their school visits. Should they start to show signs that they do not enjoy the experiences, the volunteer would be free to stop at any time.

However, there are also some limitations of this approach. Firstly, demand for a visiting dog often far outweighs supply. Organisations depend upon volunteers, and in some regions, there may be fewer people volunteering, meaning long wait times for schools to be allocated a team. Most organisations will rightly have strict regulations regarding how long a dog can work in a school for during the week, and so there will be limits to how many sessions can take place. This can result in long waiting lists for children within a school. It can also mean that the dog has more novelty value and each time the dog visits, there may be a need to settle children. Timetabling can be challenging because there is likely to be less flexibility around when the dog is present, children may miss the same in-class sessions every week, which has potential to create gaps in learning.

Relying on volunteers can also be challenging from the school management perspective. For example, in one study, schools reported:

> It can be frustrating, so far this year our volunteer has taken three weeks in term time for a holiday and had difficulties with transport meaning they missed a session. Whilst we are grateful that they come in and volunteer this has meant children who would really benefit from regular sessions have missed out.

(Lewis, 2022)

Furthermore, volunteers are also generally not trained as teachers or counsellors. Whilst they are not coming to school in such a role, understanding how to talk to and interact with children from diverse backgrounds and with diverse needs may not come naturally to some of them. This means that careful planning and briefing at a school level are needed so that, for example, individual pupils' needs are very clear, and appropriate safeguarding process understood. This can sometimes be challenging to schedule given demands on time of both volunteers and school staff.

ADVANTAGES AND DISADVANTAGES OF A PERMANENT SCHOOL DOG

There are a growing number of schools choosing to have a permanent dog on their staff team (Lewis et al., 2022). There are several possible benefits to such an approach. Over time the dog may become comfortable in the school as this becomes a familiar working environment for them. This is beneficial as dogs generally respond best to familiar environments and predictable people and behaviours. The main handlers of the dog should be able to match the dog's personality and behaviours with children's needs given that they should have a deep understanding of both individuals. The dog may be less of a novelty to students, teachers, and the wider community, thus being less of a distraction and so the impact of interventions may be greater. The more regular presence of the dog will allow more children to receive the potential benefits that such interactions bring. There is also suggestion that a school dog may enhance parental engagement with the school (e.g., Lewis, 2017) and boost attendance.

However, there may be overwhelming demands on the dog's time, which can pose a risk to their well-being. Long days in school, and working in multiple classrooms and with multiple people can place an emotional and physical strain on the dog. The main handlers of the dog need to have time to develop a deep understanding of their dog so that they can identify when they are showing any stress signals (see Chapter 9). Whilst there will be dogs who thrive in these situations, there may be others for whom this causes stress, overexcitement, and anxiety. Indeed, one respondent in a survey of educators involving dogs in schools noted:

> We did have a school dog, but it didn't work out as they got excited and sometimes overwhelmed by the children. I think there is an awful lot to consider when deciding on a school dog.
>
> (Lewis et al., 2022, p. 10)

Managing children and adults with allergies, phobias, or other reasons to not wish to interact with the dog can be more challenging if the dog is permanently on site. There are also potential misconceptions, such as the age with which a dog should start to visit school. Whilst many teachers feel that a young dog needs to gain experience in a school as soon as possible, the counterargument to this is that puppies are not yet socially, neurologically, or developmentally mature enough to participate in any AAI setting as they have not yet developed strategies to react to stressful situations (Schmidt, 2019).

Furthermore, some schools now have multiple dogs on site. This takes careful consideration and management, as this adds additional personalities, needs, and wants into the environment.

Teachers are experts in educational practice; however, the presence of a dog will place additional demands on their attention in what is already a demanding context. Chapters 8 and 9 explore tensions such as this in more detail.

CONCLUSION

In previous chapters, we have outlined the potential benefits that human-animal interactions can bring. However, much research in the field focuses on the benefits for the human rather than the animal. Indeed, Horowitz (2021, p. 49) suggests: 'The lives of the contemporary human animal and other non-human animals are surprisingly antithetical'. For example, we rarely hear of such names as Krasavietz, Beck, Milkah, Ikar, Joy, Tungus, Arkleekin, Ruslan, Toi, and Muraska. And yet, these were some of Pavlov's laboratory dogs and are amongst the most famous canines in history (Hollin, 2021). Whilst Pavlov remains one of the most cited psychologists of all time, the dogs who were part of his experiments are rarely accorded recognition as individuals (Adams, 2020). We know little about them in terms of their needs, wants, and interests, and indeed, in Pavlov's laboratory thousands of dogs suffered in the name of science. Yet when we explore Pavlov's writing further, it becomes apparent that he did recognise that each dog had a character of their own, something which presented him with something of a moral dilemma.

Amongst others, Menna et al. (2019) suggest a One Health framework for AAI where human benefits and animal health and well-being are considered, and under which circumstances the animals could benefit from such interactions. This chapter aligns with the One Health concept in that it proposes approaches that recognise that human and animal health, as well as their environment, are interconnected. From a One Health perspective, and from the pre-conditions and principles we outline, ethically justifiable AAIs should generate added value in health and well-being for all participants, humans, as well as non-human animals.

School dogs are silent participants in our interventions, often with little choice about the nature, duration, or people that they will interact with. The key message from this chapter is the importance of establishing a sound animal-assisted pedagogy underpinned by relationships between all those taking part in such educational activity, including the dogs themselves.

NOTE

1 https://www.peta.org/teachkind/humane-classroom/whats-problem-classroom-pets/

REFERENCES

AAII (2022) Animal Assisted Intervention International Standards and Competencies, Nijmegen, Netherlands. https://aai-int.org/wp-content/uploads/2022/07/AAII-Standards-and-Comp-June-24-2022-.pdf

Adams, M. (2020). The kingdom of dogs: Understanding Pavlov's experiments as human–animal relationships. *Theory & Psychology, 30*(1), 121–141. https://doi.org/10.1177/0959354319895597

Albuquerque, N., Mills, D. S., & Guo, K. (2022). Dogs can infer implicit information from human emotional expressions. *Animal Cognition, 25,* 231–240.

Alexander, R. (2004). Still no pedagogy? Principle, pragmatism and compliance in primary education. *Cambridge Journal of Education, 34*(1), 7–33.

Bekoff, M. (2019). Dogs watch us carefully and read our faces very well. *Psychology Today.* 13 April. https://www.psychologytoday.com/gb/blog/animal-emotions/201904/dogs-watch-us-carefully-and-read-our-faces-very-well

Berkoff, M. (2018). *Canine confidential.* University of Chicago Press.

Carr, J. (2019). Paws for thought: Why an academy trust spent £12k on dogs to tackle pupil anxiety. *SchoolsWeek,* 29 November, https://schoolsweek.co.uk/paws-for-thought-why-an-academy-trust-spent-12k-on-dogs-to-tackle-pupil-anxiety/

Coughlan, S. (2019). *Every school 'needs dog as stress-buster'.* 21 March, BBC News. https://www.bbc.co.uk/news/education-47655600

Derrida, J. (2008). *The animal that therefore I am.* Fordham University Press.

Didau, D. (2015). *Pedagogy? I hate the word.* 30 September. https://learningspy.co.uk/featured/pedagogy-i-hate-the-word/

Elliott, J., Stemler, S., Sternberg, R., Grigorenko, E., & Hoffman, N. (2011). The socially skilled teacher and the development of tacit knowledge. *British Educational Research Journal, 37*(1), 83–103. https://doi.org/10.1080/01411920903420016

Farnsworth, V., Kleanthous, I., & Wenger-Trayner, E. (2016). Communities of practice as A social theory of learning: A conversation with Etienne Wenger. *British Journal of Educational Studies, 64*(2), 139–160.

Fein, J., Bogumil, D., Upperman, J. S., & Burke, R. V. (2019). Pediatric dog bites: A population-based profile. *Injury Prevention, 25,* 290–294. https://doi.org/10.1136/injuryprev-2017-042621

Fredrickson-MacNamara, M., & Butler, K. (2010). Animal selection procedures in animal-assisted interaction programs. In A. H. Fine (Ed.), *Handbook on animal-assisted therapy: Theoretical foundations and guidelines for practice* (pp. 111–134). Academic Press.

Freire, P. (1970). *Pedagogy of the oppressed.* Continuum.

Giroux, H. (1997). *Pedagogy and the politics of hope: Theory, culture, and schooling.* Westview Press.

Glenk, L. M., & Foltin, S. (2021). Therapy dog welfare revisited: A review of the literature. *Veterinary Sciences, 8*(10). https://doi.org/10.3390/vetsci8100226

Grigg, R. (2022). *Becoming an outstanding primary teacher.* Routledge.

Hamilton, D. (1999). The pedagogic paradox (or why no didactics in England?), Pedagogy. *Culture and Society, 7*(1), 135–152. https://doi.org/10.1080/14681369900200048

Hayes, D. (2010). *Encyclopedia of primary education.* Routledge.

Hollin, C. R. (2021). *An introduction to human–animal relationships: A psychological perspective.* Routledge.

Horowitz, A. (2021). Considering the "Dog" in dog–human interaction. *Frontiers in Veterinary Science, 8.* doi: 10.3389/fvets.2021.642821

Howie, A. (2015). *Teaming with your therapy dog.* Purdue University Press.

Husbands, C., & Pearce, J. (2012). *What makes great pedagogy? Nine claims from research.* National College for School Leadership.

Jakeman, M., Oxley, J. A., Owczarczak-Garstecka, S. C., & Westgarth, C. (2020). Pet dog bites in children: Management and prevention. *BMJ Paediatrics Open, 4.* https://doi.org/10.1136/bmjpo-2020-000726

James, M., & Pollard, A. (2011). TLRP's ten principles for effective pedagogy: Rationale, development, evidence, argument and impact. *Research Papers in Education, 26*(3), 275–328.

Kahn, R. (2009). *Critical pedagogy, eco-literacy, and planetary crisis: The ecopedagogy movement.* Peter Lang.

Kim, L. E., Jörg, V., & Klassen, R. M. (2019). A meta-analysis of the effects of teacher personality on teacher effectiveness and burnout. *Educational Psychology Review, 31*, 163–195. https://doi.org/10.1007/s10648-018-9458-2

Kokocińska-Kusiak, A., Woszczyło, M., Zybala, M., Maciocha, J., Barłowska, K., & Dzięcioł, M. (2021). Canine olfaction: Physiology, behavior, and possibilities for practical applications. *Animals (Basel), 11*(8), 2463. https://doi.org/10.3390/ani11082463

Kurdek, L. A. (2008). Pet dogs as attachment figures. *Journal of Social and Personal Relationships, 25*(2), 247–266. https://doi.org/10.1177/0265407507087958

Langford, M. (2020). How Betty is top dog with Ofsted school inspectors. 16 February, *East Anglian Daily Times.*

Lave, J., & Wenger, E. (1991). *Situated learning: Legitimate peripheral participation.* Cambridge University Press.

Leach, B., & Moon, J. (2008). *The power of pedagogy.* Sage.

Lewis, H. (2017). Puppy dog tales: The benefits of dogs in early years settings. *Early Years Educator, 19*(6), 46–48.

Lewis, H. (2022). *Thinking of a school dog?* Presentation at Osiris World Education Summit (online).

Lewis, H., & Grigg, R. (2021). *Tails from the classroom. Learning and teaching through animal-assisted interventions.* Crown House.

Lewis, H., Grigg, R., & Knight, C. (2022). An international survey of animals in schools: Exploring what sorts of schools involve what sorts of animals, and educators' rationales for these practices. *People and Animals: The International Journal of Research and Practice, 5*(1), Article 15. https://docs.lib.purdue.edu/paij/vol5/iss1/15

Marzano, R., & Brown, J. (2009). *A handbook for the art and science of teaching.* ASCD.

McConnell, P. B. (2002). *The other end of the leash: Why we do what we do around dogs.* Ballantine Books.

Menna, L. F., Santaniello, A., Todisco, M., Amato, A., Borrelli, L., Scandurra, C., & Fioretti, A. (2019). The human-animal relationship as the focus of animal-assisted interventions: A one health approach. *International Journal of Environmental Research and Public Health, 16*, 3660. https://doi.org/10.3390/ijerph16193660

National Health Service (NHS). (2015). NHS Digital Provisional Monthly HES for admitted patient care, outpatients and Accident and Emergency Data April 2014 to February 2015: Topic of interest: Admissions caused by dogs and other mammals [online], 2015. Available: https://files.digital.nhs.uk/pdf/h/6/animal_bites_m12_1415.pdf

Nayak, P., & Jaramillo, D. (2020). Re-imagining difference in the pedagogical encounter. *Curriculum Inquiry, 50*(5), 373–377.

OECD. (2018). *Education at a glance 2018: OECD indicators.* OECD.

Pedersen, H. (2004). Schools, speciesism, and hidden curricula: The role of critical pedagogy for humane education futures. *Journal of Futures Studies, 8*(4), 1–14.

Phuong, A. E., Nguyen, J., & Dena, M. (2017). Evaluating an adaptive equity-oriented pedagogy: A study of its impacts in higher education. *The Journal of Effective Teaching, 17*(2), 5–44. https://files.eric.ed.gov/fulltext/EJ1157447.pdf

Rosenshine, B. (2012). Principles of instruction: Research-based strategies that all teachers should know. *American Educator, 36*(1), 12–19.

Russell, W. M., & Burch, R. L. (1959). *The principles of humane experimental technique.* Methuen.

Şahin, A. (2021). Humor use in school settings: The perceptions of teachers. *SAGE Open, 11*(2). https://doi.org/10.1177/21582440211022691

Sandlin, J., Schultz, B., & Burdick, J. (Eds.). (2010). *Handbook of public pedagogy.* Routledge.

Schmidt, J. R. (2019). Evidence against conflict monitoring and adaptation. *Psychonomic Bulletin & Review, 26*(3), 753–771. https://doi.org/10.3758/s13423-018-1520-z

Shulman, L. (2005). Pedagogies of uncertainty. *Liberal Education, 91*(2), 18–25.

Tedeschi, P., & Jenkins, M. (2019). *Transforming trauma: Resilience and healing through our connections with animals.* Purdue University Press.

Thomson, P., Hall, C., Jones, K., & Sefton-Green, J. (2012). *The signature pedagogies project: Final report, culture, creativity and education*. https://www.creativitycultureeducation.org/publication/the-signature-pedagogies-project/

Van Fleet, R., & Faa-Thompson, T. (2017). *Animal assisted play therapy*. Professional Resource Press.

Wallace, S. (2015). *A dictionary of education*. Oxford University Press.

Watkins, C., & Mortimore, P. (1999). Pedagogy: What do we know? In P. Mortimore (Ed.), *Understanding pedagogy and its impact on learning* (pp. 1–18). Paul Chapman/Sage.

Weller, C. (2015). 'Why every school should bring dogs into the classroom' (Weller, 2015), The Insider, 21 August. https://www.businessinsider.com/why-every-school-should-bring-dogs-into-the-classroom-2015-8?r=US&IR=T

Challenges and Achievements around the World

CHAPTER 4

THE UK AND MAINLAND EUROPE

With contributions from Nicky Barendrecht-Jenken,
Katja Renaud Løvnes, Mojca Trampuš, Sara Karlberg, Geraldine Foley,
Ceri Littlewood and Vicki Cutting.

This chapter is based largely on the contributions of practitioners and other professionals in education working in the field of animal-assisted interventions (AAIs) across Europe. Dogs are brought into schools for a range of purposes, from supporting children's reading to helping develop social and emotional competencies. For example, Lleó XIII is a multilingual charter private school in Barcelona. The school partners with the Affinity Foundation, which was set up in 1987 to promote the benefits of pets in society. To mark International Day against Bullying,[1] students in 6th Grade primary and 3rd Grade Educación Secundaria Obligatoria (ESO), the compulsory secondary education stage (for 12–16-year-olds), participate in the 'Respect Me' anti-bullying programme. Through interacting with the dogs, they learn about respecting others and develop social and communication skills in sharing their ideas with the local media.

The contributors to this chapter are among those who responded to the authors' request on social media for information on any involvement of dogs in school. Their stories do not necessarily represent what is happening more widely in the featured countries. However, they are authentic voices on a range of specific issues including perceived challenges, successes, and attitudes towards bringing dogs into school. None of the contributors refer to large scale studies in their response to being asked about the impact of dogs in school. But they do offer snapshots to illustrate the value of their efforts. Participant perspectives are an important source for qualitative research because they help us understand different orientations, actions and contexts (Morse, 2006).

THE NETHERLANDS

This perspective draws on the work of Nicky Barendrecht-Jenken, founder of Stichting AAI-maatje.[1] This is a non-profit organisation based in Gouda (South Holland), which Nicky set up in 2019. Its main goals are to promote responsible collaboration with dogs in an educational setting and Dog Assisted Reading in line with Reading Education Assistance Dogs® (R.E.A.D.). This international programme was originally designed in 1999 by the Intermountain Therapy Animals (ITA) in the United States. It now operates in each of the 50 American states and more than 27 countries through partner organisations such as Stichting AAI-maatje.

By 2022, there were there 32 officially registered R.E.A.D. teams in the Netherlands. Teams comprise a skilled handler and their certified therapy dog(s), such as Nicky and her dog Soef. All handlers receive at least a basic AAI training and

DOI: 10.4324/9781003257073-7

are sometimes also a dog assisted coach or teacher. Upon successful completion of the training, the dog becomes a certified therapy animal. The dogs are expected to interact with children, and not be afraid of them running around or playing games. Among its goals, Stichting AAI-maatje focuses on helping children to improve their literacy skills and read for pleasure. Its vision is to have a R.E.A.D team in every school 'so we can help more children experience the magic of reading to a dog. We believe that teamwork makes the dream work'.

The R.E.A.D. Programme

The R.E.A.D. programme is primarily designed for children aged between 6 and 9, although on occasions younger or older children participate. Adults also take pleasure from reading out loud to dogs. The programme is very flexible. It is designed for schools and libraries, but there are also programmes implemented around the world at other locations like bookstores, kindergartens, juvenile detention centres, hospitals, shelters for victims of abuse, or asylum centres. Library sessions are primarily designed for enjoyment and open to all. Once or twice a month, a team of handler and dog enters the library for a reading activity with children. The children can sign up for the activity and all experience the unconditional pleasure with the dog and show him their favourite book. In the school context, children are mostly selected by their teachers, such as those experiencing language or reading difficulties, or low self-esteem. Those selected follow a 10-week programme and work with a small team to build children's confidence and trust.

Sessions are always one-to-one (one team of handler and dog, together with one child) and typically last about 20 minutes for each child. Beyond this time, most children (and dogs) lose their focus. To ensure the dog's well-being, a limit is placed on the time spent in each location – no longer than two to two-and-a-half hours (including breaks) whilst the maximum number of child readers is fixed at six, one at a time. This is considered important so that the reading experience is enjoyable and safe for both the dog and the child. Nicky points out that reading aloud '... can be a terrifying thing for some children, but the dog doesn't mind when you make a mistake. He will listen to you no matter what and won't mind when you read a bit slow or quiet, or when you are easily distracted by other things'.

In Practice

Nicky uses such words as 'magic', 'special', and 'magnificent' to describe the experiences of children reading to the dog. She attributes this to the dog's 'calm and relaxed attitude and presence'. The fear associated with reading (especially out loud in front of peers) which some children face is removed or reduced significantly as the child is no longer seen as the one with the reading 'problem'. Instead, the emphasis shifts to seeing the child as an active learner or agent who can become the dog's teacher and reading companion.

When the handler asks questions about the book, Nicky explains that they are always asked 'through the eyes of the dog'. The handler has the responsibility of noticing slight changes in the dog's body language and movement which are then communicated to the child through skilful prompts and questions (Figure 4.1).

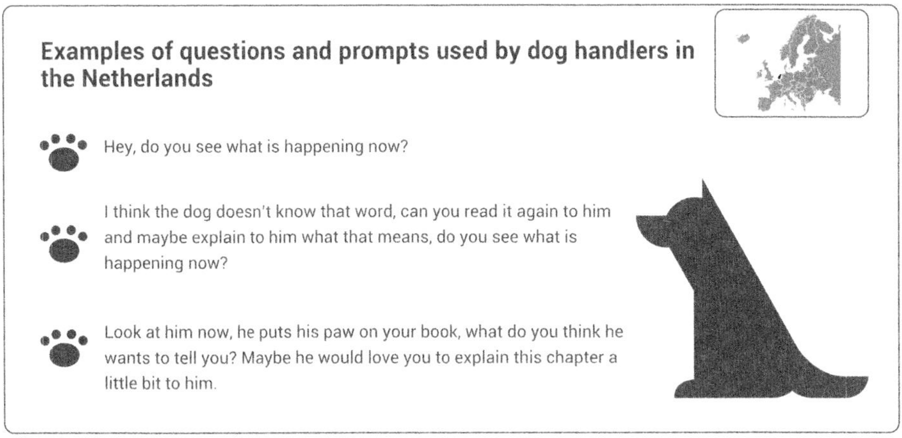

Examples of questions and prompts used by dog handlers in the Netherlands

🐾 Hey, do you see what is happening now?

🐾 I think the dog doesn't know that word, can you read it again to him and maybe explain to him what that means, do you see what is happening now?

🐾 Look at him now, he puts his paw on your book, what do you think he wants to tell you? Maybe he would love you to explain this chapter a little bit to him.

FIGURE 4.1 Prompts used by stichting AAI-maatje dog handlers.

Addressing Challenges

Such interventions are not without their challenges. Initially, Nicky describes how schools were a little sceptical about reading to dogs and how this might be organised. However, such doubts soon dissipate when teachers see the impact on children to the extent that, in Nicky's view, the greatest challenge her organisation now faces is meeting demand. Aside from growing interest in the R.E.A.D. programme across the country, other AAIs are attracting attention in the educational system.

That said, schools in the Netherlands have also experienced increased regulatory paperwork associated with a return to in-person teaching following the COVID-19 pandemic. One consequence of this is that Dog-Assisted programmes and their necessary procedures are seen in some cases as too much additional work, 'yet another thing to worry about'. Schools are under no obligation to sign up to and implement such voluntary arrangements. There are also legitimate concerns over whether a dog might bite a child and other risks, whilst children with allergies also pose challenges. This is despite efforts to reassure schools that all handlers bring their own blankets and ensure that their dogs are clean before entering the premises.

Stichting AAI-maatje provides, with relevant permission, contact information of schools already successfully working with their teams so that new schools can talk through any queries. The organisation also participates in as much scientific research as possible to add weight to its work. For example, it participated in a European Erasmus+ project 'Read4Succeed', which has focused on how to improve the reading skills of children from a migrant, refugee, or deprived neighbourhood through an Animal Assisted Reading programme.[2] Such engagement with research aims to build trust in the organisation's reliability and, more broadly, the credibility behind AAIs.

The Netherlands, like many other countries, does not have mandatory government requirements before anyone can work with a dog or bring a dog into the school. As Nicky explains, 'everyone who has a 'nice' dog can do it'. The lack of such regulation raises a range of difficulties, particularly around protecting the dogs' welfare and well-being. Unfortunately, Nicky's experiences of hearing stories of puppies being brought to school and spending whole days there, in the mistaken belief that 'it is so good for the children', have been reported by other contributors to this book. Such ignorance pays no regard to the dog's sentience, basic needs, likes and dislikes. As Nicky put it, 'the school is not a puppy playground or doggy day care centre'.

Impact

Despite these challenges, operating at various levels, Nicky is firmly of the view that the R.E.A.D programme positively impacts children's reading development. She relates several anecdotes that illustrate this in relation to individual attitudes towards reading. Some children have been inspired to take up reading at home: 'one child even emptied his piggy bank after one session with the dog to buy a book, something his parents never ever seen before'. Children practise reading at home in preparation for their next meeting with the dog and even read aloud to the family pet, whether this is a rabbit, cat, fish, horse, or guinea pig! Teachers feel that the sessions have improved students' reading fluency and comprehension, in addition to social and communication skills. For their part, children tell Nicky that they like reading to a dog more than reading to their parents or peers (Photo 4.1). Their knowledge and understanding of dog body language and signals have also increased. Reflecting on impact, as Nicky acknowledges, the difference that dogs make to children's experiences are sometimes not measurable. As Nicky explains, 'sometimes "all" we do is bring some fun, joy and cuddles in the activity which mostly also lead to more talking about things going on in their mind'.

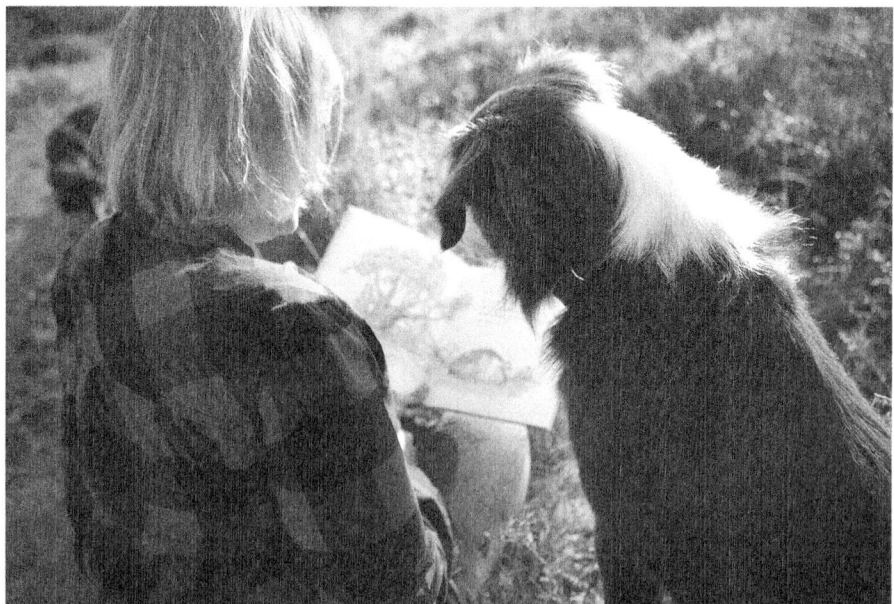

PHOTO 4.1 Soef sharing Storytime.

Reprinted by permission of Nicky Barendrecht-Jenken.

Moving Forward

Stichting AAI-maatje takes the view held by many organisations in the field, which call for regulations around AAIs in all countries. In relation to puppies, for example, Nicky maintains that they should not 'work' when they are still exploring the world and learning new human behaviours. She insists that, depending on the maturity of each dog's breed (typically 1, 3, or 5 years), dogs should only be introduced to and experience their future workplace occasionally. Moreover, both dog and handler should reach a certain level of training before they should be working in the school system. Nicky adds that dogs should not be expected to 'work' more than two or three half days a week. She feels strongly that dogs should not be in the classroom all day, only interact with individuals or small groups rather than whole classes, and the handler should be aware or the likes and dislikes of his dog, their body language and needs. For Nicky, the dog's well-being should be at the forefront of any intervention. She is working with other professionals in the Netherlands to raise the bar to safeguard both the welfare and well-being of dogs and children who participate in AAIs. Hence, they have introduced a register for professionals and providers of AAI training. Those registered professionals and providers are measured against the international standards of the European Society for Animal Assisted Therapy (ESAAT) or the International Society for Animal Assisted Therapy (ISAAT). This provides a level of assurance for schools or other interested parties who are looking for a reliable professional or provider.

NORWAY

Norway has around half a million dogs, which form an important part of Norwegian culture and heritage. Indeed, when archaeologists uncovered a 78-foot-long Langskipet (a Viking warship) in 1880 beneath a hill on a farm near Oslo, they found that it was stocked with everything needed for the owner, a great warrior, or chieftains, to make the journey into the afterlife. Among the treasures buried with him were the skeletal remains of six dogs, similar in size and stature to the Norwegian Buhund.

This case study draws on the experiences of Katja Renaud Løvnes, who works as a teacher in an All-Age school (Grades 1–10) of approximately 300 pupils and 45 teaching staff in the Municipality of Vegårshei. She has taught in the school for 11 years, across the age ranges. Katja's currently has three dogs working with her in school, an 8-year-old Jack Russell terrier Idun, and two Australian Cobberdogs, Uno and Nemi. The Australian Cobberdog may be an unfamiliar breed to readers. In the late 1980s, Wally Conron received a request for a hypoallergenic guide dog for a blind woman whose husband was allergic to dogs and decided to cross a carefully selected poodle with a working guide dog Labrador and the first 'Labradoodle' litter was born. After the new crossbreed came to the public's attention, the demand for this new 'designer dog' skyrocketed and to Conron's dismay, became a victim of its own success. Demand meant anyone could breed a Labradoodle with no regard for their hereditary quality. This led to dogs with widely varying characteristics, even between puppies within the same litter. Poor breeding techniques have resulted in some significant health concerns, including hip dysplasia, eye disease, epilepsy, and allergies. For these reasons, some concerned breeders went back to the origins and long-term vision for the Labradoodle to start again, this time with strict breeding regulations and registration criteria in place. A new name was required to distinguish it from the Labradoodle, and thus the Australian Cobberdog was developed.

Katja lives on a farm and previously had frequent visits from children to interact with the cats, rabbits, horses, dogs, and cows living there. Katja saw the benefits of these approaches for children's well-being, and so began to explore how to develop a more sustained programme based on the school involving her dogs. She undertook training and prepared a rationale for school leaders, and the programme began in 2019. Katja's dogs attend training courses, and she receives ongoing guidance from Dyrebar Omsorg (one of Norway's providers of research, education, and provision of animal-assisted interventions). Katja has also completed a course at the Norwegian University of Life Sciences in Ås and studied AAIs.

In Practice

Katja has established a 'Dog Room' in the school. This was originally designed to allow the dogs a space of their own where they could rest. Having a separate room is also beneficial for many students who do not fit into the regular classroom. Katja notes that they enjoy the lessons in the dog room, telling her:

> It's quiet here, nothing resembling a classroom, lots of pictures on the walls that we can look at, laugh at, talk about. This acts as an ice breaker for new students. Here, together with the dog, we can find peace. I can also adapt and change things and facilitate the individual student and find working methods that suit them individual best. Here the students are seen!

Working with several dogs can make the most of their individual personalities. Katja explains that each of her dogs have different things they are good at, just like humans. Some can spin the wheel of fortune, some can do many tricks, but the most important thing is that they like to lay close to the students on the sofa/duffel bag. They can fetch, lie still, stay, sit, lie down, roll over, dance, crawl, and high five. They can also fetch balls and pick up objects. They are all happy to work in varied environments across the school, from the yard, library and gym, as well as classrooms and the Dog Room itself.

Katie regards her dogs as more than 'pedagogical tools' – they are her closest colleagues. She is careful to ensure that she monitors each dog, ensuring breaks for them during the working day, and she makes sure there is a regular rest day once a week where the dogs are not in school. Students are prepared in advance of working with the dogs. Katja talks to them about animal welfare and the dog's body language. These are not just dogs who come to school, they have been carefully trained and selected.

Impact

Katja is convinced that the dog is a great aid when building relationships with a student, and it can be particularly helpful to have a dog present during difficult, painful conversations that her students sometimes need to have. She says this is because 'The dog does not judge, she does not laugh. She just is'. Katja notes that the dogs help give the students peace of mind, and natural breaks from their schoolwork or issues that might be causing concern. Suddenly the dog does something funny, or needs a walk which can provide a welcome distraction. Students may have the chance to do some trick training or make treats for the dog, as a reward after finishing their work.

Katja feels that the students really appreciate being in the dog room. They value the fact that even when they are having a bad day they are welcomed by the wagging tails of the dogs every time they enter the school, they know the dogs are happy to see them. Katja also works with the dogs in classrooms. If, for example, a secondary school student with restlessness issues is directed to watch a film, one of the smaller dogs jumps up on the desk as a companion. The student then cuddles and strokes the dog whilst they watch the film together. The dog's calmness is contagious, and the student can sit quietly for longer than usual.

The dog can also be involved with students who have difficulties on a social level in, for example, the school yard. Katja explains:

> If a student with few friends brings the dog in the school yard during recess (along with me), then we are an automatic draw for other students. Then the student with the dog gets to practice social skills together with the dog and often with the dog as the focus. And not himself.

Katja can also meet pupils with issues relating to school refusal on the way to school and go to school with them; or, meet them at home and follow them all the way. This arrangement provides a good start to the day.

Katja notes very few challenges other than those related to phobias and allergies. She is aware that not everyone is used to or likes dogs. She has had students who were afraid of dogs in the past, but over time, and through gentle, structured interactions with the school dogs, such as simple games (Photo 4.2), they are no longer afraid.

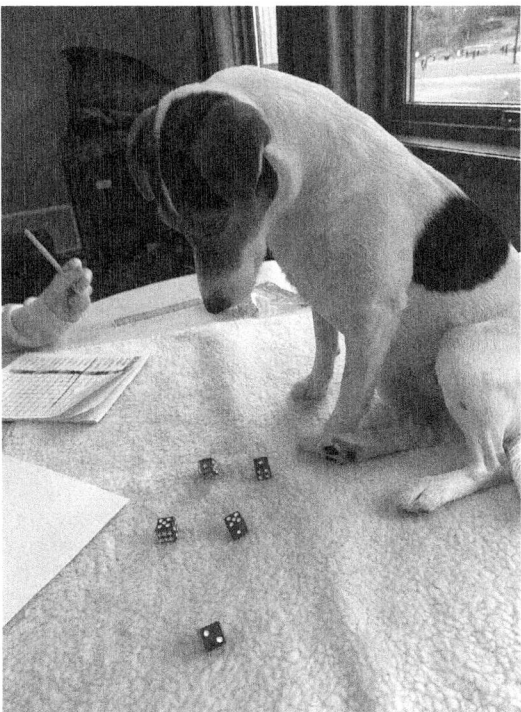

PHOTO 4.2 Idun concentrating on a mathematical game.

Reprinted by permission of Katja Renauld-Løvnes.

SLOVENIA

This case study draws on the experiences of Mojca Trampuš, who is a member of Tačke Pomagačke, the largest Slovenian volunteer association of therapeutic dogs. Mojca has also taught for 30 years as a high school teacher of mathematics. Her experiences here based on teaching at the Secondary School of Education, Gymnasium, and Art Gymnasium, in Ljubljana. The school has around 100 teachers and most of its 950 students live at home with their parents or in nearby dorms. They are typically admitted from primary school with above-average attainment, whilst most leave the school to attend university.

Mojca reports that attitudes to dogs in Slovenia are like those elsewhere in Europe. In her experience, most dogs are well cared for as family pets, and their owners act responsibly. She points out that many caregivers attend 'dog schools' and engage in various sports and activities with their dogs, such as agility classes, scent training, trailing, and search and rescue. However, she adds: 'Unfortunately, outside of the cities and around the rural areas, one can still find dogs tied up, but animal lovers are pushing for legislation to ban this practice'. Slovenia has almost no stray dogs, and animal shelters exist throughout the country. Increasingly, in recent years, dogs are allowed to go in with their handlers to hotels, cafes, shops, and other public areas. Mojca feels that whilst most Slovenians like dogs, there is a lack of specific understanding of dogs' needs and behaviours. She cites examples of people's ignorance of the problems associated with puppy mills or lack of understanding dogs' body language. Of course, both are global problems, which is why education programmes around animal welfare and support from policymakers are so important in raising public awareness and taking action to improve living experiences for dogs. This has wider social and environmental implications. For example, one study (Torkar et al., 2020) of Slovenian adolescents in upper primary and secondary schools showed that the more students report caring for their dogs, the better they are at practising more environmentally responsible behaviours.

In Mojca's case, she and her Golden Retriever Šapa (meaning 'paw') have worked hard since they completed their therapy dog training in 2012 to raise awareness of the benefits dogs can bring to those in hospitals, nursing homes, youth homes, schools, and kindergartens. In Mojca's school, until recently, Šapa worked with a group of 15–19-year-old high school students and prospective preschool teachers, which also involved working with a group of preschool children (ages three to six). The outbreak of COVID-19 meant that lessons were conducted online and Šapa was besides Mojca at home, participating in the online classes. As COVID-19 restrictions eased, Šapa came to school only occasionally. Precautions to prevent the spread of infection changed the conditions at school. Mojca is always mindful of Šapa's own well-being, given her age, reduced agility, and the need to rest most of the day. Both students and colleagues miss her presence.

Part of Šapa's original training at the Tačke Pomagačke Association required Šapa to attend various institutions. Mojca noticed how well she adapted to different environments and circumstances: 'Watching her, I started to really want to include her in my work as a teacher. Šapa seemed ideal for such work – appropriately lively, extremely sympathetic to acquaintances and strangers, eager to please, calm when necessary'. Although at the time there were a few therapy dogs regularly attending

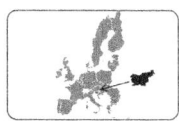

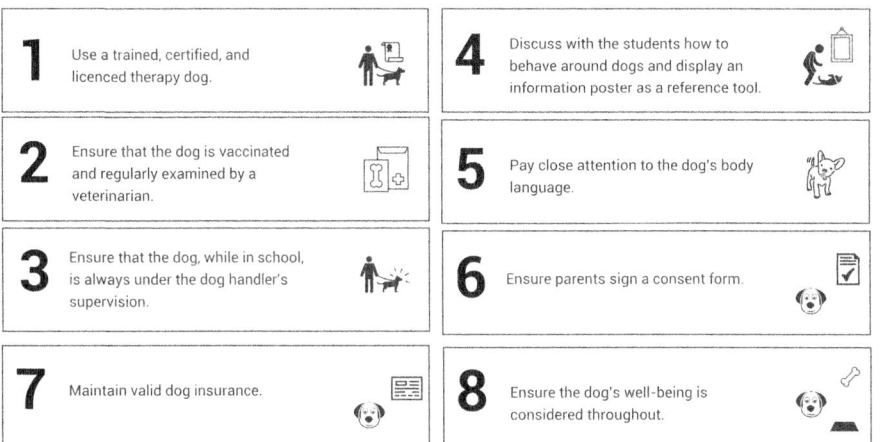

FIGURE 4.2 Mojca's risk management in Slovenia.

schools in Slovenia, they were all owned by external visitors. Šapa was the first Slovenian therapy dog to attend classes taught by their handler.

This was only possible because Mojca worked closely with her school principal and the National Education Institute to agree on the necessary planning and preparation. The fact that Šapa was a fully trained, licensed therapy dog was key to reassuring the school and wider community that this was a well-considered intervention with appropriate risk assessment to ensure the safety and well-being of all participants (Figure 4.2).

All dogs, including those who have received extensive training as therapy dogs, can react unpredictably. Hence, Mojca ensures that her students are taught how to behave around dogs, and she pays close attention to Šapa's body language to address any discomfort. Communication with students, parents, and colleagues is also key to success. Mojca presented the plans to her class at the beginning of the school year, sent an extensive letter of consent to the parent, and prepared a short presentation to her colleagues setting out arrangements. The principal's support can also be a decisive factor in the success of any intervention. In Mojca's school, the principal helped ensure that the logistics were manageable by organising lessons in the same classroom (normally, teachers move to different classrooms each hour). It helped enormously that the principal was fond of dogs, which of course is not always the case.

In her preparation, Mojca first brought Šapa to school a few times during the holidays, so she could get to know the stairs, the hallways, and the classrooms. Gradually, Šapa was introduced to Mojca's colleagues. At first, Šapa was only brought to meet students when there was another teacher in the class. This allowed Mojca to pay focused attention to Šapa's behaviour and body language. Since she showed no signs of stress, after a month, Mojca started to include Šapa in her regular classroom.

Before COVID-19, Šapa was usually in school twice a week. She would stay with Mojca all morning during her classes. Šapa rested next to the teacher's desk, in her own bed, with a water bowl and toys. Mojca is fully aware that it would be exhausting for any dog to act as a therapy dog all morning long, so rest is essential during the lesson: 'She often sleeps soundly during class, and she even entertains the students sometimes when she snores especially loudly'. Mojca agreed with her students that they would not disturb Šapa when she was resting. During breaks, when they wanted to play with her, they called her to them. Mojca recalls: 'It could be very lively then. Many students wanted to pet her or offer her a treat. At the same time, they often confided in me, telling me many things that would otherwise remain private'. Although Mojca's students have always proven to be gentle and considerate of Šapa, she displays a reminder in the form of an information poster above Šapa's bed. This gives basic instructions on how to interact with dogs.

Aside from classes in general socialisation, Mojca works with Šapa on a specific programme for students who are training to teach in preschool settings. Mojca takes the theme of 'The Child and the Dog' and helps students prepare a visit with a therapy dog to a kindergarten or preschool setting. They discuss how to teach children to socialise safely with dogs. The emphasis is placed on fostering a respectful and gentle attitude in regards to animals and nature. Once prepared, Mojca and Šapa, along with other therapy dogs and their handlers, accompany the students to their preschool settings. The key messages to students are the importance of prioritising safety first, observing closely the dog's behaviour and the need to respond quickly to any signs of discomfort. During the visits, students learn how strongly dogs can affect preschool children. They also gain experience in how properly trained and qualified dogs can be incorporated into completely different contexts working with children. Their feedback often signifies students' willingness to include some type of work with therapy dogs in their future teaching careers (Photo 4.3).

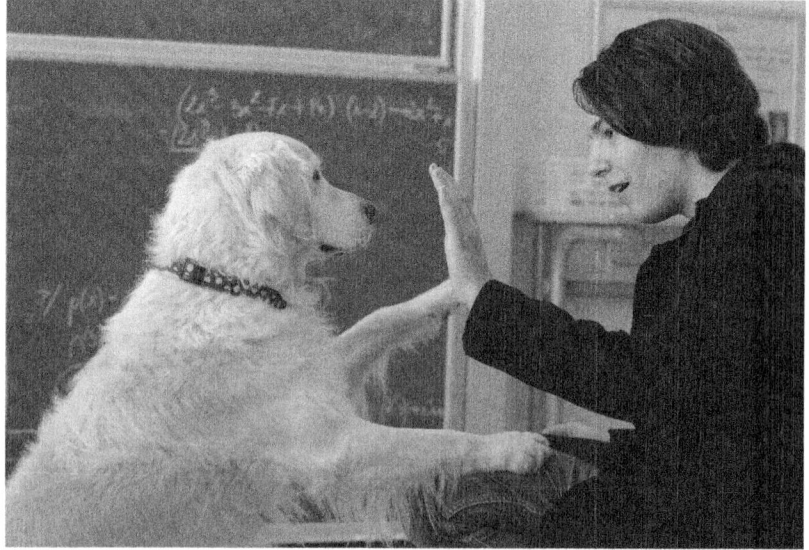

PHOTO 4.3 Šapa in conversation with a student.

Reprinted by permission of Mojca Trampuš.

Šapa has also made an important contribution to the life of the school in many informal ways. She has accompanied teachers on school excursions and hikes and acted as a morning wake-up call for residential students, running to the students' dorms and awakening them with a loud 'Woof!' Outside of Mojca's mathematics lessons, Šapa has also inspired students' work in other areas of the curriculum. In English, students prepared speeches about dogs, in psychology lessons they compared the learning processes of dogs with those of children, whilst in biology lessons they learned about anatomy of dogs, and so on.

Impact

In reflecting on Šapa's impact in school, Mojca feels that Šapa brought 'so much laughter, kindness, and affection to our class'. After visits to preschool, she points out that children always get a stamp in the shape of a paw on their hand. However, during the times of COVID-19, the kindergarten teachers asked Mojca 'to stamp them somewhere higher up on their arms, because otherwise the children didn't want to wash their hands!' It is important not to underplay this emotional impact. Parents have also reported that their children started talking about dogs at home and liked teaching their parents something new about what they had learned. For example, around New Year's Eve, they educated their parents that dogs don't like fireworks because they, like most animals, are afraid of them.

In terms of challenges, Mojca maintains that these have been relatively few. She attributes this to careful preparation. In fact, the main challenge has been meeting the demand for school dogs – 'we would need at least five therapy dogs working in the school if we wanted to fulfil all the wishes of our students'. As with most environments, there are physical challenges, such as having a place to leave Šapa alone for a whilst. Moving around a school where classes are held on different floors without an elevator, can be tiring for an older dog, which is why Mojca decided to curtail such activity.

Over the past 10 years, the number of dogs participating in Slovenia's educational institutions has increased markedly. However, in 2017, the lack of a central overview of this type of work in Slovenia prompted Mojca and two other teachers to set up an informal group known as the School Dog Network.[1] This facilitates the sharing of news and experiences, whilst providing an educational programme open to schools, kindergartens, and other educational institutions to participate, as long as a trained therapeutic dog with a handler regularly attends. The handler can be one of the teachers or an external collaborator. The School Dog Network currently connects 35 institutions, and this number is steadily increasing. Mojca knows that other untrained dogs do go to schools but asserts that 'no one can professionally review and vouch for the education of their handlers or the character and behavioural characteristics of the dog. I think this carries unnecessary risks and can be unfair, unpleasant, or unsafe for the dog'.

SWEDEN

This perspective draws on the experiences of Sara Karlberg who lives in Sweden where she is the Chief Executive Officer of a national organisation called Svenska Terapihundskolen (The Nordic Schools for Therapy Dogs). Dogs have a long and revered place in Swedish history. Some breeds such as the Swedish Valhund have a history dating back over 1,000 years ago and just like in other countries archaeological digs have unearthed remains of high-status members of society buried with their canine companions. With over one million dogs registered in Sweden in 2022, perhaps it is unsurprising that the interest in dogs in schools is gaining attention in Sweden.

The Nordic Schools for Therapy Dogs is a commercial organisation operating in Sweden and Finland which trains teams of dog handler and their dog to work in schools, therapy, and other care facilities. The organisation also run a higher vocational training programme for teachers working with dogs in schools. Sara has a background as a dog trainer and behaviourist, having studied anthrozoology, ethology, and public health. Her experiences with dogs in educational settings began in 2008, when she began taking her own dog into kindergarten settings. From here, Sara developed a programme called 'Sponsordogs', which aims to support children develop a sense of empathy and respect towards nature and all living things through a range of activities. This led onto Sara establishing her own programme, training other pet owners to learn how to implement such approaches in their schools.

Training and Regulation

One unique element to the approach taken in Sweden is that any programmes are conducted by handlers for whom this is a paid role, there are no volunteers. The National Board of Agriculture requires an assessment of all dogs who visit a setting more than three times.

To become accredited, Sara's organisation has detailed training and assessment processes in place. These are tailored for the types of activity a dog may undertake. The educational material is aimed both at people who will work in schools or health care, and teachers, can take an extra suitability test with children to continue their work with dog-assisted activity and children. The programme consists of 155 study hours, online and physical meetings and supervision by both head teacher and basic skills instructor. There are some key pre-requisites to acceptance on the programme. The dog handler must have completed an education in upper secondary school or equivalent and should have knowledge within the target group they intend to work with.

Sara's organisation does not mandate on breed of dog, but rather they consider whether an individual dog is suitable, for example, thinking about whether they enjoy spending time with strangers or whether they prefer to be petted by only the family. How well the dog adapts to different environments and whether they can regulate their behaviour to switch between being active and passive are important components of selection process. The dog must have good basic obedience, for example, they must demonstrate that they can sit, stay still, lie down, lie down, walk nicely on a leash, and handle encounters with other dogs appropriately. Online materials cover content such as canine body language and legal requirements, whilst face-to-face training explores matters such as how handlers communicate effectively with their dogs. A strength of this approach is the specific programme for those wishing to have a school dog. This involves detailed training about lesson planning, risk assessment, and documentation and explores how to adapt sessions to meet the needs of child, dog and timetable. The programme is not recommended for dogs under 18 months of age, and the initial assessment explores how they interact specifically with children. Once qualified, handlers are recommended to work for a maximum of 2 hours per day with a longer break in between (e.g., one hour in the morning and one in the afternoon) approximately 3–4 days a week.

Impact

Sara currently works with her dog Stella (Photo 4.4), a 2-year-old Golden Retriever who loves to play and fetch. Stella has completed over 500 hours of training, as well as aptitude assessments to see how she responds to both adults and children. In Swedish schools. Pupils are selected in agreement between the teacher and the dog handler. The handler has responsibility for maintaining safe interactions and will not be left alone with the children. Clear guidance regarding expectations for sessions is provided, for example, there should be a resting mat for the dog to go to if the dog needs a break, water is always present for the dog.

Sara explains that interactions are as natural as possible: 'We work with as little obedience as possible, letting the dog choose how to work. In that sense, we have discovered that the stress signals are less, and the dog likes to work longer sessions'. She emphasises that it is very important to invite the dog into the session, ask for permission from the dog to join in, and allow the dog to choose what game to play.

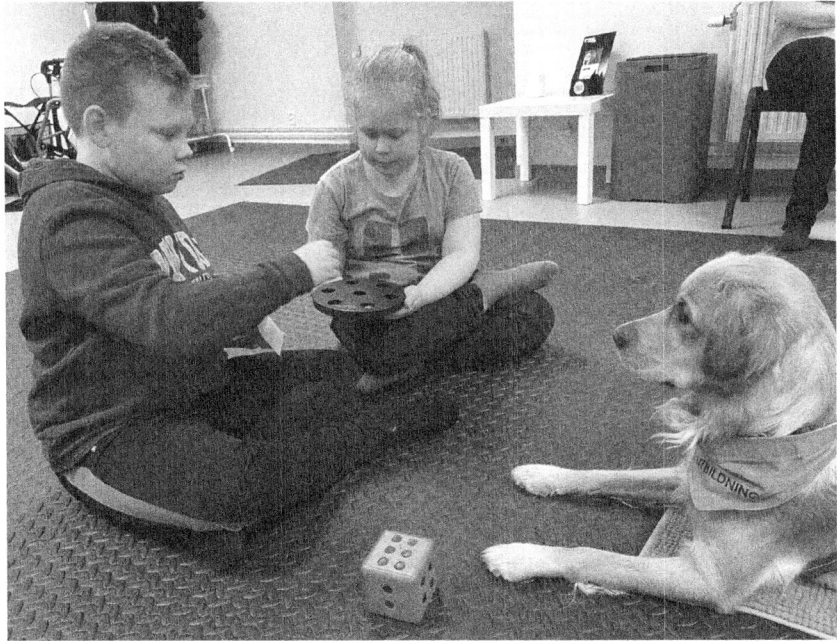

PHOTO 4.4 Stella playing with children during a session.

Reprinted by permission of Sara Karlberg.

Sara has seen the impact that Stella can have on children many times over. For example, recently she began working with two autistic children Benny and Peter. Benny suffers from panic attacks during the evenings and bedtime when he has had a bad day in school. On their first meeting, the boys played a treat game combined with a dice counting how many treats to hide in the game together. Whilst Benny has usually difficulties saying what he wants and talking to strangers this was not a problem this meeting. Later that evening, Sara received a text message from the mother of Benny: 'My son went to bed for the first time without catastrophic thoughts. A nice and anxiety free evening thanks to you and Stella'.

WALES

Dogs are embedded in Welsh culture, from the legendary medieval wolfhound Gelert to the late Queen Elizabeth II's famous Pembroke Welsh Corgis. Both the Pembroke and Cardigan Corgis were originally used to help farmers fetch and drive stock. Welsh sheepdogs have long served a similar purpose and continue to be kept busy given that Wales has approximately three sheep for every one person. Dogs can be found in around one in four Wales and UK households (PDSA, 2022).

The two perspectives from Wales are based on how two primary schools draw inspiration from dogs to support children's all-round well-being and teach about different aspects of the curriculum. The first perspective is that of Geraldine Foley, who is headteacher of Marlborough Primary School, an urban school located in the city of Cardiff. She has been a headteacher for 18 years, more than a decade of which has been at Marlborough. The school has 525 pupils, including a base for 30 children with severe and complex needs, and serves a vibrant, diverse and multi-ethnic community. Since 2019, Geraldine has brought into school Rollo, her family's Sprocker-poo (a cross between a Springer, Cocker Spaniel and Poodle). Rollo was introduced after attending pre-puppy socialisation classes, followed by 8-week puppy training.

Wales has no local or national statutory regulations regarding AAIs. Nonetheless, Geraldine discussed and gained support for the intervention from the school's Governing Body, the Estates Manager (who leads on Health and safety) and the Local Authority Health and Safety Officer. Pupils with Additional Learning Needs and Wellbeing Needs have had regular sessions with Rollo before and throughout the pandemic. During lockdown, Geraldine arranged twice weekly local walks ('Rollo's Rambles') around the school catchment area. Once children returned to school, they had access to Rollo at playtimes. Rollo also 'led' a weekly 'Rollo's Round Up' in the weekly virtual assembly. Since the children have returned to in-person lessons, a rota has been introduced for Rollo to spend time in different classes.

Geraldine has noted that Rollo working with small groups has been more effective and suitable than his presence in whole classes: 'Rollo can be overstimulated by the classroom environment – too many new smells, noises etc that he wants to explore'. However, she believes that there is inevitably an element of trial-and-error in finding out what works best for the dog and children. She allowed the AAI to 'grow organically' and acknowledges that Rollo's role as a school dog has not been what she originally envisaged: 'It has evolved to meet the changing needs of the school community, as well as meeting Rollo's needs and playing to his strengths and what works best for him'. Geraldine values the time she invested in teaching children how to behave around dogs. She drew upon the expertise of the UK-based Dogs Trust, an animal welfare charity and humane society which specialises in the well-being of dogs.

Impact

One particularly effective strategy in creating a positive ethos has been to arrange for Rollo to welcome the children on the playground at the start of the day. As a result, they have looked forward to coming into school to see Rollo. Geraldine explains:

> Children are presenting as upset or worried coming into school, [but] he has a magical effect in transforming how they feel. They take hold of his lead, walk him to their classroom door and give him a stroke or a cuddle before they go into class. It provides a valuable opportunity to talk about their feelings along the way.

Geraldine was surprised at how quickly the community embraced the notion of having a dog in school. She has built on this by developing an imaginative approach in which Rollo accompanies children on local walks around the school neighbourhood. These so-called 'Rollo's Rambles' were first introduced as 'stay at home' restrictions began to ease during the first pandemic lockdown. Schools were only open to key workers' children and so Geraldine saw the opportunity of re-connecting with the rest of the school community. Twice weekly she published a map of where Rollo's Rambles would take place. Over the course of the Summer half-term, they documented via social media their walk around every street of the school catchment area. Maisy was the name of the school's second dog, belonging to the member of staff responsible for Pupil Well-being. She came to the school temporarily.

Geraldine explains:

> Rollo (and I) made socially distanced face-to-face contact with most of our pupils during this time. I initially thought that a few families would turn out on their doorsteps to say 'hello'. Nothing could have prepared me for the response. Families lined their streets, waiting for Rollo to walk past; it turned into a bit of a royal progress. The children were overjoyed to see Rollo and chat about how they were coping. It gave me an opportunity to find out who needed support. Most importantly, it gave our school community the opportunity to just connect, maintain contact and continue to foster a sense of belonging. I would never have dreamt of doing this without Rollo. It provided much needed light during challenging times. Personally, these are incredibly special memories I will cherish.

Parents' engagement is important to the success of any intervention in education. Geraldine kept her parents fully informed and understood those who were a little sceptical at the outset. However, as parents could see the impact on their children's motivation and overall happiness, their concerns dissipated illustrated by the following feedback:

> As a family we were slightly sceptical about how a school wellbeing dog would work but the impact on our daughter has been immeasurable. She instantly fell in love with Rollo, seeing him in the playground and visiting classes. During the lockdowns unfortunately our daughter became really anxious and understandably felt quite isolated. However, seeing Rollo in the virtual assemblies and home learning tasks that were sent throughout the lockdown really helped her. We also went out to see Rollo on one of his Rollo's Rambles and he was there on the first day back at school welcoming us at the gate. My daughter would be lost without him.

Curriculum Learning

Rollo has inspired pupils to learn new knowledge and skills across the curriculum. Nationally, recent curriculum changes in Wales have afforded teachers more professional autonomy in designing their own curricula to meet the needs of their pupils although schools must ensure all pupils are taught essential knowledge and skills, described in statements of what matters across six areas of learning and experience. Over the course of the Spring 2022 half-term, teachers planned a whole-school topic called 'Rollo and his Furry Friends'. The project had a bias towards the Science and Technology area of learning and experience, with a focus on these What Matters statements:

- Science – The world around us is full of living things which depend on each other for survival;
- Technology – Design Thinking and Engineering Offer Technical and Creative Ways to meet society's needs and wants;
- Computing – Computing is the foundation of the digital world.

The curriculum in Wales has a strong emphasis on developing learner agency. Hence, pupils in Marlborough are given plenty of opportunities to raise questions and pursue enquiries that interest them. In the project with Rollo, pupils asked questions such as 'What do animals need to be healthy?' 'How can a pet help you keep healthy? (Year 2); and 'Do animals and humans have the same senses?' (Year 3). Pupils engage in active learning of scientific and technical concepts. For instance, younger children explore which materials may be waterproof when designing a coat or hat for Rollo, whilst Year 6 pupils are set the challenge of creating an animal sanctuary to a given budget. Year 5 pupils learn to think creatively as they plan a mixture to be tinned and sold as dog's food which is nutritious, eco-friendly, and cost-effective. They are then asked to create a label for this and advertise in the form of a television advertisement.

Geraldine makes the point that the impact of Rollo in her school is 'impossible to quantify' but she is convinced that he has made a significance difference to the community, acting as 'Marlborough's mascot'. He has featured in wide-ranging aspects of school life, including setting learning tasks, starring in weekly Rollo's News Round Ups, picking up fragile pupils and staff, and featuring in school videos and concerts. Perhaps the most poignant story relates to a pupil who had suffered the bereavement of a parent. When the child returned to school shortly after the funeral, understandably, he spent a few days in the office receiving high levels of emotional support. He spent much of this time with Rollo; building dens that they could 'cwtch' (cuddle) up together in, reading Rollo stories, talking to Rollo about what had happened, and going on walks with Rollo in the local park. In his words:

> I enjoyed it when we took him to Waterloo Park to play and he loved to chase squirrels.

> It is good to have Rollo interact with him and the kids too. And to help us if we were stressed and lonely, he hugs us a lot and lots of licks and makes us happy after we are sad.

The second perspective from Wales is drawn from Oldcastle Primary school, in the town of Bridgend. The school is based in the town centre and has approximately 450 pupils aged 3–11 on roll. Ceri Littlewood, the headteacher, decided that following the COVID-19 pandemic, children's well-being needed support. After research, the senior school leaders decided that having a school dog would be an approach that might support pupils. In January 2021 they started working with a local breeder of Golden Retrievers, to find a suitable dog for the school. Barney the dog was purchased by the school shortly afterwards.

Barney underwent 3 months of training with a local trainer, part of which took place in the school itself. He is registered as an Emotional Support Animal for the school. Barney works closely with key staff members who take responsibility for him during the school day, and there is a detailed plan in place for this work, which includes ongoing training. Following his initial training, Barney began visiting the school regularly, at first whilst the country was still in partial lockdown due to the COVID-19 pandemic. Barney began working regularly in school from 10 months old, and now is a permanent member of the school staff. Sara Peters, the school's Health and Safety Manager, created a detailed risk assessment and gained approval from the Local Authority Health and Safety team. Parents were consulted, and Ceri addressed any challenges or concerns directly. Typically, these were resolved through such discussions with parents and children. For example, for the very small minority of children in the school who do not like dogs, care is taken to ensure that they are never near Barney.

Barney's role is flexible and means that he can work with any child in the school. This is done based on children's needs. Barney supports children and staff in a range of activities, for example, greeting them at the school gate, providing opportunities to gain exercise during breaktime, and a rest from the pressures of the day (Figure 4.3).

Barney supports children with specific activities such as 'listening' to them read during quiet time and providing a source of comfort for targeted vulnerable or anxious children. These include those children who participate in 'Thrive', which is a programme dedicated to supporting children's social and emotional well-being.[2] This approach uses a development model that considers children and young people's needs and provided responses and activities to engage them with life and learning. There are four pillars underpinning the approach. Barney can contribute to these, which can be viewed according to the pedagogical principles outlined in Chapter 3, as Table 4.1 indicates.

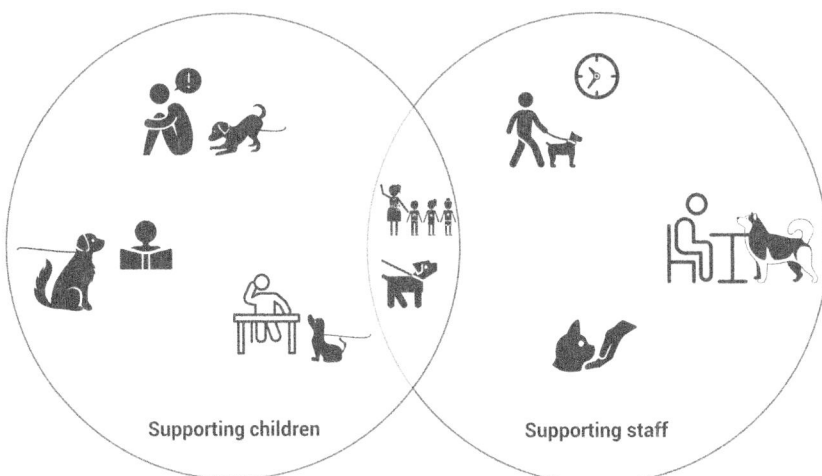

FIGURE 4.3 Examples of how dogs such as Barney support children and staff well-being.

TABLE 4.1 The four pillars of the thrive approach and how these can be supported by animal assisted education.

Pillar	What does this mean?	Pedagogical principles: How can Barney help?
Attachment Theory	Attachment theory considers how healthy attachment relationships can be formed and how these can be used to achieve better outcomes for children and young people. Research tells us that our brains prioritise attachment security over exploration, suggesting that a safe relationship is necessary before a child or young person will be ready to engage with learning.	**Positive relationships** Barney is viewed by the children and staff of the school as a 'social other', and individuals form close relationships with him. This provides safety and security for them.
Child Development Theory	The Thrive model supports teachers to identify the particular developmental gaps signalled by children and young people's behaviours. This means they can choose appropriate, targeted interventions designed to meet their needs and fill the gaps.	**Ensuring the environment is safe for all** Barney can form part of a targeted intervention, for example to support an individual child who is a reluctant reader Barney provides a safe, non-judgemental audience. Such targeted interventions can be planned to take place in a calm, safe context to also support Barney's well-being.
Neuroscience	A key development during the early years of a child's life is the establishment of the body's stress-regulation system. This lays the foundation for social and emotional development. Research has also revealed the 'plasticity' of the brain meaning it can forge new neuronal connections in response to experiences.	**Respect for all** Children develop an understanding of Barney's needs, and learn to respect these, thus promoting self-regulation, for example by learning to speak and move gently when around him.
Play, Creativity and the Arts	Play helps children interact with the world around them: it is how they learn, and how they relate. By listening, paying attention, sharing, and taking turns, a child/young person learns how to explore their own feelings, develop self-discipline, express themselves, and become empathetic to have on their peers and friends. Play also helps to develop confidence by enabling children to build the social skills needed to interact with others and form relationships.	**Creating opportunities for playful interaction** Barney interacts with children in varied ways, for example by helping children in the outdoor classroom find items hidden in the sand. Such playful activities are engaging for both children and Barney himself.

Impact

Barney has had a positive impact on many aspects of school life. For example, his presence in the school and visibility at the start of the day have been noticeable in helping children who are reluctant to come into school in the morning. Children can feel anxious about school for lots of different reasons. They might be worried about making friends, find schoolwork difficult, or find their relationships with peers and teachers difficult. Sometimes, going through difficult experiences outside of school can make it harder for a child to feel settled at school, and those with specific learning needs may find the school environment anxiety-provoking.

Oldcastle has a Family Engagement Officer, Lisa Diehl, to help tackle some of these challenges. Lisa's role is to offer support for parents, carers, and families with any issues that they have in relation to supporting their child. A major part of that role is to develop effective communication between school and home. Barney often works with Lisa to help with this, for example in the morning he will often greet and walk alongside individual children when they get to the school surrounds, to help them feel less anxious about entering the school. The school's website has a section devoted to Barney and includes news of his adventures.[3] Barney also features in the school's curriculum documentation. To help young learners make sense of the purposes underpinning the curriculum in Wales, Barney exemplifies these. For example, thinking about how Barney has modelled being healthy through his daily walk helps children begin to understand what this might mean in terms of their own lifestyles.

Overall, Barney has had an impact on pupil perceptions of dogs, pupil behaviour, and their general well-being, as nearly all of the pupils love him. Just the presence of Barney in the school can support children with fears around dogs. Ceri gives the example of one child who was required to come to the office for medical purposes and who feared dogs before Barney was introduced to the school. Ceri recalls that 'We put measures in place to ensure that Barney was in a different room when he came into the office'. Gradually, the child became increasingly interested in, and confident around the dog and is now more than happy to see Barney and will often want to stroke and say hello to him.

ENGLAND

This final contribution is based on the work of Vicki Cutting, who is an Emotional Health Worker and SEND Personalised Programme Mentor at the Kingsmead School for 11–16-year-olds in Derby. The School provides a range of care and educational provision including a Special school for pupils with social, emotional and mental health difficulties, a Pupil Referral Unit, and Hospital/Medical (EHCPs). The children's previous experiences of school life have proven to be challenging and many enter Kingsmead with Education Health Care Plans (EHCPs). These are legal documents which set out the support provided for children or young people with special educational needs, and the outcomes they would like to achieve. Other children have been permanently excluded from school and many of these have very low levels of basic skills. Some children have had very little previous school experience. One major challenge for Vicki and her colleagues is how to turnaround children's negative attitudes towards schooling and education. Her work with therapy dogs plays a key role in this regard.

Vicki has worked in the field of special educational needs and disabilities (SEND) for 30 years, in various roles across mainstream and specialist schools. For the past 20 or so years, she has worked at the Kingsmead School supporting children with social, emotional, and mental health difficulties, including those who are introvert, experience significant anxiety, or on the autistic spectrum disorder. She also provides Virtual School support within care homes. She holds a clutch of qualifications related to Animal Assisted Therapy. Vicky's first therapy dog worked mainly as one-to-one support in children's care homes and other settings, until he retired at 10 years of age. Her current dog Wilf, a male cockapoo, has been trained as a Facility (Assistance) dog with Darwin Dogs Assistance Dogs Charity, and works across several school bases. He was bought from a breeder with the specific intent of being trained as a therapy dog.

To ensure the well-being of everyone, full risk assessments are completed and shared with Vicki before she accepts any referrals. Dedicated resting spaces are set aside for the dog's well-being and Vicki is always by his side during the three half days a week he is in schools. As Vicki explains:

> This is definitely the most he is comfortable doing, although he loves being in school, it is very tiring for him. His main tasks (you need three that are specific for assistance) are play, pressure (chin on knee) and transition.

Unfortunately, in England, as in most other countries in the world, there are no mandatory requirements for school dogs. However, Vicky has worked hard with school leaders to build policies, protocols, and risk assessments for both the dog's and children's welfare and safety. The dog assists the children in play, 'pressure' (placing his chin on the child's knee) and during transitions, for example, by walking with them between sessions or to and from taxis, and supporting the introduction of new routines, ideas or resources. Wilf has worked alongside speech and language therapists delivering sessions of rehabilitation work supporting students' successful return to mainstream education. The school has developed a literacy box with animal themed books, magazines, and colouring that can be used when Wilf is not in school. Wilf has his own social media presence[8] and is followed by parents as well as their children. The school uses this channel to advertise mental health issues and school themes, and the students feel safe to write to Wilf, which staff follow up (Photo 4.5).

Impact

Vicki has seen how the presence of a trained dog has helped children and young people at school. She has noticed how 'students who have struggled to engage with any teaching and learning begin to feel safe and able to attend classes through the support of their relationship with the dog'. Students tell staff that they like Wilf because he is 'nice, loving, caring and enthusiastic', helps them with their reading and 'makes you feel welcome'.

Wilf provides a kind of 'breathing space' for those children who need time to pause in between challenges. This might mean taking Wilf for a walk around the school grounds accompanied by the handler, simply sitting alongside the dog in a quiet corner for a few minutes or participating in emotional support sessions. The

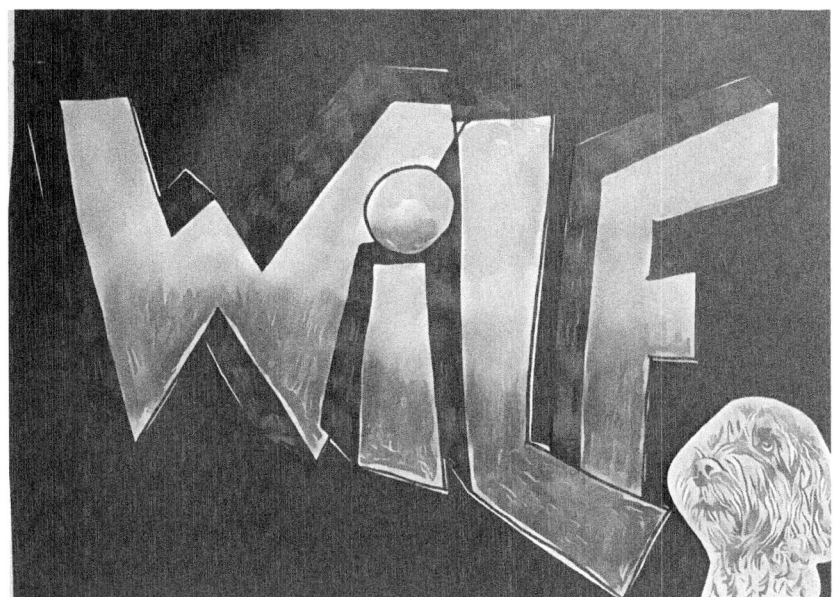

PHOTO 4.5 Pupil art work based on Wilf.

Reprinted by permission of Vicki Cutting.

children and young people enter their relationship with Wilf without fear of failure or adverse judgement. They also learn important life skills, such as caring for others, a sense of responsibility and the freedom to express emotions and act kindly. Wilf mostly works with students who find it hard to engage with agencies to help them towards the next tier of support such as arts or dramatherapy, School Health or Children and Young People's Mental Health Services (CAMHS). The staff have seen students develop confidence in being able to discuss their emotions and begin to feel safe to verbalise their emotions.

For Vicki, the success of her interventions rests on the support from managers in establishing a robust system which recognises the importance of the dog's welfare as well as the children's well-being. She also believes that sharing ideas across local schools and nationally has helped build a knowledge base and informed her reflection. The school has developed a Pawpals project where students write to other school dogs creating links and promoting a sense of community. This meant, for example, the successful delivery of Christmas Cards to 30 other schools, telling them about Wilf's experiences with the children. The school also has displays where Wilf shares his weekly thoughts and ideas – such as his favourite websites and challenges, and his Word and Joke of the Week.

CONCLUSION

Whilst the contributors to this chapter vary in the contexts within which they work, their stories illustrate several factors that are key to successful CAE. The dog needs to be trained by a fully committed and qualified dog handler. The school community needs to be receptive, including supportive senior leadership, and sufficient time devoted towards planning, preparation and commitment to ensure that the dogs' well-being is not compromised.

NOTES

1 https://lleoxiii.com/en/international-day-against-bullying-may-2
2 Find out more about the research underpinning the Thrive approach: https://www.thriveapproach.com/impact-and-research/research-behind-thrive
3 https://www.oldcastleprimary.co.uk/barneys-oldcastle-story/

REFERENCES

Morse, J. (2006). Editorial. *Qualitative Health Research*, *16*(8), 1019–1020.

People's Dispensary for Sick Animals (PDSA). (2022). PAW Report 2022. https://www.pdsa.org.uk/media/12965/pdsa-paw-report-2022.pdf

Torkar, G., Fabijan, T., & Bogner, F. X. (2020). Students' care for dogs, environmental attitudes, and behaviour. *Sustainability*, *12*(4), 1317. https://doi.org/10.3390/su12041317

CHAPTER 5

AFRICA

By Leigh Adams Tucker, Sunday Agbonika, Marieanna le Roux,
Sharyn Spicer, Helen Lewis, and Russell Grigg

> What you help a child to love can be more important than what you help him to learn.
>
> African Proverb.

Education has routinely been connected to the pursuit of freedom, as noted by the late Nelson Mandela (1990) in his iconic words, 'Education is the most powerful weapon to change the world'. However, the formal education sector in many parts of Africa has faced concerns regarding the provision of quality education that is conducive to learning and personal development while also being inclusive of students' varied needs. It is important to find innovative and sustainable ways to support young people in their educational attainment and psychosocial well-being. Animal-assisted interventions (AAIs) have been identified as one such pathway for support. This chapter provides conceptualisation and operationalisation of AAI in Africa, by drawing on experiences from South Africa and Nigeria. It is recognised that each context holds its own dynamics regarding educational practice, attitudes to companion animals, and animal-related policies and practices. The experiences presented in this chapter should not be seen to reflect a singular African experience, but rather an introduction to shared points of struggle and areas of differentiation or growth.

This chapter begins with two contextual sections: a review of education in South Africa and Nigeria, and current attitudes towards companion animals. The status of AAIs is then discussed against this background, with a focus on the provision and impact of two well-established programmes. The chapter concludes with reflections on the future direction of AAIs in Africa.

EDUCATIONAL CONTEXTS

South Africa reflects a complex past and unsteady future relating to socio-political concerns in primary, secondary, and tertiary education. The country's educational system operated along racial segregation lines prior to the 1994 democratic processes. Despite the passing of legislation designed to provide a more equitable system, many young Black people continue to face educational deprivation. In practice, this means that across the provinces, there is considerable variability in the quality of educational provision. Moreover, national standards of literacy and the number of young people with basic qualifications remain significantly below international averages (Howie et al., 2017). In 2020, 15% of 25–34-year-olds in South Africa had a tertiary qualification compared to 47% on average across OECD countries (OECD, 2022).

Nigeria faces similar challenges to South Africa. In particular, the country suffers from low literacy rates, high inequalities in terms of educational access and outcomes

DOI: 10.4324/9781003257073-8

between and within groups, and 'an age-grade system centred on class or curriculum completion rather than knowledge acquisition' (Adeniran, 2022). Further, for centuries children with special educational needs (e.g., Autism and other neurodevelopmental diagnoses) were severely stigmatised. It was commonly believed that such disorders were caused by an evil spirit possessing the child or that either the child or his/her parents were witches. While these specific beliefs do not tend to hold the same weight today, the stigma of caring for a child with special needs persists. In extreme cases, parents have been known to lock their children away in their homes, to avoid the perceived judgment of outsiders.

ATTITUDES TOWARDS COMPANION ANIMALS

Historically, animals have served a safety and security function in Africa. In South Africa, dogs have assisted in hunting, personal protection, guarding property or stock, and keeping feral cats away (McCrindle et al., 1999). In Nigeria, hunting dogs, mostly the local breed dogs, could be seen accompanying the hunter on their adventures, without any form of restraint or control, knowing what is required and executing their part of the hunt masterfully. These dogs were catered to by the hunter's family and lived harmoniously as members of the family structure.

Broader global transitions and social forces have altered attitudes towards animals, where people in communities across Africa do share closer relationships and emotional bonds with their animal companions. The emergence of pet enthusiast groups is fast becoming a trend in Nigeria, with people of various age groups, socio-economic status, religion, and cultures, joining such groups because of the shared love for animals, especially dogs. These groups, and the activities they often engage in, such as dog walks, dog shows, dog carnivals, and dog play dates, further help to portray dogs and other animals in a positive light. As the popularity of these activities grows, more people are made aware of responsible pet practices and the positive advantages of human-animal companionship.

The pet care industry has expanded considerably in South Africa, with an increase in animal guardianship during the COVID-19 pandemic and a range of different pet product offerings entering the market (Thukwana, 2022). South Africa's pet industry is worth 7.1 billion Rand (over $400 Million) and is expected to grow 2.5% between 2021 and 2026, according to data by Euromonitor International (as cited in Thukwana, 2022). It is against this backdrop that a receptivity towards animal-assisted, and more specifically canine-assisted, interventions would be anticipated. However, one of the biggest barriers to involving dogs in therapeutic efforts in places across Africa is the negative attitude towards dogs, largely through their association with risk and systemic violence.

Over the decades, and as exotic breeds of dogs began to make an appearance in Nigerian homes, the lack of awareness about optimal animal care, health and vaccination, training, and feeding led to various cases of dog bites, which were sometimes fatal. These stories spread rapidly, causing a fear of dogs among many Nigerians and limiting the potential for positive interactions with a dog. Many Nigerians lacked the understanding that breed selection and associated factors like general temperament and energy level, blended with family/home dynamics or lifestyle, can determine the eventual outcome of the Human-Dog relationship. South Africa is currently in the midst of a heated debate regarding the banning of pit bulls as domestic pets, following a series of dog attacks and deaths, many of which involved children. Outcry over human deaths has prompted petitions, calls for breed specific legislation, as well as acts of mob violence, resulting in the stoning and burning alive of pit bulls in communities (SPCA Cape of Good Hope, 2022). A disproportionate number of attacks have taken place in Black communities and the pitbull issue has become racialised on social media and has polarised South Africans. These attitudes and actions must be contextualised. Pitbulls are the breed of choice for the Black underclass and dogs, like their owners, are stigmatised and discriminated against (Kay, 2015). The majority of pitbull advocates, activists, rescuers, and denialists are White.

Notions of race and class, and order and disorder have underpinned dog management discourse in South African towns and cities, as early as the 1800s (Mackenzie, 2003). The fear of rabies, along with urbanisation, constructed dogs 'into new social problems' in various parts of the world (Irvine, 2017, p. 3). Tropp (2002, p. 460) notes how African people's dogs came to be viewed as 'trespassers, predators and vermin' by colonial administrators. This resulted in the mass killing of Black people's dogs, specifically 'Native' dogs that had been constructed as a 'sub-species which could be controlled and destroyed' (Doble, 2020, p. 70). The state-sponsored dog culls that took place throughout both the colonial and Apartheid period demonstrate the intersectionality of race, animals, and inequality. Throughout the Apartheid era, dogs were trained and conditioned to be 'racist' and to protect White privilege (Adebayo, 2021; Baderoon, 2017; Doble, 2020). Consequently, many Black South Africans fear dogs, especially breeds like German Shepherds, which are still commonly used for police work.

The way individuals relate to animals is also connected to broader cultural and personal values, including the place of religion. Islam is one of the largest religions in Nigeria, representing approximately 50% of the national population (World Population Review, 2022). Traditionally, dogs are considered haram or forbidden in Islam as they are thought of as 'dirty' and at risk of transmitting disease like rabies. Individuals may be considered impure or unclean, and unable to perform sacred acts of prayer, if touching a dog's saliva. Conservative Islam advocates an avoidance of dogs, while moderates recommend engaging but avoiding the animal's mucus membranes, such as their nose or mouth (Campbell, 2014). Islamic beliefs may influence the keeping of dogs as pets and limit interactions with dogs in various settings such as schools for children (neurotypical or neurodivergent). Having a dog for other purposes such as guarding or hunting remains more acceptable. There is, nonetheless, a growing population of Muslims in Nigeria who are increasingly interacting with dogs in fond ways, as a result of changes in perception or tolerance.

THE STATUS OF AAI IN AFRICA

AAIs is a developing field of study and practice in Africa. As such, it inevitably faces challenges. Globalisation and social media have increased awareness of this form of intervention and its ability to positively impact human and non-human lives. While there are no statistics available to account for all organisations in Africa that operate under the umbrella of AAI, there is a growing public awareness of the professionals and organisations in Africa who are working to formalise and support the practice of AAI. Two such examples include Pets as Therapy (PAT) (South Africa) and Dogalov Human Support Initiative (Nigeria), which provide the case studies for this chapter.

In South Africa, there has been a growth in the number of organisations that offer AAI, more specifically canine visitation support programmes that fall within the ambit of animal-assisted activities (AAA). Most of these organisations that practice AAA within South Africa are accredited non-profits that comply with basic standards and monitoring procedures, as stipulated by the national Department of Social Development. However, in the absence of a shared protocol for AAA in South Africa, operating standards and procedures may differ across these organisations. The typical components that are shared by these organisations include formal application processes for volunteer teams, veterinary health and behavioural assessments for the animal companion, and the inclusion of indemnity insurance for volunteers. These AAA organisations are located across South Africa, with differing levels of reach. In many cases, these organisations are managed by volunteers who may lack the time and capacity to readily engage with new evidence-based practice standards for AAA, as generated internationally. Further to this, there are concerns that the volunteers within these programmes are skewed towards a White female demographic, which is not reflective of the broader community that is being served. Organisations like Pet Partners in the United States openly acknowledge the need for greater diversity in their volunteer recruitment, to reach the varied populations that they serve (Pet Partners, 2022).

Many countries in Africa, South Africa and Nigeria included, do not have professional boards governing AAI, creating difficulties in the monitoring and regulation of this practice (Lubbe & Scholtz, 2013; Thompson, 2013). There is also an absence of many of the elements that could make for a successful AAI practice, that is in line with global standards. Some examples include a lack of insurance cover for companion animals; external organisations that are dedicated to assessing and certify animals for therapy or service; locally derived legislation or guidelines for the practice of these interventions; and an absence of organisations or a central body that certifies animal trainers and holds a database of credible animal trainers.

Concerns also emerge regarding the professional training made available for AAI in Africa. Currently, AAI-related courses and training opportunities are being facilitated by private academies of learning and individual practitioners, which has implications for assessing and moderating the quality of information that is disseminated. The growth of online distance learning has increased the accessibility of international AAI programmes for scholars and practitioners in Africa; however, students may lack the practical, in-person experience of these online programmes or face other barriers such as the financial costs relative to the local exchange rates.

Finally, published peer-reviewed research surrounding AAI, both in theory and practice, is scarce within the African context. The small body of local scientific evidence for AAI that does exist, primarily from South Africa, faces many of the same methodological limitations that have been expressed internationally (Lubbe & Scholtz, 2013; Thompson, 2013). This includes the promotion of intervention efficacy based on anecdotal evidence that is the result of weak study designs with small, homogenous samples, lack of randomisation, no control groups, and vague detail regarding intervention design and delivery (Fine et al., 2019; Johnson et al., 2002). Figure 5.1 sums up the developmental needs for CAE within Africa, although these are not confined to this continent.

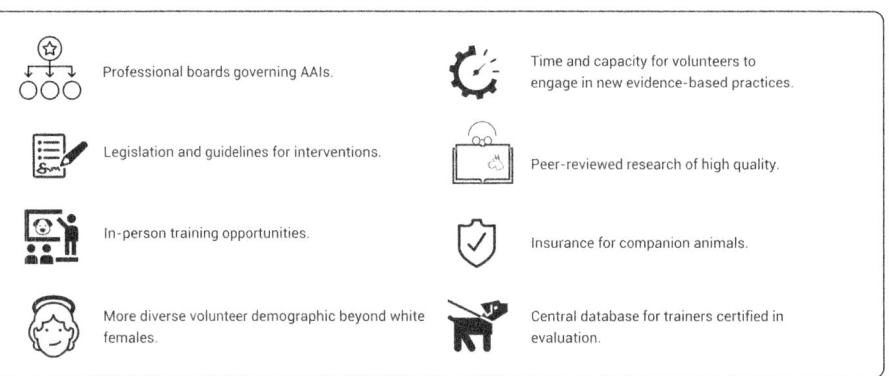

FIGURE 5.1 Developmental needs for CAE in Africa.

CASE STUDY: THE LEES-UKUFUNDA-READ PROGRAMME (SOUTH AFRICA)

The Lees-Ukufunda-Read programme is an animal-assisted education (AAE) programme hosted by volunteers within the organisation PAT, South Africa. The programme is designed to be rolled out in schools or libraries, and currently operates in a small number of schools across the Western Cape in South Africa. The aim is to assist children, primarily Grade 3 students, to improve their reading skills. The general premise is that a child is provided with a space to sit and read a book to a PAT therapy dog, with support and without fear of judgement.

Each reading interaction involves a child, the PAT dog, and the PAT handler.[1] Children are called from their classrooms, individually, to a room where they can interact with the PAT team. Care is taken to refer to this as an activity, and not a lesson, to remove or minimise the pressure of academic performance. At the start of the interaction, the PAT handler introduces the dog by providing a bit of background information about the dog and his/her breed and providing an opportunity for the child to give dog treats, as supplied and supervised by the PAT handler. Each PAT dog wears a yellow bandana, which is not only part of the branding but also a way to soften the appearance of the dog. Children may project fears and uncertainties about dogs, as communicated by family and the broader community system. For example, one of the first children who started the programme nervously asked a member of the PAT team, 'Sal die hond vir my blaf as ek verkeerd lees?' ('Will the dog bark at me if I make a mistake while reading?').

At the start of the interaction, a PAT handler will place a blanket on the floor to create a physical and symbolic frame for the child and PAT team. During the reading activity, the dog lies on the floor next to the child, with the PAT handler in proximity. Once all parties are comfortable, the child is encouraged to begin reading his/her chosen book to the dog. The child shares a physical closeness with the PAT dog and can stroke the dog's fur while reading. These exchanges last for approximately 15–20 minutes, which is an appropriate duration as per the attention levels of the youth.

The PAT handler does not need to be an educator or trained in special education methodologies, as they are not actively assessing or correcting the child's reading abilities. However, volunteers benefit from the familiarity with children, to understand developmentally appropriate ways of responding. The PAT handler plays a fundamental role in interpreting the dog's behaviour and answering any questions or uncertainties that the child may have about the process. For example, the child may be encouraged to explain or expand on parts of the story that is being read, by suggesting that the PAT dog would like to learn more.

It is also not uncommon for PAT dogs to fall asleep during the session. If a dog falls asleep, this may be perceived negatively as the dog becoming bored or potentially disliking the child. The PAT handler therefore needs to have the flexibility and tact to be able to interpret behaviours in an affirming and reassuring way.

Using the example previously stated, the PAT handler may remind the child that dogs listen better with their eyes closed. PAT volunteers learn these different response strategies through their initial training, as well as ongoing mentorship and support by members of the PAT organisation. This emphasises the important role that the handler has in any interaction between dog and child, something which is explored throughout this book.

Existing PAT members with approved therapy dogs need to attend an additional workshop, pass an open book test, and be registered with the R.E.A.D.® programme of Intermountain Therapy Dogs in Utah, USA, to become part of the Lees-Ukufunda-Read intervention.

Dr. Marieanna le Roux (2013) studied the efficacy of a PAT reading programme on the reading and spelling skills of students in an elementary school in a low socio-economic community in the Western Cape. The study was the first known investigation into the effect of an animal-assisted reading programme in South Africa. It was based at an Afrikaans-medium school with a predominantly Black student population. The intervention involved the participation of nine PAT teams, including four Golden Retrievers and five other breeds (Boxer, Weimaraner, King Charles Cavalier, Poodle, and a Jack Russell cross). PAT teams visited the schools once a week for the term (10 weeks). Each child who completed the programme received a READ certificate from the volunteer.

The study employed a pretest-posttest control group design. Grade 3 students with poor reading skills ($n = 102$), as assessed by the ESSI Reading test, were randomly assigned to one of three intervention groups. The 'Dog' group ($n = 27$) read to a dog with a facilitator present, the 'Adult' group ($n = 24$) read to a facilitator only, while the 'Teddy Bear' group ($n = 26$) read to a teddy bear with a facilitator present. The Control Group ($n = 25$) continued with their normal school activities. Once a week during the 10-week animal-assisted reading programme, the participating children read for approximately 20 minutes from a grade 1, grade 2, or grade 3 level Afrikaans reading book, which they chose from a selection of texts. The students' reading rate, reading accuracy, and reading comprehension were measured by the Neale Analysis of Reading Ability. The word recognition and spelling tests were measured by the ESSI Reading and Spelling Tests. Collection of data took place before the start of the reading programme (Time 1), directly after completion of the programme (Time 2), with a follow-up measurement eight weeks after completion of the programme (Time 3).

At Time 1, 75% of the participating Grade 3 students were reading below required standards, at a Grade 1 level. By Time 3, 24% were still reading at a Grade 1 level; however, the balance of the group showed reading improvement, including five children who were now reading at a Grade 5 level. Analysis revealed that the reading comprehension of the 'Dog' group improved significantly compared to that of the other three groups (le Roux et al., 2014). During Time 2 and 3, the 'Dog' group also performed significantly better in word recognition, as measured by the ESSI Reading Test, than the other three groups (le Roux et al., 2015). Children in the 'Dog' group were also less absent from school during the programme than the other three groups.

CASE STUDY: DOGALOV (NIGERIA)

Dogalov Human Support Initiative is a Nigerian Non-Profit Organization, founded by Dr. Sunday Agbonika. The aim of Dogalov is to spread the awareness of Human Animal Interactions (HAI) across Africa and grow the population of AAI practitioners and beneficiaries in countries with low or no HAI presence, especially in Nigeria. Dogalov has been conducting AAA in special education schools across Abuja, Nigeria's capital, since 2018.

The journey towards Dogalov began in 2004 when Joshua, Dr. Agbonika's nephew, was born. As Joshua grew, it appeared that he struggled with achieving some of his developmental milestones. There were no medical professionals or tests that could reveal what was wrong, as neurodevelopmental diagnosis and awareness were absent in much of Nigeria, at the time. Joshua passed away in 2013. Dr. Agbonika graduated from veterinary school and was navigating through life and career options when he came across a documentary by Nathan Selove, lecturer and disability activity, recounting his experiences of Asperger's Disorder and his parents' decision to introduce an Autism Service Dog. This video inspired Dr. Agbonika with the thought of helping other children like Joshua in Nigeria to experience this kind of healing.

In 2017, Dogalov hosted a children's club in Cornerstone Montessori School, teaching children aged 5–10 years old about the basic care of and ethical relationship with animals. The weekly programme used a combination of relatable animal cartoon characters, pictures of animals, and then finally, after demonstrating knowledge of animal handling and ethical relationship, introducing live dogs. During the few sessions with the dog, the children took turns to play with the dog and to demonstrate some of the previously taught lessons about the appropriate care and handling of dogs. When Dr. Agbonika proposed the initial idea for the children's club, the idea seemed new and different, and was in fact turned down by two other schools. The school that gave Dogalov the opportunity to host the club indicated that it would only continue past the first meeting if the children loved it. Fortunately, the children responded positively, and the club thrived for an entire school year, until Dogalov decided in 2018, to focus more on school visitations to special needs schools.

In the first AAA assessment trial in 2018, the Dogalov team visited CADET Academy (Comprehensive Autism and related Disabilities Education and Training), also known as DewDrops Community Centre for Special Needs Children. Two dogs were included in the programme, Ceecee, a 1-year-old Lhasa Apso, and Tish, a 1-year-old

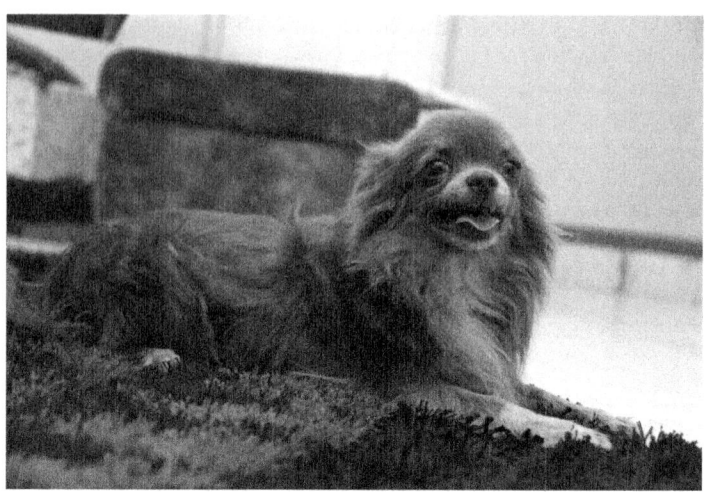

PHOTO 5.1 Tish the chihuahua.
Reprinted by permission of Sunday Agbonika.

Chihuahua (Photo 5.1). Eight children were present in the assessment trial, as well as three on-site staff – two therapists and a teacher. The parents were pre-informed about the meeting, and only children whose parents granted consent were allowed to participate. The interaction in the assessment meeting was largely unstructured. It began with basic introductions, where the staff and students were able to greet the dogs and hear from the handlers about the dogs' personality, likes, and dislikes. For example, Mish and his brother Tish were both imported from Ukraine in 2017. Tish is described by Dr. Agbonika as the low energy, sweet, and affectionate one, who connects easily with people, especially children. Tish enjoys having his tummy tickled. On the other hand, Mish had high energy, was quite affectionate, and was often feisty and less suited to this type of work.

At the start of the programme, the young people spent approximately 15 minutes playing with the dogs, during which the staff and Dogalov team observed to see if there were any adverse reactions from both the children and dogs alike. The children were then given another 20 minutes in which each child had an opportunity to interact with a dog one-by-one. During this time, the school staff were asking questions or giving the children tasks based on what they had been previously taught, that relates to animals, animal care, or social interaction. The session ended with 5 minutes of unstructured group interaction.

The teachers and therapists present during this visit reported that the session could benefit all the children who participated. However, it was the experience of two boys who showed 'breakthrough potential' after interacting with the dogs. These boys were rarely excited or motivated at school, which proved a challenge for the teachers. Yet, when Dogalov came in with the dogs, these same two boys were ready and engaged to do whatever was asked or required of them (Photo 5.2).

One of the boys is still at the Centre and is always excited when the Dogalov team visit with their animals, especially the dogs. One of the issues he presented with in 2018 was communication delay and social interaction difficulties. Today,

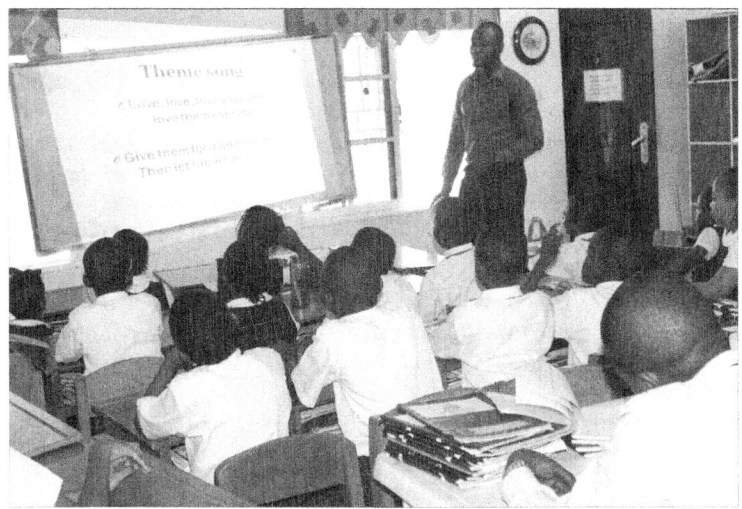

PHOTO 5.2 Dr. Sunday Agbonika singing the Dogalov club song with children at Cornerstone Montessori School, Abuja, Nigeria (2017). The song is sung to the tune of the popular nursery rhyme: 'Row, Row, Row your boat, …'.

Reprinted by permission of Sunday Agbonika.

when the Dogalov team visits, the young man is communicative and filled with joy when he speaks about his dog, who his parents got for him following the positive feedback from the Dogalov assessment trial, back in 2018. The AAA visits continue to be unstructured interactions between the children and the animals, typically lasting from 30 to 45 minutes. However, there are plans to work with onsite teachers and therapists to include more structured, goal-oriented interactions.

The Patrick Speech and Language Centre, founded by Mrs. Dotun Akande, was one of the first centres to provide services for children with autism and other neurodevelopmental disorders in Nigeria. The centre uses evidence-based methods to provide individuals living with autism and other related developmental disorders, the opportunity to identify their needs and achieve their full potential. The Centre, on learning about the power of HAI, decided to trial incorporating animals in their premises and gave opportunities for the children to interact with animals, as well as care for the needs of the animals. The Centre began with rabbits and later added three goats on the premises. The presence of the animals was found to have positive effects on the children. In one case, a 3-year-old boy diagnosed with Autism and having communication and social interaction difficulties was reported to have developed spontaneous speech and better social interaction, credited to the presence of and his interactions with the rabbits. These skills were later transferred to the classroom and immediate environment. Today, he speaks three languages and is integrated into society. In another example, a young boy diagnosed with Autism with severe communication delay and social interaction issues, was reported to have shown spontaneous speech and improved self-regulation, which was credited directly to the introduction and presence of the goats.

THE FUTURE OF AAIS IN AFRICA

Considering the realities and difficulties experienced by young people, and the individuals who teach them, schools are well-placed to address academic issues and to support and foster physical and psychosocial well-being (World Health Organization, 2007). AAE initiatives, like the Lees-Ukufunda-Read programme (Photo 5.3), have the potential to address barriers to literacy by decreasing rates of absenteeism and fostering a culture of positive reading habits (le Roux et al., 2014, 2015).

To maximise impact, AAE in South Africa should target at-risk populations that include boys, young people in remote rural areas, and informal housing settlements, as well as those learning in African languages (Howie et al., 2017). AAA like those facilitated by Dogalov have the potential to provide psychosocial and emotional support to youth in various schools (neurotypical and neurodivergent) while also reconstructing the narrative around stigma and neurodevelopmental disorders in Nigeria.

There is a need to continue to promote public awareness of human-animal interaction across Africa and grow the population of AAI practitioners and beneficiaries in countries with low or no AAI presence. Initiatives like the 2021 and 2022 Animal-Assisted Interventions in Africa Conference, as hosted by Dogalov, is one such mechanism for increasing this visibility. In terms of literature, the limited amount of published peer-reviewed research that does exist in Africa suggests that AAI can

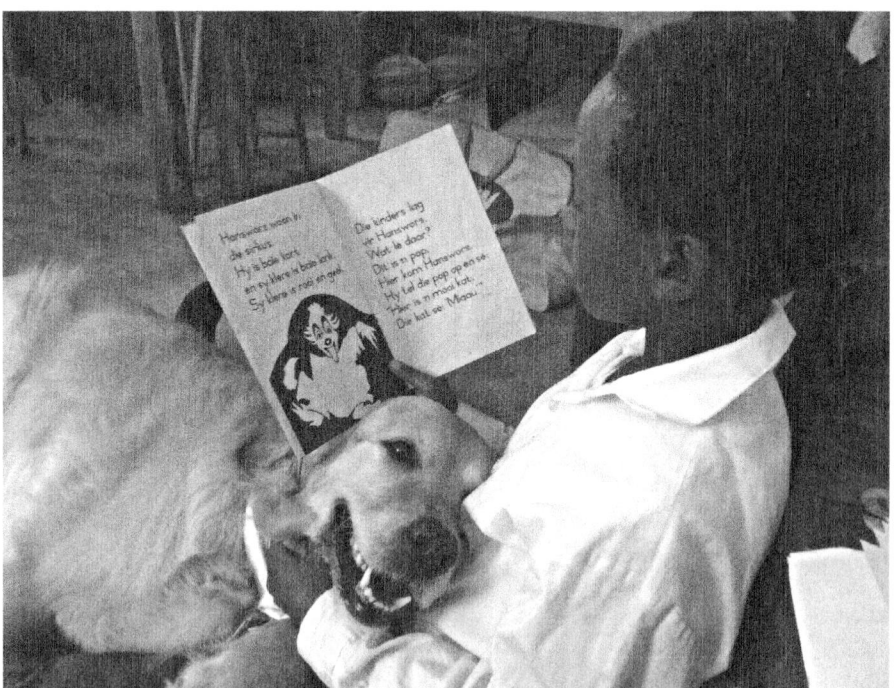

PHOTO 5.3 A Pets as Therapy volunteer interacting with a child during a Lees-Ukufunda-Read session (2012).

Reprinted by permission of Leigh Adams Tucker.

improve health outcomes for various populations including children (le Roux et al., 2014, 2015; Lubbe & Scholtz, 2013; Van Loggerenberg & VanFleet, 2021), but more needs to be known about how animals are incorporated in these interventions, and how those benefits are achieved. There is a need to understand the mechanisms within this practice, as a lack of structure may be ethically problematic and cause harm to both humans and animals alike (Ng et al., 2015). Further needs include the communication of accurate information by reputable bodies, the formalisation of accreditation to undertake AAI, and the recognition of a professional body to regulate and monitor minimum standards.

In summary, there is a need for local, comprehensive, and evidence-based frameworks that will guide the development of AAI in Africa. Africa should be represented in the conversation regarding human-animal relations, to add to the dynamics and cross-cultural realities that guide these exchanges. There remains a need to educate and provide an awareness of the significance of human-animal interactions, where individuals have different values attached to animals. Contemporary views about dogs in many African societies are tainted by cultural beliefs, myths, and negative past experiences. To promote happy, healthy, and impactful interactions, the introduction of AAIs needs to be cognisant of these tensions as to how class, race, gender, and species shape human-animal interactions and entanglements. This includes opening conversations about the diversity of practitioners and volunteers involved in the design and delivery of AAI.

NOTE

1 The terms 'PAT handler' and 'dog' are used to describe the human volunteer and the non-human animal, respectively. It is not to be conflated with ideas of power and ownership.

REFERENCES

Adebayo, S. (2021). *Dogs are racists only if their owners are.* Mail & Guardian. 10 October. https://mg.co.za/africa/2021-10-10-dogs-are-racists-only-if-their-owners-are/

Adeniran, A. (2022). Five ways to build resilience in Nigeria's education system. 15 September. https://oecd-development-matters.org/2022/09/15/five-ways-to-build-resilience-in-nigerias-education-system/

Baderoon, G. (2017). Animal likenesses: Dogs and the boundary of the human in South Africa. *Journal of African Cultural Studies, 29*(3), 345–361. https://doi.org/10.1080/13696815.2016.1255599

Campbell, C. (2014). A Guy Held a Dog-Petting Event and Got Death Threats from Muslim Hard-Liners. 23 October, *Time Magazine.* https://time.com/3533236/malaysia-islam-muslim-dogs-canines-religion-syed-azmi-alhabshi/

Doble, J. (2020). Can dogs be racist? The colonial legacies of racialized dogs in Kenya and Zambia. *History Workshop Journal, 89,* 68–89. https://doi.org/10.1093/hwj/dbaa003

Fine, A. H., Beck, A. M., & Ng, Z. (2019). The state of animal-assisted interventions: Addressing contemporary issues that will shape the future. *International Journal of Environmental Research and Public Health, 16*(20), 3997–4015. https://doi.org/10.3390/ijerph16203997

Howie, S. J., Combrinck, C., Roux, K., Tshele, M., Mokoena, G. M., & McLeod Palane, N. (2017). *Progress in international Reading literacy study 2016: South African Children's literacy achievement.* Centre for Evaluation and Assessment. https://www.up.ac.za/media/shared/164/ZP_Files/pirls-literacy-2016_grade-4_15-dec-2017_low-quality.zp137684.pdf

Irvine, L. (2017). Animal sheltering. In L. Kalof (Ed.), *The Oxford handbook of animal studies* (pp. 97–112). Oxford Handbooks.

Johnson, R. A., Odendaal, J. S., & Meadows, R. L. (2002). Animal-assisted interventions research: Issues and answers. *Western Journal of Nursing Research*, *24*(4), 422–440. https://doi.org/10.1177/01945902024004009

le Roux, M. (2013). *The effect of an animal-assisted reading programme on reading skills of Grade 3 children from a Western Cape school.* Unpublished doctoral dissertation, Stellenbosch University South Africa.

le Roux, M. C., Swartz, L., & Swart, E. (2014). The effect of an animal-assisted reading program on the reading rate, accuracy and comprehension of grade 3 students: A randomized control study. *Child & Youth Care Forum*, *43*(6), 655–673. https://doi.org/10.1007/s10566-014-9262-1

le Roux, M. C., Swartz, L., & Swart, E. (2015). Die effek van 'n troeteldier-ondersteunde leesprogram op woordherkenningsvaardighede van graad 3-kinders. [The effect of an animal-assisted reading programme on word recognition and spelling skills of grade 3 children.]. *Tydskrif vir Geesteswetenskappe*, *55*(2), 289–303.

Lubbe, C., & Scholtz, S. (2013). The application of animal-assisted therapy in the South African context: A case study. *South African Journal of Psychology*, *43*(1), 116–129. https://doi.org/10.1177/0081246312474405

Mackenzie, K. (2003). Dogs and the public sphere: The ordering of social space in early nineteenth-century Cape Town. *South African Historical Journal*, *48*(1), 235–251. https://journals.co.za/doi/pdf/10.10520/EJC93488

McCrindle, C. M. E., Gallant, J., Cornelius, S. T., & Schoeman, H. S.. (1999). Changing roles of dogs in urban African society: A South African perspective. *Anthrozoös*, *12*(3), 157–161. https://doi.org/10.2752/089279399787000228

Ng, Z., Albright, J., Fine, A. H., & Peralta, J. (2015). Our ethical and moral responsibility: Ensuring the welfare of therapy animals. In A. H. Fine (Ed.), *Handbook on animal-assisted therapy. Foundations and guidelines for animal-assisted interventions* (pp. 357–376). Academic Press.

OECD (2022). *Overview of the education system (EAG 2022).* OECD. https://gpseducation.oecd.org/CountryProfile

Pet Partners (2022). *Diversity, Equity & Inclusion.* https://petpartners.org/about-us/dei/ SPCA Cape of Good Hope (2022) *Pit Bulls Killed and Set Alight by Mob.* 21 November. https://capespca.co.za/inspectorate-news/pit-bulls-killed-and-set-alight-by-mob/

Thompson, J. A. (2013). *Exploring best practices in animal–assisted therapy with children in the Western Cape* [Unpublished doctoral dissertation, North-West University].

Thukwana, N. (2022, 16 January). *Pet ownership in SA rose during the pandemic, and it's fuelling the R7.1 billion pet goods sector.* Business Insider South Africa. https://www.businessinsider.co.za/increased-pet-ownership-in-south-africa-has-created-a-pet-market-boom-during-the-pandemic-2022-1

Tropp, J. (2002). Dogs, poison and the meaning of colonial intervention in the Transkei, South Africa. *Journal of African History*, *43*(3), 451–472. https://doi.org/10.1017/S0021853702008186

Van Loggerenberg, M., & VanFleet, R. (2021). The healing power of playful animals. Animal assisted play therapy as an intervention for childhood bullying in South Africa. In S. Jennings, & C. Holmwood (Eds.), *International handbook of play, therapeutic play and play therapy* (pp. 384–392). Routledge.

World Population Review. (2022). *Muslim Population by Country 2022.* https://worldpopulationreview.com/country-rankings/muslim-population-by-country

CHAPTER 6

THE UNITED STATES OF AMERICA

With contributions from Jen VonLintel

This case study is based on the experiences of Jen VonLintel, who since 2008 has worked as a school counsellor at B.F. Kitchen Elementary in Loveland, Colorado. This is a small public elementary school with around 200 enrolled students from kindergarten through 5th grade (roughly 5–11 years). As a Title 1 School, a large percentage of the students qualify for free or reduced lunch. Most of the students who follow the AAI programme are selected through the school's Response to Intervention (RtI) process. This identifies students who may be having difficulty with certain academic skills, and (or) social and emotional aspects of behaviour; and aligns their needs with interventions that are offered in the school.

In the United States, school districts are empowered to establish their own policies before animals enter school, although these are not mandatory. In Colorado alone, there are 178 school districts. Typically, such policies require proof of the handler's registration with a recognised animal certification organisation; proof from a licenced veterinarian that the therapy animal is in good health and proof of insurance. Across the United States, there are many different organisations who support the training and licensing of dogs for work in schools. For example, Pet Partners,[1] a national non-profit organisation, lets schools post volunteer opportunities (aligned to their goals for pet therapy) and matches them with local volunteers. The Alliance of Therapy Dogs[2] deploys fully insured volunteer teams to schools at no cost.

The dogs who work at B.F. Kitchen Elementary School in Colorado's Thompson district must be registered or certified with a therapy dog organisation, such as Pet Partners, Alliance of Therapy Dogs, Love on a Leash, Human-Animal Bond of Colorado (HABIC), and Canine Community Heroes.

Such regulations are primarily designed to ensure health and safety. About a year into the programme at BF Kitchener School, a local newspaper reporter published a story about its work. Jen recalled:

> The day after it was published, I received an email from the district risk management department. They said we could no longer provide interventions. I submitted a large packet of information to risk management that outlined Copper's training, vet records, my professional development in AAI, permission forms, and insurance. There wasn't much research published at that time but I would add it to a packet today if it was requested. This packet was about 2 inches thick and changed the perception of risk management. They realized that this wasn't me bringing my pet dog into school but a very well thought out and documented program. They then allowed me to continue. I now work closely with risk management when we have new teams in the district to ensure we are all meeting high standards and building safe and research-based foundations for our programs.

Working in partnership with school districts or local authorities is key to the success of AAIs. The school district provides space for therapy dog training. A trainer with

DOI: 10.4324/9781003257073-9

Canine Community Heroes offers classes on Thursday evenings in B.F. Kitchen Elementary school's gym. This is important because it allows dogs to train in a school environment, hearing announcements over the loudspeaker, experiencing lockdown drills, taking tours of the school, and exploring classrooms. Jen feels that this localised training is essential because for example, when you have lunches lined up in the hallway, it is important to know that the dog will not be distracted and poke his head in everybody's bag. Once potential therapy dog teams reach a particular level of expected behaviour, they are introduced to volunteer students whose parents sign permission documents for them to attend the training. The students bounce balls in the gym, sing and dance, read books, and play on the playground while the dogs and their handlers learn how to interact with them.

Jen first became aware of AAIs in 2010 when she participated in the Human-Animal Bond in Colorado (HABIC) research project at Colorado State University. The school had one therapy dog team as part of this research that would work with individual students in 30-minute sessions once a week for about 10 weeks. The child participants were identical twins: one student met with the therapy dog team and the other student met with a social work graduate student. Jen started seeing positive results with the student who was working with the therapy dog team after the second session, having previously worked with the student for several weeks with little observed growth. This sparked Jen's interest in why this intervention appeared to have such a positive and immediate impact.

Through their training and interaction, Jen and her team of handlers can identify the strengths of each dog, even within the same breed. For example, Cavalier King Charles Spaniel Toby's strengths involve helping students with empathy goals, literacy tasks, and feeling comfortable talking about issues and problems. Dottie, who is also a Cavalier King Charles Spaniel, has the trait of moving close to students and lying next to or resting her head on a student's lap or hand. As a result, Jen has observed that Dottie has made several strong connections and opened conversations about difficult topics. She has also started more active work with students and featured in a presentation to a 5th grade class about animal communication. Jen reflected: 'The presentation was delivered by a student who had self-esteem goals and became motivated to speak in front of his class because he thinks Dottie is the best thing that has ever happened to him in school'.

The school motto for the AAI programme is 'Dogs First, Students Always'. The team considers the needs of the animal first, on the basis that they can always find another modality to help their students. Having intimate knowledge of each dog's needs is key to their well-being. Murren, a seven-year-old Bernese Mountain Dog, has food allergies, which means that the students need to be aware of only using treats that Georgia, Murren's handler, has provided. Murren specialises in working with students who have self-esteem goals. Jen learnt through her training at the Hearts and Horses Therapeutic Riding Center[3] how individuals value communicating with large animals who listen to what they have to say in a calm manner. Students learn different cues and communicate with Murren by asking her to do different things. They then teach these cues to peers or staff members and may present this information in front of their class. Such activities build students' self-esteem and confidence. The slow, gentle movements of Barnie, a St Bernard, helps students overcome any initial hesitancy in approaching and interacting with such a large dog. Due to his size, the teams are careful to screen students to ensure that they are comfortable in his presence. They provide a second short lead so students can take him for a slow, leisurely walk, whilst maintaining a safe environment for all.

Of course, small dogs can also bring out the best in children and young people. Bug, a Chihuahua mix, enjoys participating with students in a school-adapted version of the game 'Rally' created by the American Kennel Club.[1] Bug and the students navigate a course side-by-side through different signs, each of which provide instructions on the next skill to be performed. The emphasis is on teamwork although students who have focus and attention goals benefit considerably.

Each team that is interested in volunteering comes to the school for a Meet and Greet experience. During that time, Jen talks about different interventions at the school and takes the volunteers on a tour of the building and outside area. They discuss what preferences the dogs may have, activities that they enjoy, experiences working with children, and any requests from the handlers. The therapy dog paperwork and insurance are reviewed, alongside any specific rules and potential interventions that may be a good fit for that team. This also gives the school an opportunity to see how the team navigates being in a school setting. In a few cases, teams display strong stress signals during this Meet and Greet time. Jen acknowledges that she has had therapy dogs growl at students and points out that some dogs may love working with different populations like volunteering at a nursing home or hospital but not a school setting. The fit must be right for all parties.

Jen works with her own dog, Toby, for a half day, once a week. This model has a wider impact beyond the classroom as Toby interacts with students in the hallways, before and after school, during intervention time, and at recess. She keeps a close eye on Toby's schedule to ensure that his needs are met. For example, she plans for multiple breaks outside, time without student interactions, and times to nap. Moreover, Toby's schedule can change during the school year. This calls for flexibility and a willingness to adapt to each dog's changing needs. For example, in the case of her older dog Copper, Jen had to adjust by reducing the demands especially towards the end of the school year 'when the environment at school had more energy and dysregulation' (Photo 6.1).

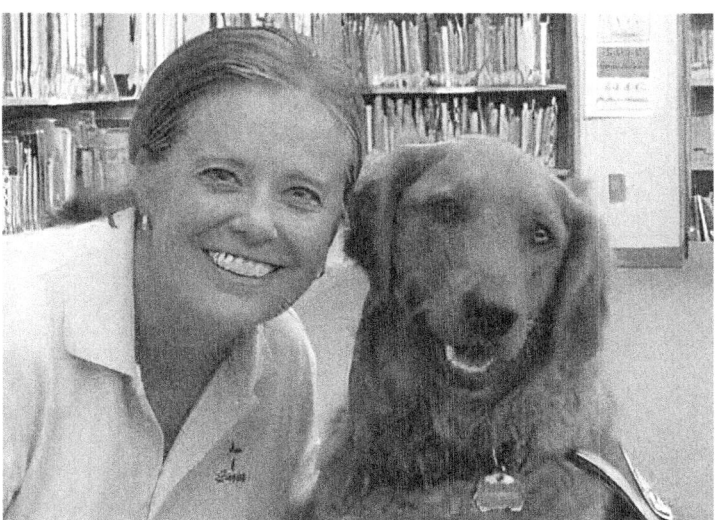

PHOTO 6.1 Jen and Copper.

Reprinted by permission of Jen VonLintel.

IMPACT

Over the last decade or so, Jen has worked with 19 therapy dog teams. She recognises that each team has something unique to offer and hopes that integrating those strengths and preferences helps her students, handlers, and the animals they work with enjoy their time together. She has developed a good understanding of what each dog enjoys and dislikes (Figure 6.1), which is an important consideration that can be overlooked when the focus is on the potential benefits of AAIs to children.

Jen suggests there are cases of dogs who benefit in specific ways. Java, a Labrador retriever, had originally been assigned to train as a seeing eye (guide) dog but she was reassigned from the programme due to a lack of confidence. However, she has flourished since she has worked as a therapy dog in school. Java was one of the first to return when COVID-19 protocols started to allow outside mental health supports back into the building. Reflecting on Java's impact, Jen notes:

> Because of her positive enthusiasm, she consistently works with our students who have significant trauma histories. I have not seen her turn away from a student or remove herself from an interaction. She has an innate ability to connect with students and Lynn, her handler, helps bridge those connections to others around them. She has demonstrated the ability to change her energy to match the student she is working with. She can be actively playing with one student and then the next student comes in, Java reads the energy, and they rest quietly on the floor.

More generally, the impact of the interventions on students' learning and well-being has varied because of several factors. Jen suggests that there have been differences between a volunteer team and the more comprehensive model offered when the intervention is led by a member of the school staff working with their own dog. This may be due to the time the animal is in the environment, the nature of the interactions, and the number of students and staff who participate.

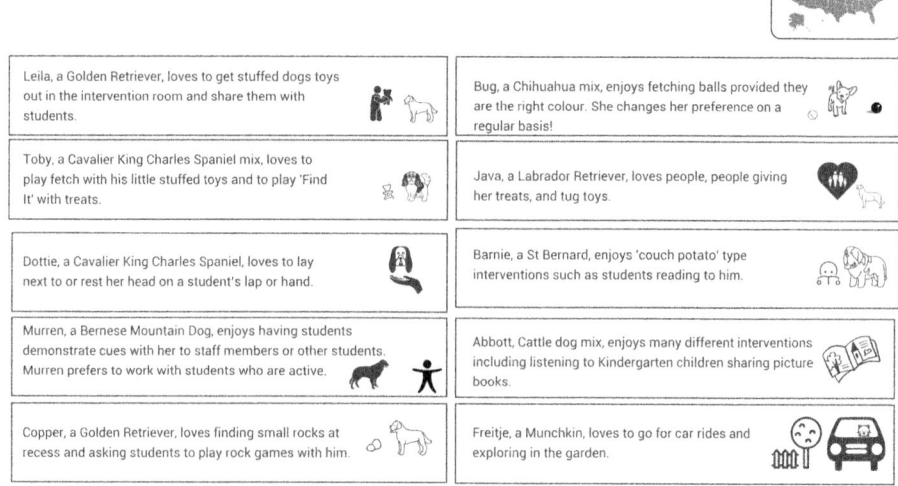

Leila, a Golden Retriever, loves to get stuffed dogs toys out in the intervention room and share them with students.

Bug, a Chihuahua mix, enjoys fetching balls provided they are the right colour. She changes her preference on a regular basis!

Toby, a Cavalier King Charles Spaniel mix, loves to play fetch with his little stuffed toys and to play 'Find It' with treats.

Java, a Labrador Retriever, loves people, people giving her treats, and tug toys.

Dottie, a Cavalier King Charles Spaniel, loves to lay next to or rest her head on a student's lap or hand.

Barnie, a St Bernard, enjoys 'couch potato' type interventions such as students reading to him.

Murren, a Bernese Mountain Dog, enjoys having students demonstrate cues with her to staff members or other students. Murren prefers to work with students who are active.

Abbott, Cattle dog mix, enjoys many different interventions including listening to Kindergarten children sharing picture books.

Copper, a Golden Retriever, loves finding small rocks at recess and asking students to play rock games with him.

Freitje, a Munchkin, loves to go for car rides and exploring in the garden.

FIGURE 6.1 Dogs and cat behaviour in B.F. Kitchen Elementary School.

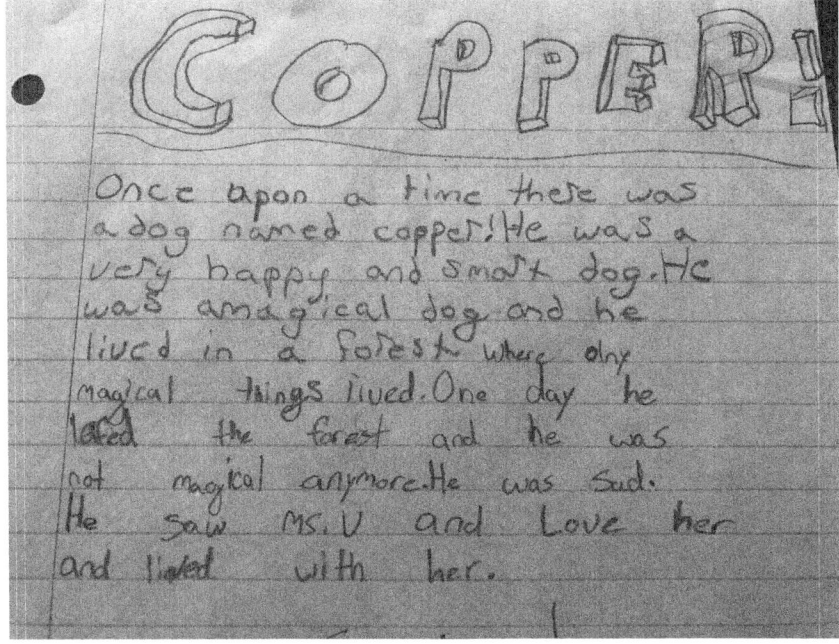

FIGURE 6.2 Story writing about Copper.

The team tracks how students are responding to interventions. This includes data for students' attendance data, behaviour referral, and grades. In recent times, the school has used a commercial programme[5] to capture data on students' social and emotional needs and how they are progressing in response to the intervention. Their evaluation also draws on the views of teachers and parents, and the pupils themselves, who frequently draw or write about their experiences. This can be a letter to say thank you to the dog, or may inspire some writing where the dog is the main character (Figure 6.2).

Some dogs, such as Toby (Cavalier King Charles Spaniel mix), like close companionship but do not like constant petting. Copper, her recently retired Golden Retriever, not only enjoys retrieving small rocks to play games with the students but also enjoys rolling in dead grass and wood chips on the playground, while kicking his legs in the air. Jen and her students call this his 'happy dance'. She adds that he excelled at helping students with regulation goals as they practise skills and co-regulate with Copper when it is time for active play and when to slow down. Copper also loved attending after school Yarn Club when students learn skills, such as crocheting, finger weaving, and latch hook. He would frequently carry skeins of yarn around whether they were attached to a project. This created laughter throughout the group and increased student participation in extracurricular activities. Jen learned to look to his guidance when working in crisis situations. Copper would identify individuals needing support while Jen may not have been aware of the need. For example, when she visited a different school as part of a crisis response, Copper led her to a student that was sitting in class. They sat with the student for several minutes and then Copper moved to other individuals. In speaking with school staff after the visit, Jen learned that the student Copper identified had recently lost a close family member.

Occasionally, parents make direct requests for their children to participate in the AAI programme because they have heard of its success with other children. In one case, the advice of an allergist who was treating a child was acted upon: grooming protocols were increased, hands washed before and after, the student made no physical contact with the dog, and the interaction occurred in a room not previously used by the AAI team to limit the allergens in the environment. Such efforts proved successful because the student exceeded the goals set, parents were happy, the teacher thrilled, and the student looked forward to the next session. Such individual stories demonstrate what is possible through preparation, commitment, collaboration, and a personalised approach to AAIs.

In terms of her counselling role, Jen believes that working with a dog has enabled her to make 'faster and stronger connections' to her students and families. The team use a bridging model in their crisis work where an individual impacted by a traumatic situation first interacts with the dog, then that connection is passed to the handler, and finally to a mental health provider that can support the individual. The school only allows positive reinforcement methods because so many students have significant trauma histories. The focus is on kindness to others and healthy relationships, which can be demonstrated through force free interactions with the animals.

The dogs also act as a highly requested behaviour and academic incentive. Jen notes that teachers can submit names of students who have done outstanding work or made a really good decision as far as being responsible, respectful, or excelling. As a reward, they might get to take a dog on a walk or teach them a new trick (Photo 6.2).

The handlers themselves also derive much pleasure from bringing their dogs into school. Lynn, for example, loves to see her working with students. On a personal level, Jen has found interacting with dogs has brought her joy, decreased stress levels, and increased her oxytocin daily. This has improved her mental health because she is involved in AAI daily at work.

When Jen introduced dogs into school, she wondered whether she was seeing such positive results because this was something new. However, over a decade later, she and her team are convinced that the students are deriving considerable benefits from the programme. They noticed that during COVID-19, in general students' mental health dipped. When some students returned to face-to-face lessons, they displayed old behaviours after interventions have ended, which had not been seen prior to the pandemic. Jen's data showed that they were not making as much growth, compared to similar interventions held prior to COVID-19. As an example, prior to COVID-19, she would have expected to see a 30% increase in emotional regulation following an intervention. However, after COVID-19, that number changed to around 10%. She has found that things are steadily improving however now and feels that with time the success of the interventions will return to pre-COVID-19 levels.

This case study illustrates several important factors that contribute to successful dog-assisted interventions. Dog charities need to work in close partnership with school districts or local authorities towards achieving shared goals. But these should not focus exclusively on what children might get out of the dog's visit. Each dog needs to be treated as a sentient individual with their own strengths, likes, dislikes, and foibles. The dog then needs to be carefully matched with the child, and the

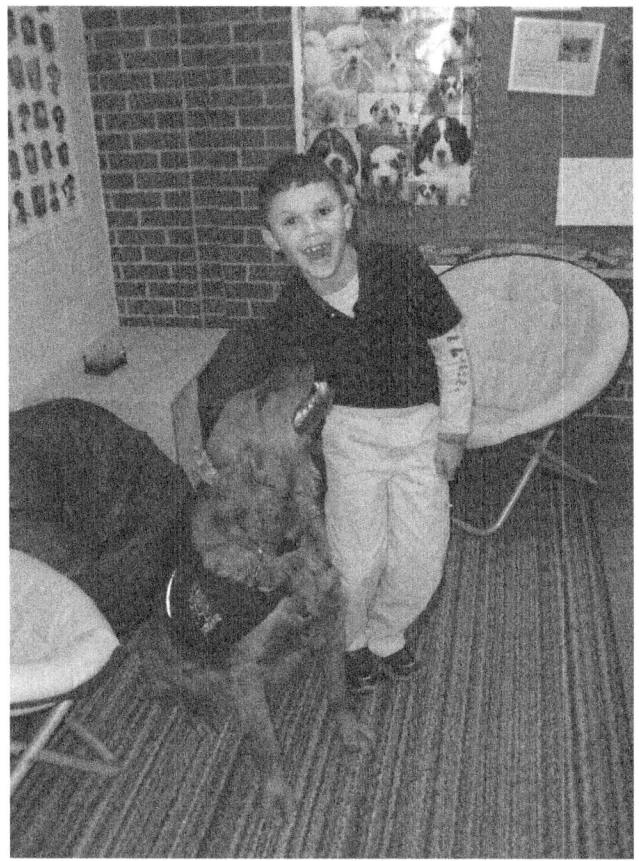

PHOTO 6.2 The joy an interaction can bring.
Reprinted by permission of Jen VonLintel.

kinds of activities that are going to be expected to be undertaken. Preparation time is needed in the school environment so that dogs become familiar with school settings and that humans learn from observing the dogs where adjustments are needed. This ensures that the animal leaves the school having benefited from the interactions as much as the children have.

NOTES

1 https://petpartners.org/
2 https://www.therapydogs.com/
3 https://www.heartsandhorses.org/
4 https://www.akc.org/sports/rally/
5 https://www.bloomsights.com/

CHAPTER 7

ASIA AND AUSTRALIA

*With contributions from Adele Lau, Nurstasha Arifin Wong,
Debbie Ngai, Poorvaja Kuma, and Roz Rimes*

This chapter is based on the contributions of those engaged in dog-assisted interventions in Singapore, Hong Kong, India, and Australia. Their stories cannot be taken as representative of what is happening in the world's largest and smallest continents. But they do highlight the importance of social and cultural factors in planning interventions and provide a sense of the challenges and opportunities that these contributors face. What they have in common is a passion for dogs, alongside a clear commitment to their well-being. They also share a belief in the contribution to children and young people's quality of life dogs can make.

SINGAPORE

Adele Lau is the founder of Animal-Assisted Interactions Singapore (aaisg), which is the country's first social enterprise specialising in the field of animal-assisted interventions and interactions (AAI). Its mission is to foster mutually beneficial and life-giving interactions between humans and animals, in growing healthier communities together. Nurstasha Arifin Wong is the Director of Animal-Assisted Interactions Singapore. Owing to the multidisciplinary nature of AAI (Arkow, 2000), aaisg employs a collaborative approach to building an ecosystem surrounding our three key initiatives: (1) AAI services and programmes for a variety of target populations such as children, elderly, and healthcare workers; (2) education and training; and (3) research and development of public guidelines.

The creation of aaisg was motivated by perceived gaps in the Singaporean context. Specifically, there is a rising demand for AAI, but a lack of standardised guidelines, as well as poor awareness of best practices for protecting the health and well-being of beneficiaries and animals involved in AAI. These gaps pose risks to public health and safety, animal welfare, and the reputation of the growing field of AAI. This case study discusses the challenges and how aaisg aims to address these while offering practical guidance on how to introduce canine-assisted programmes to facilities with concerns about having dogs on site.

The Landscape of AAI in Singapore

Singapore is a small country in South-East Asia with a population of close to six million (Strategy Group, 2022). Compared to other countries, aaisg faces unique challenges in the implementation of animal-assisted programmes (Figure 7.1).

DOI: 10.4324/9781003257073-10

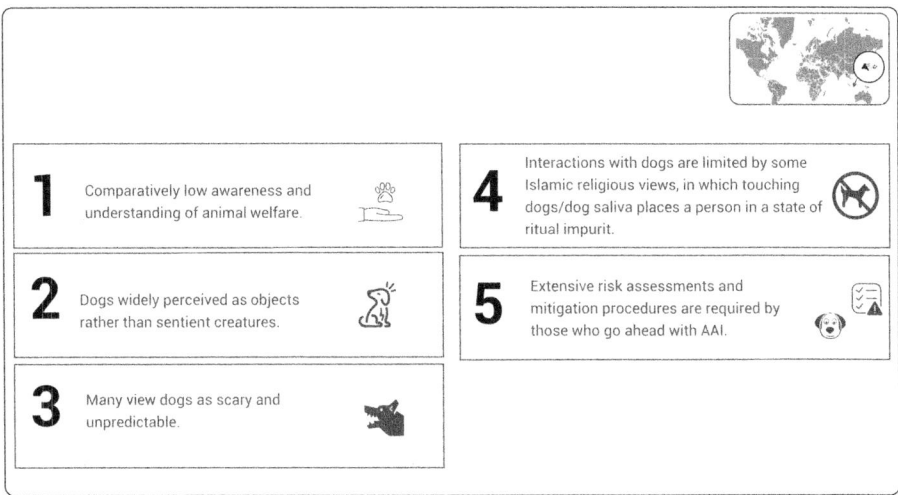

FIGURE 7.1 Challenges facing the introduction of AAI in Singapore.

Firstly, animal welfare regulations in Singapore have been slower to develop compared to other countries. In the 2010s, there was an increasing awareness of the need for better animal welfare standards in Singapore, and a public push for stronger regulations (Retnam et al., 2016). Compared to most western countries that have much earlier incorporated a legal duty of care towards animals, a person's duty of care towards an animal in Singapore was only made mandatory via the Animals and Birds Act in 2015. Prior to this, people were not obliged to provide minimum standards of care for animals in their possession, and authorities were only able to take enforcement actions against an individual after the act of cruelty had been committed. As a result of arguably lower awareness and understanding of animal welfare in Singapore, there is a greater risk of individuals seeing dogs as 'objects', or 'just a dog', rather than our partners. Related to this is also a lack of understanding and receptiveness of the benefits of the human-animal bond and AAI. Through its educational activities, this is something that aaisg aims to change.

Secondly, even though dog ownership is less common in Singapore than many other countries in the world, the number of households applying for dog licenses is steadily increasing (Ministry of National Development, 2022). It is possible that comparatively lower levels of dog ownership in Singapore and an intersection of numerous other structural and societal factors are in part responsible for a perception of dogs as objects or property rather than sentient beings or companions with personalities and individual preferences. However, additional research is necessary in order to draw more conclusive claims.

Thirdly, children and young people who have had little exposure to dogs from an early age tend to have poor awareness of canine body language and behaviour and are more likely to view dogs as scary or unpredictable. While aaisg's programmes are run on an opt-in basis, the organisers are conscious that a significant proportion of the potential client population may not feel sufficiently comfortable interacting with dogs. This may mean that they do not receive the fullest therapeutic benefits of the human-animal bond.

Fourthly, Singapore is a multi-ethnic and multi-religious country, and there is strong societal consensus on the importance of ethno-religious harmony for social cohesion. Around 15% of Singapore's population identify as Muslims, including those who follow the rulings of prominent Islamic scholars and jurists t whereby contact with dogs and/ or their saliva places a person in a state of major ritual impurity. Although there are different views about dogs amongst members of the Muslim community, those who sub-scribe to the latter religious opinion (Hukum) tend to avoid sensory contact with dogs or dog saliva. Many organisations and institutions have opted not to run canine-assisted programmes, out of respect for the Malay-Muslims present at their facilities.

Finally, although organisations have gone ahead with canine-assisted pro-grammes, they are required to conduct extensive risk-assessment and mitigation pro-cedures. This can include devising concealed access routes into facilities or placing signages in publicly accessible areas that announce the presence of dogs. Such pro-cedures, while necessary, can prove time-consuming and expensive.

Aaisg's Programmes for Children and Young People

All the programmes offered by aaisg are designed to consider the preferences of Malay-Muslim young people. To date, that cultural or religious concerns have not prevented these participants from enjoying the therapeutic benefits of aaisg's canine-assisted programmes. However, some accommodations and modifications to programming are occasionally necessary to ensure that their participation remains consensual and that they feel comfortable and respected throughout.

The various aaisg programmes are underpinned by the fundamental belief in fostering mutually beneficial and life-giving interactions between humans and animals in Singapore, beginning in early childhood. The programme objectives vary depending upon the participants and educational focus. The most popular programme is called 'Doggie Detectives' with a target audience of children aged 6–12 years old, who assume the role of 'Sherlock Bones' for the day. The emphasis is on inquiry-based and hands-on learning to achieve a range of objectives (Figure 7.2).

While aaisg's emphasis on teaching children how to read canine behaviour and body language is not unlike human- or animal-assisted education programmes run in other societal contexts, the difference lies in staff sensitivity to the possibility that most of our child participants and perhaps even their parents have never interacted with dogs before.

Bearing this in mind, the Doggie Detectives programme has three prominent features. Firstly, a low child to adult facilitator ratio is deployed, typically groups of five children to one dog-handler team. An additional team of three staff and two vol-unteers (who are not handling dogs) are deployed to oversee a session involving only 20 child participants. While this arrangement is labour intensive, it ensures timely interventions if a child or dog is exhibiting behaviours of stress or discomfort.

Secondly, rather than assuming that the child participants know what a 'happy' or 'relaxed' dog looks like, staff try to point out a dog's positive signals. This is help-ful for reassuring children who feel uncertain about the presence of dogs, as they understand that the dog in front of them is non-threatening, or that they know to pretend to be a 'tree' (standing still with arms tucked) if they want a dog to leave them alone. This is also a useful opportunity to teach children about establishing

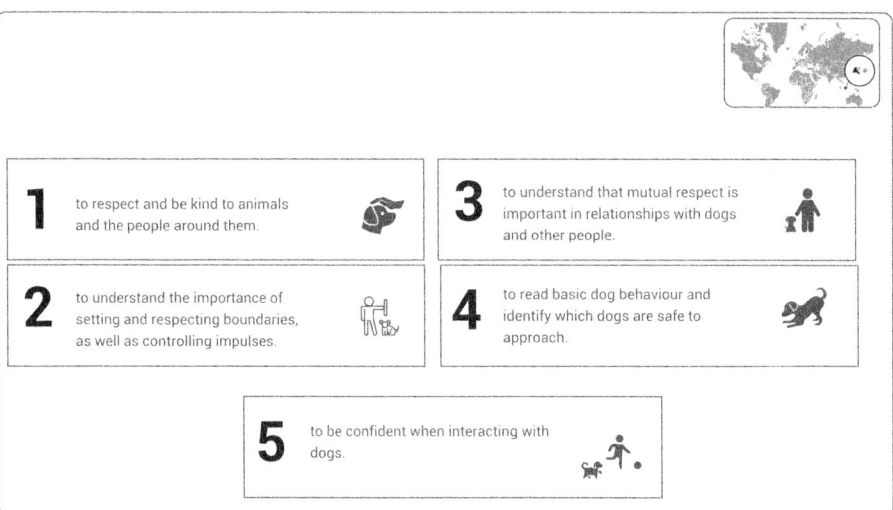

FIGURE 7.2 'Doggie Detectives' programme objectives.

and respecting boundaries. Such activities also facilitate inquiry-based learning as children are encouraged to ask the handlers questions about what makes each dog feel 'happy' or 'sad'. The aim is to help children recognise that they share a range of emotions with dogs, and that most dogs can be expected to respond positively if we treat them like our friends and treat them with kindness.

Thirdly, while the entire Doggie Detectives programme is 90 minutes long, the actual duration of interactions between children and dogs is capped at 60 minutes. Although parents often request for the interaction time to be increased, aaisg do not want to compromise animal welfare by involving the dogs to the point where they no longer enjoy, but merely tolerate interactions with the children. In this way, the aaisg team actively advocate on behalf of the dogs. Staff report a general lack of awareness on AAI best practices, and parents carry the expectation that canine-assisted programmes are 'safe' so long as the dogs involved do not bite. Upon reflection, the programme was tweaked to give the children some pre-programme reading time while they were waiting for the other children to join and settle in, allowing them to spend 60 minutes interacting directly with the dogs.

Over time, staff decided to make the Doggie Detectives programme one that had the option of including parents. In doing so, the intention was to allow parents to come alongside their child's journey in learning to be kind and respectful to animals and the people around them, to continue this conversation even after the end of the programme, and perhaps learn a little something themselves. This was a successful element of the programme.

Take a Paws

The 'Take a paws' programme promotes free and easy interactions with aaisg dogs, with the hope of reducing participants' stress, anxiety, and improving their mood. AAISG staff work with partner organisations to identify young people who they think would benefit from with dogs. Public access rights for dogs in Singapore are extremely limited, and so aaisg work closely with facility managers to erect signages or posters indicating that there are dogs on the premises, so as not to cause alarm.

Although the programmes are not recommended for individuals with extreme fears or aversion towards dogs, aaisg has had success with several young people who overcame their mild fears through gradual, controlled, and positive exposure to the dogs. During a session at a sheltered home for female youths, several participants surfaced worries about touching dogs with their bare hands or coming into contact with dog saliva. Even so, they were eager to take part in the activities, some even insisting on meeting particular dogs they found to be 'cute'. One solution was to offer the young women surgical gloves to wear during the session and red clay soap for them to perform ritual cleansing (*sertu*) afterwards (Ahmad & Shariff, 2016).

Adele and Stasha are keen to point out that aaisg prepare their dogs carefully to ensure that they are comfortable with the smell or sensation of latex or rubber gloves. This is an aspect of careful consideration and preparation to specific contexts that is crucial in ensuring effective practice. These measures might not always be applicable in all settings, however, as other Muslim beneficiaries may deem these measures inconvenient or insufficient for maintaining ritual cleanliness. Nevertheless, aaisg highlight the importance of direct consultation with individual beneficiaries to assess their levels of comfort with the activities, as opposed to excluding them from canine-assisted programmes outright or relying on assumptions based on broad generalisations of Malay or Islamic culture.

In line with this, the aaisg handler training programme includes a module on cultural competence. This emphasises how 'culture' is not static or homogenous; individuals who identify with the same social group may also have varied beliefs or responses to cultural norms typically associated with this group. It is important to acknowledge that culture fundamentally shapes human experience and involves processes 'through which ordinary activities and conditions take on an emotional tone and moral meaning to participants' (Kleinman & Benson, 2006, p. 294). Handlers are introduced to cultural competence as a way of doing AAIs that involves asking good questions about how each beneficiary would like to be visited. This means asking questions that facilitate (1) understanding the beneficiary as a unique individual rather than a representative of a group; (2) understanding what aspects of the AAI experience matter most to the beneficiary; and (3) closing the cultural distance between handlers and the beneficiary, in order to create and grow meaningful relationships (Napier et al., 2014).

As this case study shows, there are challenges associated with AAI in Singapore, which is very much in its infancy. As of 2023, Adele knows of only two qualified animal-assisted therapists, individuals who have professional qualifications in mental health as well as certifications in AAI. Despite the lack of expertise and other challenges, however, Adele and Stasha are sure that the potential gain for participants warrants further interest and support from educators and policymakers.

HONG KONG

Over recent years, there has been growing interest in dog-assisted interventions within Hong Kong's educational settings (Ngai et al., 2021). For example, since the

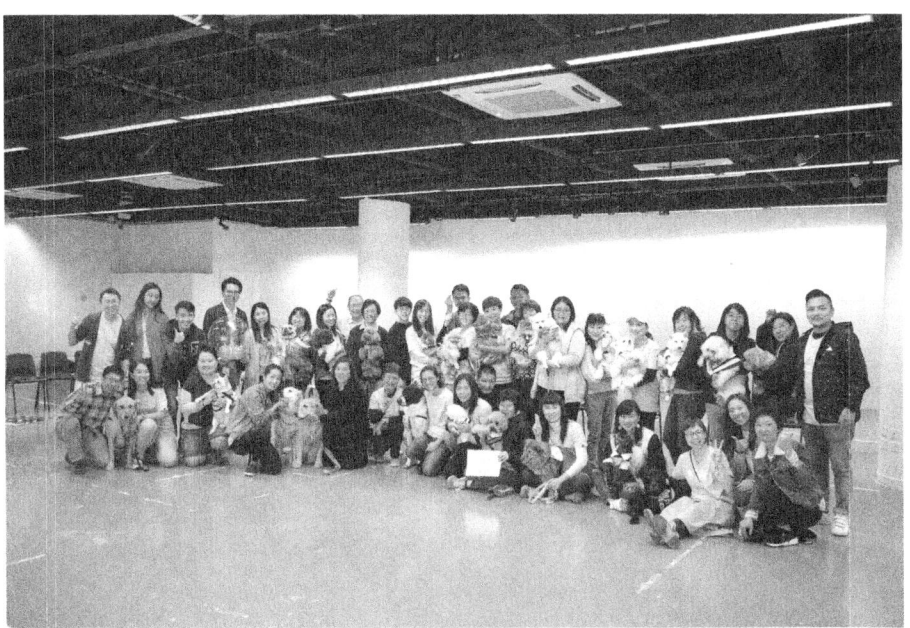

PHOTO 7.1 HKAATA Therapy Dog Team.
Reprinted by permission of Debbie Ngai.

early 1990s, the Animals Asia Foundation through its Dr Dog programme has sent therapy dogs to support children and the elderly with specific cognitive needs (Ye, 2016). This case study is based on the work of Debbie Ngai, who is a trained and certified Animal-Assisted Therapist and registered Social Worker. Debbie is the founder and director of the Hong Kong Animal-Assisted Therapy Association (HKAAT) and has been working in social work and student support for 18 years, covering primary and secondary schools and higher education. Her focus is supporting children and young people with special education needs (e.g., Autism and Dyslexia) or with emotional difficulties (mainly depressive mood/depression and anxiety). Debbie has also initiated a non-profit organisation, which develops professional Animal Assisted Intervention (Services) in Hong Kong. She leads a team of AAT therapists, practitioners, training and certification of Therapy Dogs Team (Photo 7.1).

Debbie's own dog, Pearl (Photo 7.2), is a toy poodle who was rescued from puppy mills as the owners considered she was too weak and sick to have healthy puppies. According to the breeder, Pearl was no longer 'productive'. Malnourished and abused, Pearl was adopted when she was 2.5 years old. She received some humane and holistic-based training to help her relax, regain trust from people, and to build a bond with Debbie. Pearl received 9 months training before she had the therapy dog team assessment and each year since then she has had update training. The goal is to help build up her confidence and socialisation, strengthening the team. Pearl's involvement in this work has promoted her well-being, as she has been offered a new and enriched life.

The association has many different breeds of dogs working across 70 or so teams. These include golden retrievers, poodles, mixed breeds, Shiba Inus, Pomeranians,

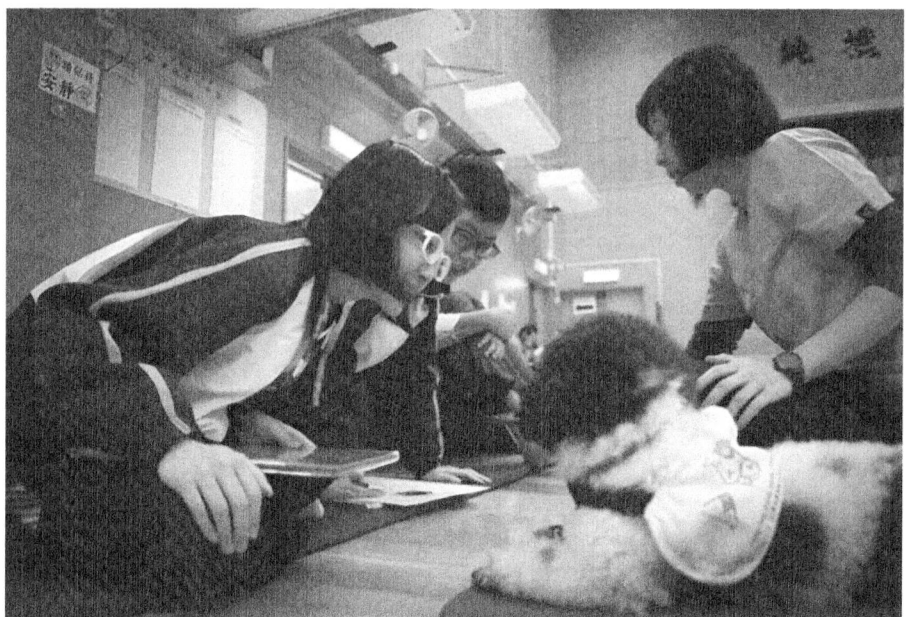

PHOTO 7.2 Ther@Pearl 'listening' to student's reading with her handler, Debbie.
Reprinted by permission of Debbie Ngai.

corgis, Shinshu, and pugs, ranging in age from 2 years to 15 years. This range of breeds and ages demonstrates that there is no one-size-fits-all breed of dog, something discussed further in Chapter 8. For dogs to be certified and for the certification to be renewed annually, dog handlers must attend training including workshops, fulfil certain services hours, and pass an annual assessment. However, neither the central nor local authorities have mandatory requirements that need to be met before a dog can be brought into school.

The dogs are monitored closely to ensure their well-being needs are met. For example, each dog will only work for one or two sessions a day. These typically last between 60 and 75 minutes each. The dogs are not used in consecutive sessions. To safeguard both the welfare of the dog and students, participant numbers are limited during each session, depending on the type of interaction taking place. In Animal-Assisted Therapy groups, the maximum number of participants is six, whereas in Animal-Assisted Activity sessions, the typical group is between 8 and 14 participants. Discussions are held with school staff on logistical matters such as preparing the rooms and flooring, as well as health-related issues such as preventing zoonoses.

The Programmes

The Association offers a range of programmes to suit the different needs of school-children and university students. For the preventive programme, which is dedicated to building resilience and compassion, there is no specific screening of participants. It takes the form of a Life education talk delivered by Debbie (Photo 7.3).

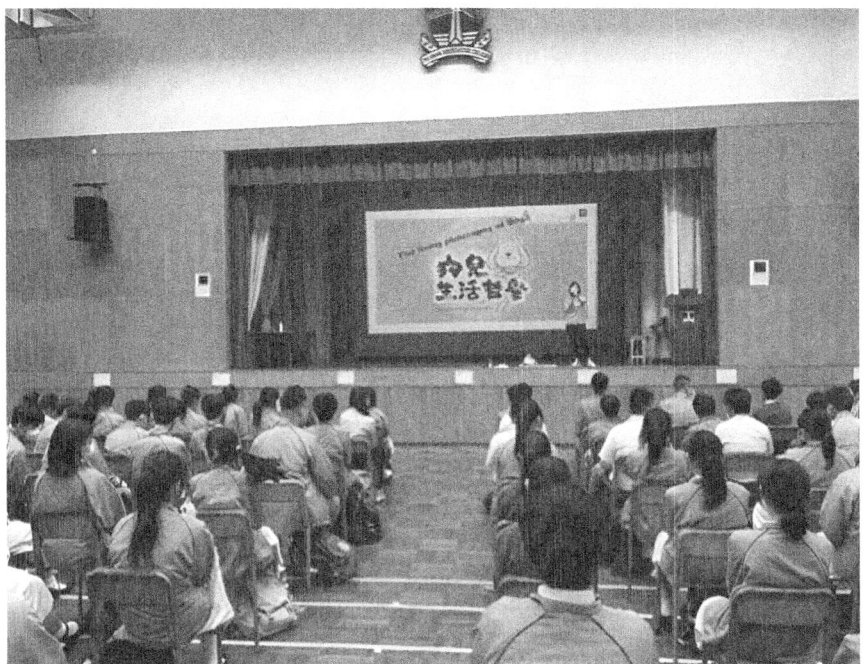

PHOTO 7.3 Ther@Pearl & Debbie on stage delivering the Animal Assisted Life Education Talk to students.

Reprinted by permission of Debbie Ngai.

For the therapeutic and training-based intervention, teachers, social workers, counsellors, and other professional select the participants based on their social or emotional needs, interest in animals and sometimes because they have not responded as well as expected to other training or therapy programmes. Parents are required to sign a health consent confirming that their children do not have allergies to dogs.

Impact

Based on her own experiences and observations, Debbie believes her programmes are making a positive difference in children and young people's lives. She cites examples from her team's work with students who have ADHD/ASD, the Reading Assisted programmes, which support children with dyslexia, and interventions that focus on supporting students with anxiety. Students with dyslexia are motivated to write storybooks featuring a therapy dog based on their Animal-Assisted Reading Programme (Photo 7.4).

Debbie is convinced that her programmes are having a positive impact based on feedback from participants and her own observations. She notes:

> I think bringing dogs to school is very eye catching and always popular with students, parent and teachers. Under delicate guidance and facilitation, the therapy dogs always help to bring out the strength and empathy of the students.

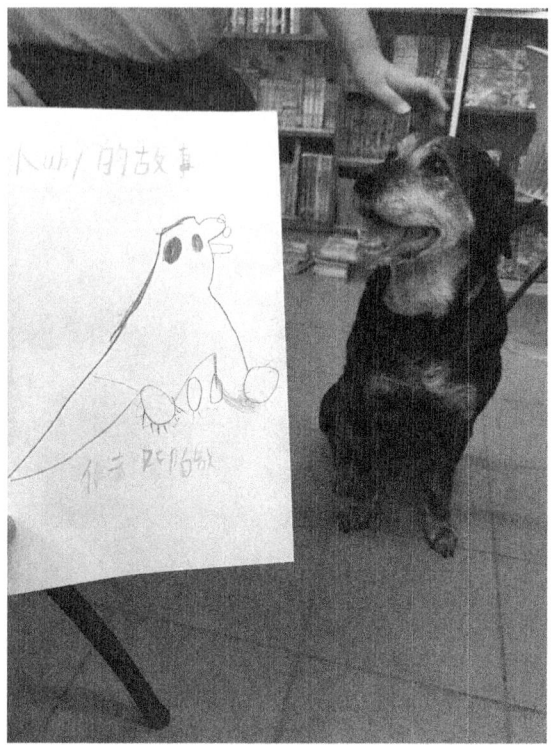

PHOTO 7.4 Sample of students' work with Ther@Ruby.
Reprinted by permission of Debbie Ngai.

In terms of student feedback, Debbie explains that they all enjoy the sessions and look forward to the therapy dogs coming each week. The gains relate to children's feelings of self-worth and attachment to dogs. For teachers, the biggest surprise for many has been how those identified as 'troubled students' show patience and their gentle side in front of the therapy dogs. In some cases, children who were previously withdrawn gradually become more conversant and socially adept in sessions. Significantly, teachers report that the children then show such prosocial behaviours during their classroom lessons as well without the presence of the therapy dog.

However, Debbie has also found that there is a tendency amongst some school-teachers and other professionals to think 'my dog can do that as well' when they hear reports of the success behind the association's therapy dog programmes. In most cases and in contrast to HKAAT's team (Photo 7.5), these dogs are not certified, and neither teachers nor social workers receive training. This inevitably raises concerns around animal welfare and making the most educationally from such experiences. The lack of appreciation for the importance of training is not peculiar to Hong Kong, as other case studies in this book show. But if schools and other educational settings are serious about impact, then they need to allow for well-designed interventions, noted in Chapter 10. This includes investing in training for their staff. They also need to balance the needs of students and the characteristics and strengths of the individual dogs who must be viewed as partners.

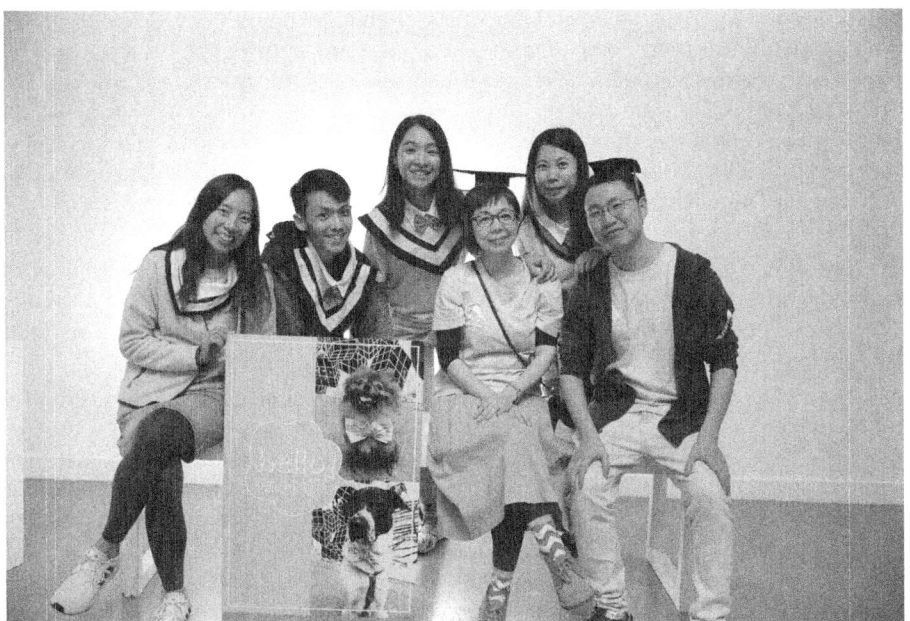

PHOTO 7.5 HKAAT's highly qualified therapy team.

Reprinted by permission of Debbie Ngai.

Like all such interventions, Debbie and her team have faced challenges. One of these comes from unrealistic expectations from cooperating schools who push for longer working hours and greater group numbers based on the misguided notion of being cost-effective. Requests to increase the number of children in a group would jeopardise the dog's welfare and is potentially self-defeating because these limits the interaction individuals can have with the dog. The association does not compromise on its protocols and seeks to educate schools on animal welfare needs. In some cases, schools have turned to other more accommodating organisations, although Debbie feels that more school leaders are willing to respect their values and revise their expectations accordingly.

INDIA

Animals are central to Indian culture, steeped in its literature and the ancient religious traditions of Hinduism, Buddhism, and Jainism. Certain animals, such as the elephant and monkey, are associated with deities while Hindus have long venerated the cow as the country's most sacred creature. Modern-day attitudes towards dogs, however, are more ambivalent. On one hand, there are regular reports of dog cruelty, abandonment, abuse, and neglect, while on the other hand, there is a rise in the number of organisations that are rescuing dogs, human feeders in colonies, and medical aid provided by some local governments.

Community dogs have also been a part of Indian families, where entire settlements fed and took care of them while they lived in the streets and guarded communities. There is some debate over whether bringing such dogs into peo-ple's homes is the right move. Their genetic make-up requires them to be on the streets for mental stimulation. Yet the rising population of street dogs, estimated to be around 35 million, raises other public health concerns. Anti-stray sentiments are largely based on the spread of rabbis and dog attacks on people. Public killings of stray dogs in 2015–2016 and reports of rewards being offered for such killings caused out-rage amongst animal welfare groups, while further anti-dog sentiments were raised in 2022 following a reported rise in dog bites (Sebastian, 2022).

The aim of this case study is to describe the introduction of AAI in India, set in this wider social and cultural context. The focus is on the efforts of Poorvaja Kumar, a Veterinary Assistant, Canine Behaviourist and Trainer, practising Animal-Assisted Therapy in New Delhi.

During her experience as a researcher, Poorvaja observed a positive response amongst people of varied age groups towards alternate forms of therapy such as music therapy and dance therapy in the presence of dogs. This inspired her to spe-cialise in the field of mental health and canine-led programmes in schools and other institutions. In 2016, Poorvaja established 'Humans of Canines', with the aim of improving the relationship between humans, pet-parents, and dogs. Its educational focus is on contributing to children and young people's well-being, which aligns to the government's education improvement plan (Ministry of Human Resource Devel-opment, 2020).

Such interventions need to be set in the wider educational context. Although India has a proud and long history of learning, the educational system faces endur-ing challenges in areas such as securing equal access to education, improving basic Infrastructure and facilities, maintaining an up-to-date curriculum, and ensuring pedagogy meets the needs of learners in the modern world (Lall, 2005; Vedasnee, 2023). There are no quick-fix solutions to such macro-level challenges. However, in recent years, there have been significant improvements (e.g., the country has well-respected universities and colleges) and the Indian government recognises the importance of developing students' wellness as central to educational experiences and outcomes.

It is in child development and learning that Poorvaja believes dogs can play a key role. She offers several services including canine-assisted activities, canine therapy, and canine-led education. Since the concept of AAIs is new to the Indian educa-tional system, Poorvaja first opted to conduct short-term workshops in a range of educational institutions, drawing on students and staff from varied backgrounds, perspectives, and working conditions. Prior to the pandemic, Humans of Canines began running short-term initiatives. These comprised:

- 'fun' workshops to introduce primary-aged children to their new classrooms;
- sessions for older students which focused on interacting with dogs to relieve stress ahead of examinations; and
- activity-based workshops for children with special needs such as Autism, Attention deficit hyperactivity disorder (ADHD) and learning disorders.

The overall theme of most workshops was supporting children and young peo-ple's emotional well-being and respect for animals. The learning focus for younger children (3–5 years) included developing their listening skills, respect, empathy, and friendship. For secondary school students (16–19 years), the focus moved to reducing stress, anxiety, and academic pressure.

Teachers selected and grouped the children based on age, emotional needs, or educational background. Two trained dogs were used, a 4-year-old golden retriever called Leo, who loves to fetch and likes cuddles from people, and a 5-year-old beagle called Murphy, who enjoys performing tricks for an audience. In selecting these dogs, temperament and size were key factors. Younger children or adults with limited previous experience interacting with dogs tend to prefer the beagle because they are smaller than the golden retriever. The children particularly like the fact that someone is listening to their instructions. Older students and adults in a mental health setting respond better to the golden retriever, finding comfort through petting him and setting tasks that an assistance dog would do.

Poorvaja carefully designs each programme to meet the diverse needs of the target population. For example, if the school or other setting wants an academic focus, she invites the dog to perform tricks, which require the children to calculate or learn new vocabulary with the dog. For life skills or mobility-related needs, she includes activities such as leash walking and training the dog with assistance-related tasks. For emotional needs and well-being, activities involve interaction such as petting, storytelling, or reading to the dog. Reflecting on the sessions, Poorvaja identifies several key takeaways (Figure 7.3).

Mixing dance, music, and dog movement helped to keep children focused and ensured it felt like a non-threatening environment. Younger children were most impressed by the dog performing mathematical tricks. Students of all ages who were afraid of dogs initially would try and interact with them and became less fearful. Those with special educational needs responded well to music,

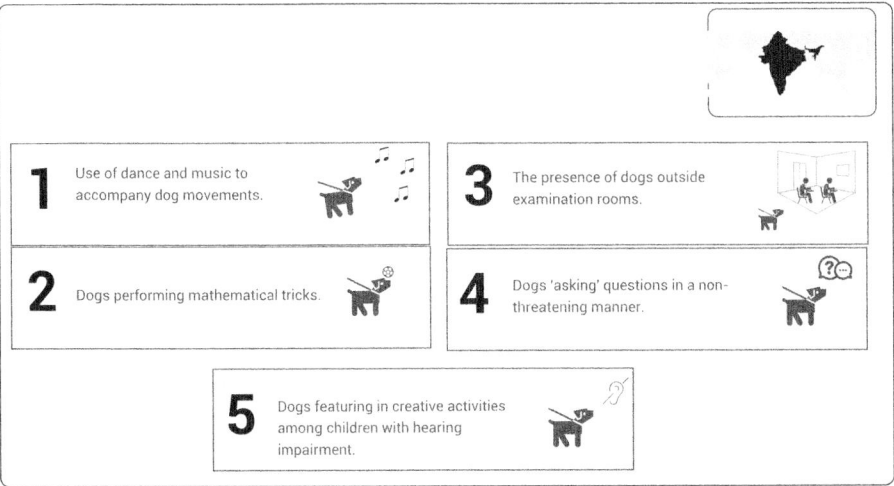

FIGURE 7.3 What worked well in maintaining children's focus.

movement, and the presence of dogs. Walking was highly effective amongst students with Cerebral Palsy, as it provided a sense of achievement, empowered them, giving them a purpose to try and walk. Care was taken to monitor the dog to ensure they were happy to work alongside a child with these types of physical needs.

Students with hearing impairment and learning disabilities benefited from both the calmness and excitement associated with creative activities featuring dogs. The presence of dogs in destress sessions outside examination rooms brought some temporary relief to children. All parents mentioned that they were happy to see their children enter an examination hall with a smile on their faces.

For Poorvaja, animal well-being is as much a priority as that of the children's well-being. Hence, she places a strong emphasis on ensuring that both dogs enjoy sessions, and she keeps an eye on noticing and responding to any signs of their anxiety. Both dogs have been tested for therapy work and have been certified. Poorvaja is accompanied by a colleague Mansi, who is also certified in AAT and dog training, to help handle the dogs during sessions so that they receive dedicated attention throughout.

Given the novelty of AAIs in educational and mental health settings and the social, cultural, and economic context of India, not surprisingly Poorvaja and her colleague have received mixed responses. She also points to the taboo associated with mental health. Yet, one survey of Indians on World Mental Health Day reported that it was their pets that brought them 'great joy and light' when experiencing tough times (Mittra, 2019). There are optimistic signs. Poorvaja refers to the rise in the number of dog trainers, the increasing use of non-coercive methods of dog training, better access to mental health care and more schools turning to non-didactic methods of teaching. She sees education and society in a transition phase, which offers some confidence to supporters of AAIs.

The outbreak of the COVID-19 pandemic meant that schools in India were shut for 2 years, and lessons were conducted online. This disrupted Poorvaja's efforts to introduce dogs to a classroom setting. Schools grappled with the issue of completing their syllabi. A few non-government organisations which supported children and adults with mental health issues decided to continue to work with Poorvaja online. She recalled that while it was challenging at first, it proved an important learning opportunity for her organisation. And so even when schools returned to face-to-face teaching, she continued to use regular online sessions and has seen some benefits.

While in virtual sessions, no one gets to be physically close to the dog, Poorvaja has noted an increase in participation from those uncomfortable with being close to a dog. Although there are limited activities that can be done online, this made Poorvaja rethink her pedagogy. She became more creative by turning many of the in-person activities into virtual ones. For example, showing tricks virtually, getting the participants to give commands online, inviting participants to move along with the dogs to music, and using self-relaxation massages with dogs.

There have been cases of individuals who have particularly benefited from interactions with dogs. Poorvaja cites the example of a young person with mental health issues, who would avoid maintaining eye contact or interacting with anyone during the in-person sessions started attending her virtual sessions. She refrained from

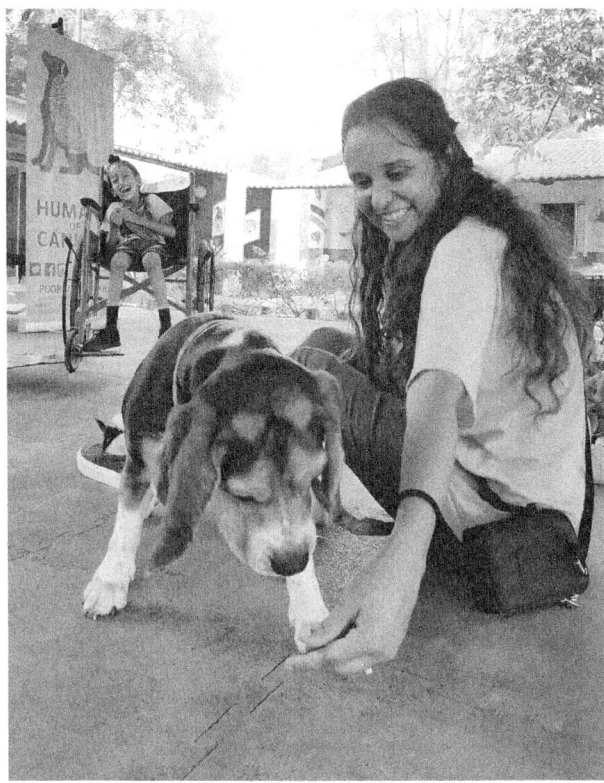

PHOTO 7.6 Poorvaja and Murphy at play.

Reprinted by permission of Poorvaja Kumar.

pushing the participant to respond (as instructed by the psychologist). However, after a long gap during the pandemic, once the virtual sessions started, Poorvaja observed a big change. She noticed him talking openly in the session and expressing how much he missed Murphy. He also drew Murphy on a sheet of paper and showed it to the other participants. The psychologists called it a 'eureka moment' and started using 'art therapy' with him. In another example, a child with Cerebral Palsy who was undergoing physical therapy took Murphy for a short walk on the leash. The child took around ten steps, but the teachers mentioned that it was the first time the child did it with a smile on in face and without having anyone push or motivate him (Photo 7.6).

Despite these uplifting stories and Poorvaja's efforts to adapt following the pandemic, her organisation and others face the major challenge of funding. As practitioners of Animal-Assisted Therapy, their work is still considered to be philanthropic activity and the services termed 'recreational', which inevitably questions the sustainability of their work. Poorvaja and her colleagues do not let such issue detract from their commitment to enhance the bond between dogs and children as they maintain school visits (Photo 7.7).

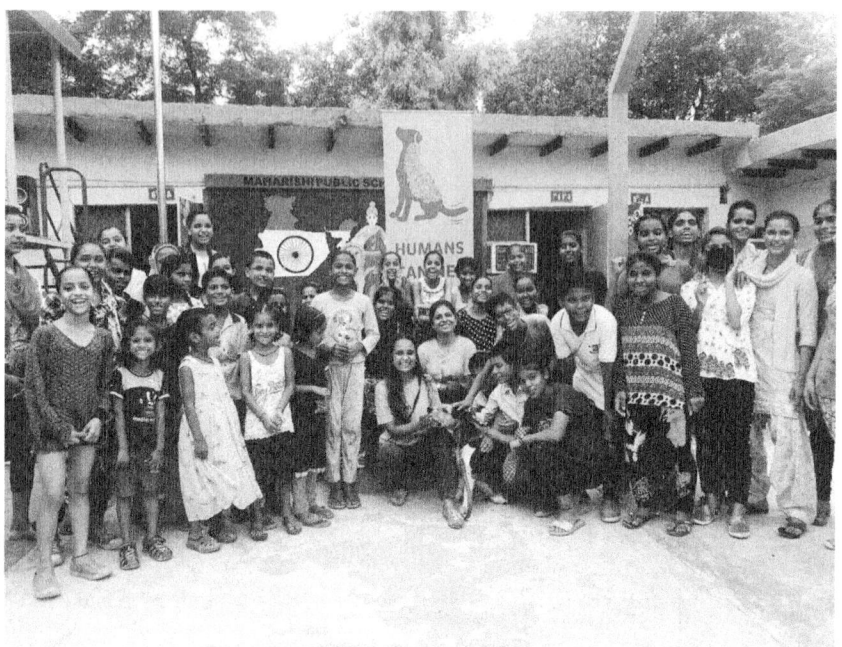

PHOTO 7.7 Poorvaja and her team.

Reprinted by permission of Poorvaja Kumar.

AUSTRALIA

The dogs of Australia and other parts of Oceania originated from southeast Asia around 3,300 years ago (Greig et al., 2018). The earliest inhabitants of the Continent passed on tales of both the companionship and threat associated with the Dingo, the native canine. Photographs from the 1920s show Aboriginal women carrying dingos as living blankets around their waists, while they also served as a source of food, hunting aids and guards against intruders (Philip, 2017). Dingos were particularly valued for their skills in detecting water both above and below ground. Although dingoes have cultural significance to many Aboriginal and Torres Strait Islander peoples, they have long suffered a negative image since European colonisation, heightened by news coverage of dingo attacks on children. In fact, such attacks are rare – one study found 52 reports in more than 120 years of newspaper coverage (Brumm, 2022).

While Australians have mixed views of dingoes and wild canines, their love of domesticated dogs is strong. It is estimated that around 40% of Australian households own at least one dog, making them the country's most popular pet (Animal Medicines Australia, 2020, p. 6). According to the 'Great Australian Dog Survey', conducted on behalf of the pet food company Scratch (2022), two out of three Aussies allow their dogs to sleep in the same room as themselves. During the pandemic, dogs were particularly valued for their companionship, with owners reporting mental health benefits such as reduced loneliness and anxiety (Oliva & Johnston, 2021). Although research does not suggest a causal relationship between dog ownership and mental health, there is general support in and beyond Australia for the view that dogs act as an important catalyst for activities such as striking up conversations and getting out of the house and walking, which provides further opportunities for socialising.

There are various Australian organisations working in the field of AAIs in education. The Delta Institute, based in New South Wales, offers a range of education programmes including Delta Classroom Canines, which is designed for primary and secondary-school students who might benefit from the therapeutic intervention of a Therapy Dog. The focus can vary from specific skills such as literacy development, pro-social skills, or motor skills, to encouraging attendance and increasing motivation.

Roz Rimes (Photo 7.8), founder of 'Live with Zest' and a qualified Canine-Assisted Educator, offers her perspective on the potential of school dogs. Live with Zest is a social enterprise and delivers programmes across primary, secondary, and tertiary educational settings in the State of Victoria. Roz has two Labradoodles, Rafa and Flash, whose main focus is on supporting children and young people's well-being.

Roz approaches her work by always checking in with school leaders (e.g., the school principal, assistant principal, or well-being lead) to ascertain the students' particular needs. Such briefings enable Roz to plan suitable activities. For example, in the case of two primary-school children living with trauma, she provides opportunities for them to talk with her and one of her dogs.

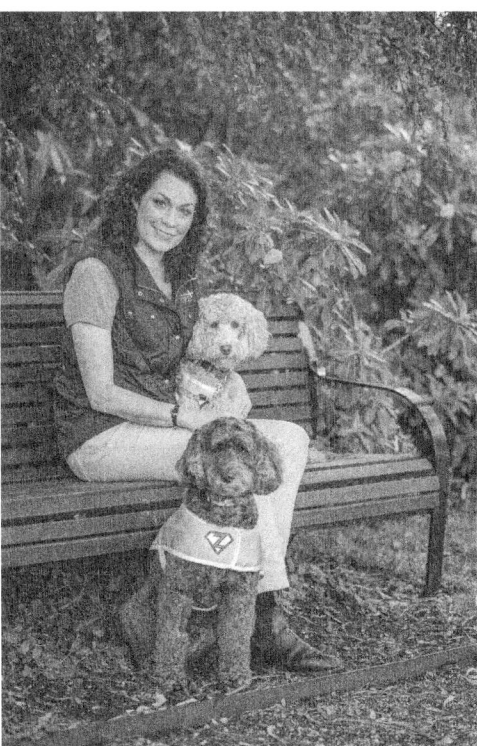

PHOTO 7.8 Roz with Flash and Rafa.

Reprinted by permission of Roz Rimes.

In reflecting upon the impact of her work, Roz believes that dogs have helped reduce children's anxiety levels and supported their capacity to regulate their own emotions. In turn, and based on feedback from teachers, this has contributed to a calmer classroom environment. Teachers feel better prepared to teach and students are more inclined to learn. Roz also thinks that each student has benefited from greater agency, for example in taking responsibility for the dog, through participating in coaching sessions. They enjoy introducing the dog to their friends/classmates and choosing which of Flash's 15 tricks they would like him to perform. The sessions are seen as 'treats' rather than therapy. Roz also relates that one school principal she works with was 'so proud of the therapy/education dog program that he planned school tours to coincide with my visits to the school'. She would see him in the school grounds with small groups of parents and prospective students at a respectful distance.

Throughout her time in school, Roz keeps a close eye on how activities impact her dogs' welfare and well-being. She is aware that some 'kids want to scream or swarm around the dog' and takes steps to prevent this, including teaching the children to read dog facial expressions and body language. While Flash is an experienced 13-year-old therapy dog, his needs are different to the more energetic 5-year-old Rafa who is in his prime. Hence, Flash participates in more physically less demanding tasks such as listening to children read stories. As the founders of Animal Assisted Play Therapy (AAPT) write, 'To the greatest degree possible, AAPT ensures the equal and reciprocal respect of clients and animals. The needs of humans and non-human animals are considered equally important' (Risë van Fleet & Thompson, 2017, p. 50). It is important to allow time and space for spontaneous play and teachable moments.

This chapter highlights some achievements and challenges associated with CAE, particularly with misconceptions such as some people mistakenly thinking that any dog could do this kind of activity. This serves to illustrate the commonly shared, and urgent need for regulations and guidance. Contributors in this chapter also share a deep commitment to protecting the well-being of the individual canine participants in their contexts, and several note specific times where they have actively advocated for their dogs. They share the view that cultivating close relationships between schools, parents and outside bodies who provide therapy dogs are key to building impactful interventions.

PART THREE
Making the Most of Relationships

CHAPTER 8

PLANNING AND PREPARING FOR A SCHOOL DOG

As previous chapters have shown, involving dogs in educational contexts brings many potential benefits. However, this should always be undertaken in an ethical manner, so this chapter explores how to plan and prepare for happy, humane, and healthy interactions. To do this, it is crucial to build strong and trusting relationships between both human and dog, and that dogs are carefully selected for the role. As Clothier (2002, p. 29) states,

> Each relationship with an animal and a human is a bridge uniquely shaped to carry only those two and must be carefully crafted by them.

Establishing this relationship takes effort and time. The humans and the dog must be recognised as individuals so that their needs, wants, and interests can be understood. Whilst educators are used to doing this for their learners, ensuring that the dog is also happy is crucial.

Selecting the right dog to bring into school needs considerable thought. A dog who is a wonderful companion in their home environment may not be appropriate for working in a school because they may not feel comfortable or relaxed in such a context. To develop strong, positive relationships, it is important to go beyond caring for the dog's physical needs and ensure that their emotional health is also considered. As Westgarth (2021, p. 42) points out:

> For a dog to reliably perform whatever task we have trained him to do, when we need him to, we must make sure the dog actually wants to do it. And the only way to make sure of this is if the dog enjoys doing it.

Schools are complex sensory environments. To ensure a dog is happy, and enjoying their work in school means careful preparation, planning and, crucially, identification of a dog who will thrive in a school setting. This chapter explores considerations that need to be made when selecting a dog for such experiences, as well as considering some of the thornier issues that exist, for example around the age a dog should start visiting a school environment. Through the chapter these debates and dilemmas are introduced via social media posts. Whilst these have been generated for this publication, all are based on genuine questions raised by teachers in school dog groups on social media sites.

PART 1: WHAT IS THE 'RIGHT' DOG TO CHOOSE?

Selecting a dog who can thrive in a school setting is the most fundamental aspect of establishing happy, healthy and humane interactions. There are many factors to consider, from appearance to sociability. In one international study of educators the temperament of the animal featured in many of the responses as the most

DOI: 10.4324/9781003257073-12

important element in selecting a suitable animal (Lewis et al., 2022). Indeed, the International Association Human Animal Interaction Organisations (IAHAIO) recommends

> Only those with the proper disposition and training should be selected for AAI. Regular evaluations should be performed to ensure that the animals continue to show proper disposition.
>
> (IAHAIO, 2018: 8)

In this book, we use temperament to mean the dog's 'usual pattern of behaviour and individual traits' (Horowitz, 2009, p. 53). Temperament is a complex interaction of genetics, environmental influences, and experiences during early development that all combine to create the individual. Temperament is demonstrated through observable behaviours. Dog behaviour is complex – it can be learned, reinforced, emotionally driven, affected by health and environment, but it is also influenced by breed. Hardly surprising then that one question frequently asked about school dogs on social media is which breed to choose (Figure 8.1).

So, are some breeds better partners in these activities than others? Whilst all dogs are individuals, knowing their breed and what they were bred to do gives us insight into how they may behave and respond in certain circumstances. As Horowitz (2009, p. 61) suggests, knowing the breed of a dog may give us

> … a first-pass entry into understanding something about the dog …… But it is a mistake to think that knowing a breed guarantees that it will behave as advertised – only that it will have certain tendencies.

Dog breeds developed to serve specific purposes and their temperament and personality can be heavily influenced by generations of selective breeding. Different dog breeds also look very different, and the impact differences such as coat texture, ear shape, or tail morphology may have on perceptions of dogs, and their suitability for school life is explored in this chapter.

Breed Type and Traits

Research (e.g., Arvelius et al., 2014) indicates a strong genetic component to dog personality. Therefore, for those thinking of a pedigree dog, researching breed type is an important part of the selection process. Different breeds were required to possess different characteristics or traits. Breeds are frequently described as having specific temperaments – the 'merry' cocker spaniel, the 'reserved' Chow Chow, or the 'aloof' Afghan hound. Although there are of course individual exceptions to every rule, different breeds have been developed because of hundreds of years of selective breeding. Some breeds have been bred to hunt, others to guard, and others to herd, and this will determine some of the drives and instincts these dogs have. For example, different breeds will have tendencies to behave differently in terms of interactions with other dogs, in sociability to new people and around other species. These breed traits impact on physical, as well as behavioural aspects of the dog's overall character, particularly if a dog comes from strong working lines.

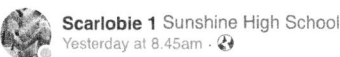

Scarlobie 1 Sunshine High School
Yesterday at 8.45am ·

Hi everyone. Just looking for some advice. I work in a high school and can start planning for a school dog from the fall. I'm wondering how many of you have small dogs who are trained? I'm wondering about small breeds vs large breeds, what are the pros and cons? Is there a breed that is best for this kind of work?

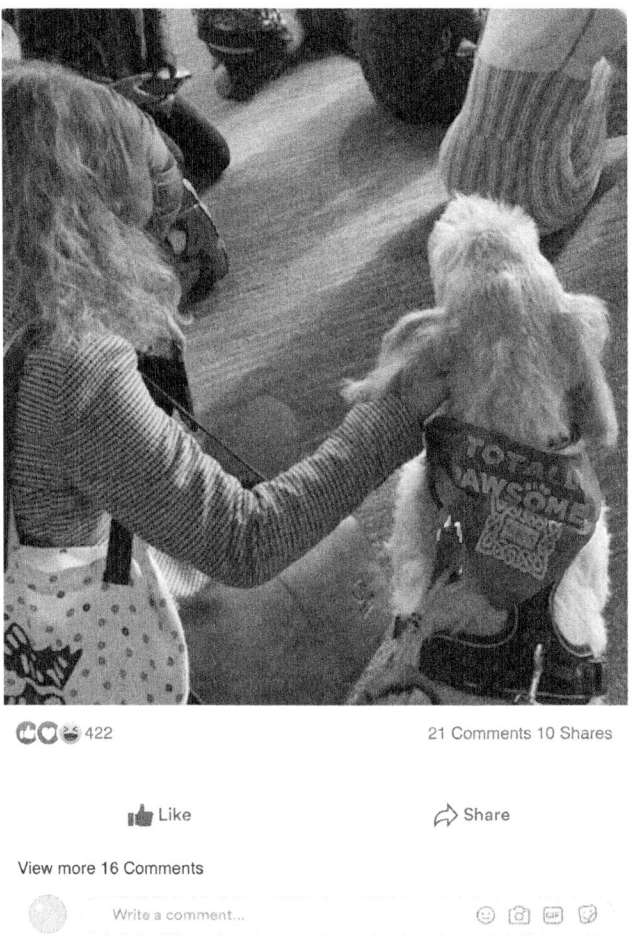

422   21 Comments 10 Shares

👍 Like   ↪ Share

View more 16 Comments

Write a comment...

FIGURE 8.1 Facebook post: breed.

When I (HL) walk my three dogs, I notice differences in how they behave and respond to the environment. This reflects the roles and desirable traits that they were bred for, and their individual personalities. When we enter our local field although all three dogs are excited, they behave in subtly different ways. For Scarlet, who is a poodle mix, the main priority is to enter the field and run, stiff legged and with her tail high, alert to any potential intruders. Once satisfied we are alone, she generally sticks close to me, gently sniffing, digging, or rolling in the grass. She does, however, keep alert to passers-by and is the first to notice anyone who might approach. Carlo, an Italian Spinone, is a gundog breed. He runs into the field, alternately sniffing ground and air, and ranging far and wide in search of birds, rabbits, or his favourite prey – squirrels. He keeps an eye on me from a distance, he will come and check in at various points, but his focus is to cover ground quickly and methodically. Obie is an otterhound, a scent hunting breed. When he enters the field, his nose drops to the ground, his tail raises like a flag, and he moves systematically around the field boundary. For the first few minutes in the field, these scents are his whole focus. He will make several circuits, and only after he has thoroughly checked these out will he join the other dogs in play.

These tendencies and traits different dogs possess can influence their suitability for animal-assisted intervention (AAI) work. For example, dogs such as collies and retrievers often respond actively to events that stimulate the movement of prey. They are more likely to chase and pounce on a ball than dogs from toy breeds who are more likely to watch the ball (Frederickson & Howie, 2000). These different responses may enhance or inhibit an AAI interaction, depending on the intentions of the activities. For instance, some children may feel rejected if a dog does not want to chase and fetch the ball for them, whilst others may feel anxious about a dog who is making quick chasing movements, and others may not wish to handle a sticky, wet ball that has been in a dog's mouth.

Although International Kennel Clubs may name and group breeds (and indeed recognise different breeds) in slightly different ways, as shown in Table 8.1, all breeds have been developed for specific purposes, which are worth bearing in mind if a pedigree dog is being considered for school-based activity.

Genetically, breeds have been selectively bred to possess certain drives, instincts, and interests, often called collectively breed traits. The traits with the highest amongst-breed heritability have been identified as trainability, stranger-directed aggression, chasing, and attachment and attention-seeking. This is seen to be evidence which is consistent with the hypothesis that these behaviours have been important targets of selection during the formation of modern breeds (MacLean et al., 2019).

Depending on how strong these traits are in any individual dog is important to consider when searching for a suitable school dog. For example, a cocker spaniel from a strong genetic line of working dogs may be very different in terms of appearance, coat type, energy, drive, and focus to a cocker spaniel from a strong genetic line of show or pet dogs.

Understanding what can be modified with training compared to which behaviours are hard-wired through genetics or the individual dog's experience is important. Some behaviours can be shaped and amended with practice and careful training, but a dog's temperament influences these behaviours as well. For instance, a very shy dog may become more at ease with familiar people over time but may never be totally comfortable interacting with new people. Training may mean that they comply and tolerate such interactions, but they may not feel truly comfortable, happy, or relaxed. From the perspective of promoting happy, healthy, and humane interactions, such a dog may not be best placed to participate in certain situations, such as in a school where they are expected to interact with a range of unfamiliar people. Training is explored in more detail in Chapter 9.

TABLE 8.1 Dog breeds and their original purpose

UK group	US group	Australian group	Purpose	Breed examples
Terrier	Terrier	Terrier	Bred for pest control, hunting vermin above and below ground, including rats and foxes. Tough and brave, often with strong personalities.	Border Terrier Jack Russell Terrier Dandie Dinmont Terrier West Highland White Terrier
Toy	Toy	Toy	Although some were originally bred for other jobs, now primarily companions, so generally small dogs who are usually sociable and friendly.	Bichon Frise Chihuahua Pomeranian Shih Tzu
Hound	Hound	Hound	Bred to hunt other animals by sight or scent. Sight hounds are fast, light framed dogs whilst scent hounds have great stamina, and heavier frames. Independent and intelligent.	Beagle Greyhound Otterhound Saluki
Utility	Non-Sporting	Non-sporting	Bred for a specific purpose (that doesn't fall into pastoral or working groups), so hard to pinpoint key traits as each breed is so different.	Chow Chow Dalmatian Keeshond Poodle
Working	Working	Utility	Developed to work alongside us, to do specific jobs such as pulling sledges, guarding or water rescue. Tend to be larger, active dogs who need a job to do.	Boxer Rottweiler Newfoundland Siberian Husky
Gundogs	Sporting	Gundog	Bred to flush, point, or retrieve game alongside their human companions. Often sociable and sensitive, these breeds thrive with regular, invigorating exercise.	Italian Spinone, Irish Setter Labrador retriever Pointer
Pastoral	Herding	Working	Herding and working with livestock. Resilient, high intensity dogs who enjoy being out in all weathers and who need a job to do.	Bearded Collie Border Collie Briard Cardigan Corgi

Selecting a dog for school needs to be a carefully considered process. As individuals, we may have preferred breeds of dog or have a fondness for 'gundog types' for example, but even within the breed groups themselves there are great differences. So, for instance in the Hound group, scent hounds like bloodhounds, and sighthounds like greyhounds were bred to hunt in very different ways. Although this has impacted their appearance, and instincts (nose to the ground, or scanning the environment) and even potentially their brain structure (Frederick, 2019), both are likely to have quite a high prey drive and may be difficult to distract once they are on the trail or have sight of quarry. So, when thinking of selecting a specific dog for working in a school, it is important to consider what role the dog will be expected to fulfil. For instance, if the school has an outdoor classroom where the dog will spend a lot of time, very small, fluffy-coated toy breeds, or a highly driven scent hound may be less suitable than a gundog breed who has been bred to work in the outdoors alongside 'their person'. And of course, within each breed, within every litter, every dog is an individual, shaped by their life experiences and personality as well as their genetics. School leaders must consider the 'job description' of their school dog, as this will help shape the selection process. This idea is explored in more detail in Chapter 9.

PHYSICAL FACTORS

Thinking about where a dog will be working, who they will be working with, and the environmental conditions are important things to consider before selecting any dog. These are practical considerations, as different breeds will have different physical characteristics. Breeding clearly impacts a dog's appearance, which raises the question of whether a dog with floppy ears, big eyes, and fluffy tails may be seen as cute – and therefore make a better school dog than those which appear more wolf-like. From a perceptual point of view, this is possible. There is some evidence that people have clear biases towards certain dogs based on how they look. In a study of how people perceived dogs with floppy ears versus those with pointy ears, floppy eared dogs were perceived to be less extraverted, more agreeable, and less neurotic. In a similar study about perceptions of dogs of different colour, dogs with yellow coats were seen as more conscientious, more agreeable, and less neurotic than their black coated peers (Fratkin & Baker, 2013).

Though this research may have little bearing on a dog's ability to work effectively in a school context, it makes a clear point that people do judge a dog simply based on the way that they look, and so some school dogs may be selected based on personal preference for appearance, rather than how suitable they are for the role. Considering the individual dog's ability to undertake the tasks they are going to be asked to do, and their connection to the children they will be working with, rather than whether they conform to perceptions of 'cuteness' is crucial – and after all, beauty is in the eye of the beholder.

COAT TYPE

Considering the coat type of the dog is important. From a practical perspective, the coat will impact on frequency of grooming, amount of moulting, and specialist care. Dogs come with short, medium, or long coat lengths and a variety of texture types,

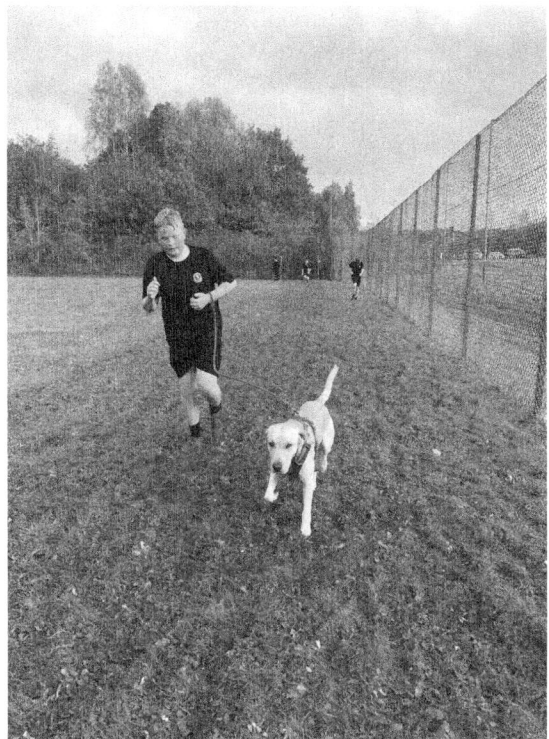

PHOTO 8.1 Cross country lesson for Rhys and Aled the dog.
Reprinted by permission of Darren Berry.

from hairless to corded. Coats were developed to serve a purpose, for example, the double-layered coat of a Siberian husky is ideal to keep them warm, even in temperatures as low as −60°C. A Labrador retriever's original job of retrieving game from water has led to these dogs being bred with very active oil glands, a factor that helps to waterproof their fur and skin.

In terms of practicalities, it is important to consider the activities the dog will undertake and children that the dog will work with. For instance, some coat types will be better suited to outdoor work. Working with teenagers in a secondary (high) school, Lewis School Pengam, in Wales, Aled (Photo 8.1) the Labrador's oily, medium length coat keeps him warm when he is outdoors and dries quickly upon return to inside the school. This is ideal for coping with the climate of the Welsh countryside – and the muddy, wet conditions he sometimes finds himself in when supporting children running the cross-country course or taking part in orienteering lessons in the woods. For example, in Photo 8.1, Aled is running with pupil Rhys Lamb (on a damp Welsh day). As a large, active dog, the physical exercise will be beneficial for his well-being, and combined with his coat type he is well-suited to these activities.

Table 8.2 highlights some of the benefits and challenges of different coat types, and facts about the breeds who have them.

TABLE 8.2 Coat types

Coat type	Benefits	Challenges	Interesting facts about breeds with these coats	Breeds include
Hairless	• May help those with allergies to fur (although not to saliva or dander). • Have been known as 'canine hot water bottles'	• Requires protection, e.g., sunscreen to prevent sunburn and jackets for warmth. • Regular baths are needed to keep the skin healthy.	• The indigenous Mexican Xoloitzcuintli was said to have been created from a sliver of the 'Bone of Life' from which all humanity sprang.	• Chinese Crested • Peruvian Inca Orchid • Xoloitzcuintli
Smooth/ medium short haired	• Less grooming is required. • Coats are easier to keep clean and hygienic. • Pests cannot hide on them very well.	• Some short-coated dogs are prone to develop contact allergies. Walking through bushes and tall grass may cause irritation.	• Greyhounds are the only breed of dog specifically mentioned in the Bible.	• Doberman Pinschers, • German Shorthaired Pointers, • Greyhounds
Long	• Long, thick coat protects the dogs, e.g., from wet or cold climates. Some long-coated breeds shed less than smooth or medium coated dogs. • The long fur can may be coarse, silky, or soft.	• Requires extra grooming to prevent knots. • May pick up debris easily.	• Legend has it that the Afghan hound was the dog rescued by Noah. More likely, the dogs came over into Afghanistan with Alexander the Great's army, rock carvings showing the distinct-looking dogs in caves in Afghanistan to support this theory	• Irish setter • Afghan hound • Yorkshire terrier

(*Continued*)

TABLE 8.2 (Continued)

Coat type	Benefits	Challenges	Interesting facts about breeds with these coats	Breeds include
Curly/ fleecy	• Tight curls serve as good insulation for water activities and protection from brambles and grasses.	• Although these breeds may shed less, regular grooming is needed to prevent mats forming. This may need to be breed specific – for example, the curly coated retriever should be combed not coat brushed to avoid frizzy hair.	• As a boy, the actor John Wayne owned an Airedale named Duke, and he would frequently take Duke to visit the local fire station. The firemen would say 'Here come Big Duke and Little Duke'. John Wayne was Little Duke, and the nickname stuck with him for the rest of his life.	• Poodle • Airedale terrier • Bichon Frise
Wiry	• Wiry coats protect the dog from elements, environment, and prey. Many wire-haired breeds are 'stripped' when groomed which removes old hair but maintains texture of new hair. Clipping eventually would soften the hair.	• Many wiry haired breeds also have beards. These can harbour a wealth of dirt.	• Wire-haired fox terriers have been favoured by many famous owners over the centuries. Edward VII owned a fox terrier called Caesar, whilst biologist Charles Darwin owned Polly the fox terrier in the 19th century, and Vicki the fox terrier lived with writer and poet Rudyard Kipling.	• German wire-haired pointer • Wire haired Hungarian Vizsla • Wire haired fox terrier

(*Continued*)

TABLE 8.2 (Continued)

Coat type	Benefits	Challenges	Interesting facts about breeds with these coats	Breeds include
Double	The double coat is made up of a topcoat or 'guard' hairs and a softer undercoat. As well as being insulating, the double coat can keep them cool by protecting their skin from the sun.	Most double coated breeds 'blow' their undercoats twice a year, which means they shed their entire undercoat in response to seasonal changes.	The Chow Chow is one of the world's most ancient breeds and is famous for being the only breed to have blue-black tongue and lips.	Bernese Mountain Dog Chow Chow German Shepherd
Corded	• Long, rope-like strands. Outer coat grows coarse as the dog ages, trapping the softer undercoat to form cords. These protect from predators and provide warmth and coverage from the harsh elements. • Puppies aren't born with cords, typically it takes up to 2 years for these to develop.	• Needs considerable grooming to keep its cords clean, neat, and attractive • Cords need special washing and drying to ensure they do not get bacterial or fungal growth like mould or mildew.	• Although many people claim to not have heard of breeds like the Komondor, the cover for Beck's 1996 music album, Odelay, features a Komondor mid-air. In the years since its release, the image has become one of the most recognisable covers of all time.	• Komondor • Puli • Bergamasco

(Continued)

TABLE 8.2 (Continued)

Coat type	Benefits	Challenges	Interesting facts about breeds with these coats	Breeds include
Oily	• The oils in the coat help repel water, provide insulation, and also allow the coat to dry off faster.	• Oily coats may have an odour, and so it can be tempting to wash these dogs more frequently. • Normal shampoos may strip the natural oils. • Stripping the coat's oils can also remove some of the waterproofing and protection, making them less able to cope with the conditions.	• Basset Hound Victoria became mayor of Concord, Ontario in 2011 sharing the responsibility with a Great Dane named Nelson. She appeared at parades, travelled to nearby towns, and helped raise money for animals in rescue shelters.	• Labrador Retriever • Newfoundland • Basset hound

HYPOALLERGENIC COATS – FACT OR FICTION?

Within Table 8.2, no reference has been made to so-called 'hypoallergenic' coats and breeds. As Figure 8.2 shows, this is a popular topic of conversation on social media school dog sites.

In fact, whilst there are some breeds which will shed less hair, research suggests that many allergies are not to the fur of the dog, but to the saliva, skin cells (dander), and even urine cells, which all dogs, regardless of coat type will shed. Educators need to beware of making assumptions about allergies. Indeed, Doodle Trust (2022), a UK-based rehoming charity, states that the belief that these dogs are allergy friendly and suitable for people with allergies is a myth. Burnett et al. (2022) report that a common misconception of prospective dog owners is the belief that some 'designer crossbreeds', such as the Labradoodle, cockerpoo or cavapoo, are hypoallergenic and therefore have a reduced risk of eliciting an allergic reaction in humans. Another study of over 800 educators with school dogs, found 28% of these dogs were identified as poodle crosses and many have been selected specifically because they were deemed 'hypoallergenic' (Lewis, 2022). There is no extant research for differential shedding of hair and the dog allergen CanF1 between designer and non-designer dogs (Nicholas et al., 2011). Furthermore, as well as possible variety amongst coat

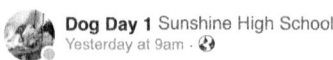
Dog Day 1 Sunshine High School
Yesterday at 9am · 🌐

Advice please - how do you manage allergies in your school? My golden
retriever has been at our school for a few years, but we have a new
colleague who is allergic. She has no reason ever to interact with the dog
and she has raised a concern. However, she literally screamed and ran
away from us in the hallway today, and we were a good ten feet from her,
and walking the other way. I'd like to find a solution and while I definitely
want her to feel heard and safe at work, I'd love some science to
reassure her that the risk to her is very low.

 121   8 Comments 3 Shares

                     Sad   Share

View more 16 Comments

   Shell ✅ I did some research on this. The two most prevalent
       proteins that cause an allergic reactions are found in saliva.
       Addressing allergies as part of your risk management plan is
       essential. Dog allergies are real, and can be mitigated with
       best practices: bathing/condition the dog, oral hygiene, don't
       allow students with allergies to touch the dog or put hands in
       mouth, use a HEPA air filter, and take responsibility for
       cleaning the learning space yourself. I have a sink in the
       learning space for students to wash their hands. There are
       no fabric chairs or rugs. All of these measures decrease the
       incidence of students with allergies having a problem. I have
       students in my classroom with dogs allergies every year
       without event.
                                                                    😮 1
       Like · Reply · 1h

   Carl ✅ Find out if the student is allergic to fur and pet
       dander or saliva. Surprisingly most dog allergies are to
       saliva so it's much easier to manage. I sat down with parents
       and asked them what they would like or need me to do to
       keep their child safe. Many parents just wanted their child to
       wash their hands after petting the dog. I've had a parent say
       their child just can't pet the dog or be licked by the dog but is
       ok to be near the dog.
                                                                    😮 1
       Like · Reply · 1h

          Jay ✅ Oh - so what is the breed of dog(s) at your
              school district? There was a time all you heard was
              hypoallergenic. If your school allows dogs that are
              NOT, how do they handle allergies?
                                                                    😮 1
              Like · Reply · 1h

   (Write a comment...)

FIGURE 8.2 Social media message: allergies.

type of puppies in a litter, as a dog ages, their coat can change, and so even if there is little reaction to the dog when she is a puppy, as she grows up this may alter (Smalley, 2009).

Therefore, countering the widespread misconception with educational messaging is of high importance, because selecting a dog as suitable because they will be less likely to cause an allergic reaction cannot be guaranteed. Yet, there are things that can be done to minimise the risk of allergic reactions in school. For example, breeds that are usually clipped should be kept in a short coat to prevent carrying allergens in on their fur. Schools can use HEPA filters to purify the air in rooms where dogs work. Brushing and washing the dog before coming to school is important. In the summer months, it is advisable to bathe the dog frequently to remove pollen and other allergens from the coat and there are wipes designed specifically to remove allergens from the coat between bathing. But frequent bathing may be unpleasant for the dog and may damage their coat by stripping essential oils, so another key consideration is what is also best for the individual animal's health and well-being.

CHILDREN'S INDIVIDUAL NEEDS

Some children, particularly those with sensory needs, may find physical interaction with dogs challenging. Physical differences between dog breeds may be something to consider if a dog will be working with children with such needs. For instance, research suggests that up to 96% of autistic children show hyper- or hyposensitivities in several senses (Watson, 2022). 'Senses' are broad, and include sight, hearing, smell, taste, touch, balance (vestibular), proprioception (body awareness), and interoception (perception of senses inside the body). So, a child with hypersensitivity might be very sensitive to texture, or dislike being dirty, and so a dog who has a wiry, coarse, or oily coat may be unpleasant for them to touch. The natural oils in some dog coats may be too overwhelming in terms of smell for some hypersensitive children.

There are other challenges relating to sensory processing. Many breeds of dogs such as schnauzers, shih tzus, and spinones have beards. These were developed to help protect dogs' faces, for example, from getting scratched by the claws of their prey. Whilst these beards can give a dog tremendous character and are endearing to look, the truth is that beards can harbour dirt, mud, bits of food and general muck. This can be off-putting to children and adults alike. Likewise, in hairless or short-haired dogs, genitals can be clearly visible, and this can be a concern for some children who may not want to interact with these dogs.

EARS AND TAILS[1]

Different breeds come with a variety of ear shapes, originally selected and designed to help them do their jobs effectively (Figure 8.3).

Are dogs with some ear shapes better suited to life in school than others? Whilst this may seem like a strange question, research suggests that animals that were domesticated by humans tend to have certain characteristics in common: curvier tails and more juvenile facial features than their wild ancestors, including floppier ears (Dugatkin in Mervosh, 2019). And there is some evidence to suggest that those

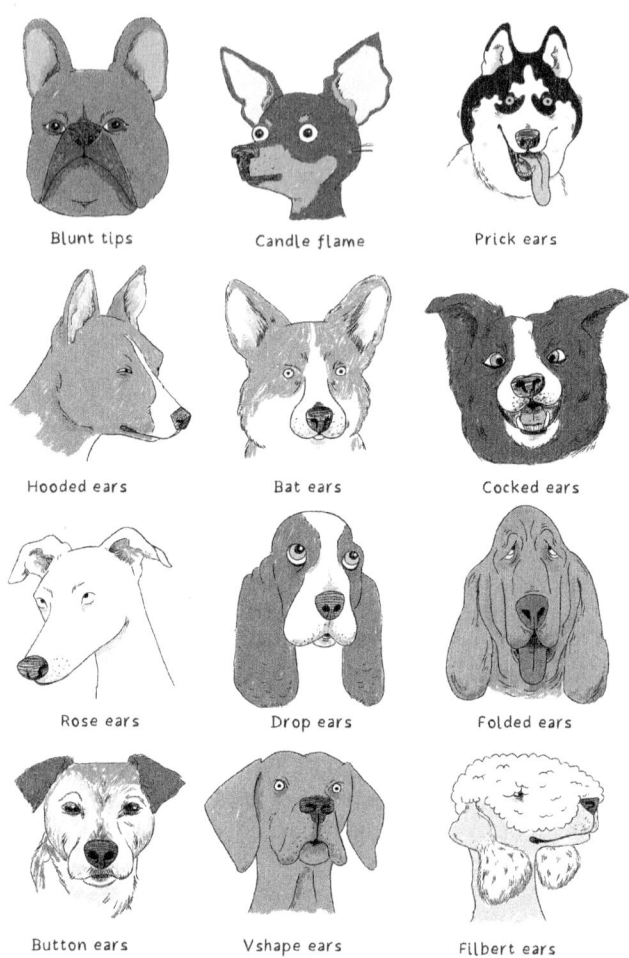

FIGURE 8.3 Different ear shapes.

Reprinted by permission of Tom Bradraw.

breeds with floppier ears appear to be less threatening than more erect ear shapes. For example, Mervosh (2019) reports that in America, the Transportation Security Administration (TSA) agency favours floppy-eared dogs over pointy-eared dogs, especially in the jobs that require interacting with traveling passengers, because floppy-eared dogs appear friendlier and less aggressive.

There may be a scientific reason for this. In the late 1950s, Russian scientist Dmitri K. Belyaev began an experiment, to replicate the process of domestication in real time, selecting silver foxes for breeding based on one characteristic: their calmness and friendliness towards humans. Within about five generations, the foxes began to act more domesticated, wagging their tails and licking people's hands. After about ten generations, they started to develop floppy ears, possibly because these animals have fewer neural crest cells, which are cells that can form cartilage. This effects ears as without so much cartilage, they cannot stand up as straight.

However, from a practical point of view, floppy or droopy ears can be an issue for a school dog. Although these ears are often velvety soft and easy to stroke, they can also be easy to pull. Dirt, water, and bacteria can easily become trapped under a floppy or creased ears meaning these breeds can be more susceptible to painful ear infections, requiring medical treatment. Long ears can get very wet when the dog drinks from their water bowl, which can be unpleasant for children. Furthermore, as we explore in more detail in Chapter 9, understanding and interpreting a dog's body language is an essential part of establishing and maintaining trusting, happy, and humane relationships. A dog's ears are used to communicate subtly, and the impact of size and shape of their ears will dictate how they can use them. This means that we need to observe our individual dogs very carefully to pick up on the signals they are providing.

The same is true of tails, the movement (speed, direction, and position) conveys different emotions from excitement, to fear and aggression. Once again, selective breeding has resulted in several tail shapes (Figure 8.4), from tufted, sickle, and otter to some cases, like some Australian Shepherds, having a tiny bob tail (no tail at all). These differences may cause challenges in interpretation, for both people and other dogs. Furthermore, a thin, whip-like tail can hurt when wagged enthusiastically against your shins, and children with particularly sensitive skin, or conditions where they bruise easily may find this painful. From a health perspective, dogs with corkscrew tails may have severe itching and discomfort around the tail, leading them to chew at their tail and drag their rears on the ground.

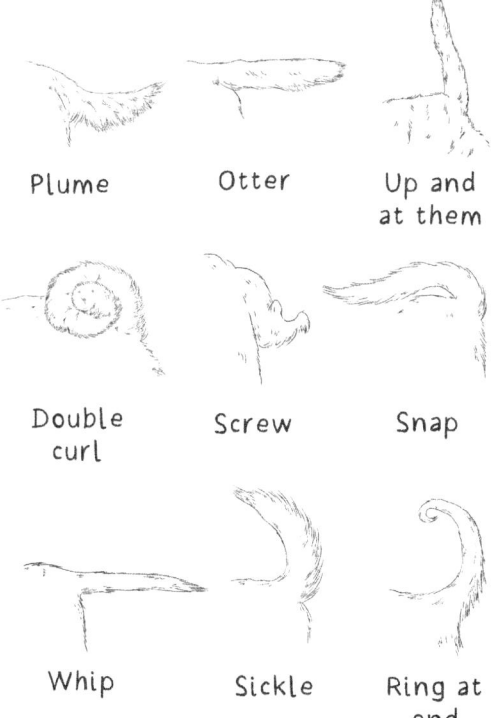

FIGURE 8.4 Different tail types.

Reprinted by permission of Tom Bradraw.

DROOL AND DRIBBLE

Dogs drool (or salivate) for a variety of reasons, such as when they are happy, excited, nervous, or feeling sick. They tend to drool even more if they are anticipating food because like humans, they have glands in their mouths which produce saliva. This is important as the enzymes in saliva begin breaking down food as the first step in the digestive process. Whilst all dogs produce saliva, some breeds, typically those with deep jowls, loose lips or a pronounced top lip that overhangs their mouth produce more than others. These include boxers, Newfoundlands, bulldogs, Great Danes, mastiff breeds, and otterhounds. Again, within each breed, there are individual differences from one dog to another. A dog who produces excessive saliva can be challenging to manage in a school setting. One shake of the head can result in thick, gelatinous drool finding its way onto ceilings, children, and teachers. Some people may not be fazed, and indeed many children may find this funny, but for others this would be off-putting, and a challenge from a hygiene perspective. As a very minimum requirement, the handler would need to have towels, bibs, and wipes to hand to manage this appropriately.

ENERGY LEVEL AND INTENSITY

Different dogs have different energy levels. Some need a lot of exercise and mental stimulation; others appear happy with a gentle stroll and a snooze on the sofa. Some of these may relate to breed and age, and some to a dog's individual personality. Energy levels can have implications for suitability for work in school. A dog with high energy levels may be less suitable for spending time in a classroom context. If their needs are not met, and their energy does not have suitable outlets then the dog may become frustrated and will search for an outlet for their excess energy – be it productive or destructive. Intense, high-drive, high-prey, working-line dogs may not be easy to manage in a school context. They demand attention and need to stay busy. These dogs will probably not be happy in a classroom or office for any length of time, and they may not feel happy in a confined context.

However, it is important to consider the type of interactions you are planning. For instance, if the child is mainly going to be sitting calmly and stroking the dog, the intervention requires a dog that is comfortable doing this, and probably a lower energy dog would be more suitable. On the other hand, if the intention is for dog and child to be actively interacting, such as walking outdoors, or engaging in playful activities the dog may need more energy and endurance. These are all factors to consider when looking at the energy level of any potential canine partner (Hamilton, 2022).

PUPPIES AND YOUNG DOGS

There is no doubt that puppies are delightful, and their joie de vivre, curiosity, and innocence are appealing. However, they are also demanding, destructive, and can add stress, cost, and concern into our already busy lives (Lewis, 2023). Considering the age that a dog is most suitable to start working in schools is an issue of considerable debate. Most organisations who train dogs for educational activities recommend waiting until a dog is at least 18 months old before starting to train them for specific work in school. At this age, many breeds are reaching maturity. Prior to this as puppies, there are many specific and natural behaviours such as chewing and mouthing that may be undesirable or dangerous around children and classroom resources. Puppies' lives have (and need) a rhythm and a routine to them, typically revolving around patterns of eating, toileting, playing, and sleeping. These routines may not fit conveniently into the rhythm of a school day. For instance, puppies need to spend long periods of time sleeping, and adequate high-quality rest can be difficult to provide in a busy school environment. A typical 12-week-old puppy needs between 16 and 20 hours of sleep, punctuated by brief periods of playing, socialising, and learning. Without this sleep, a puppy can become over-excited and over-tired, and, just like an over-tired toddler their behaviour may then become more challenging. Whilst the amount of sleep needed will decrease as the dog grows up, many adult dogs still need 12–15 hours of sleep a day, although this will of course vary from individual to individual.

Unpredictable or very frequent toileting habits can be an additional challenge to deal with in a busy classroom environment. House-training takes time and focus, and in a classroom, it may not always be possible to observe the puppy full-time, or to immediately take the puppy outdoors.

As adolescents, associated hormonal changes means that some dogs, just like some teenagers, test boundaries. These surges in hormone levels can lead to more energy and playfulness, and puppies usually become bolder and more adventurous. This can impact training, exercise, and their ability to focus. Breed impacts how quickly a dog will mature – typically smaller breeds mature more quickly. Giant breeds such as St. Bernards may not reach maturity until they are 2 to 3 years old.

Despite the challenges of meeting the needs of puppies effectively in a school environment, many teachers make the decision to bring their dogs in from an early age. Indeed, one international survey found great variation in how teachers viewed the ideal age to introduce a school dog. For example, one teacher stated: 'I've just bought a puppy and can't wait to take him to school!', whilst another was clear that puppies should not feature in any intervention as 'they need their sleep!' Some expressed 'grave concerns over the use of puppies in schools, commenting 'Puppies should enjoy puppyhood', yet other respondents perceived value in bringing in a puppy so that they became familiar with the school environment from a young age (Lewis et al., 2022, p. 10). These differences in opinion are frequently echoed by posts on social media such as Figures 8.5.

When asked, many teachers feel that they need to bring their dogs in from a young age to socialise and familiarise them with the routines of the school. It is true that dogs' early experiences (just like in humans) can affect their behaviour later in life. Hence puppy owners are encouraged to provide opportunities for their young charges to meet new people, new animals, and new environments. The term 'socialisation' refers to 'Creating as many varied, positive, safe and enjoyable experiences for your puppy as you can, as soon as possible in their life to build "social" immunity' (Mann, 2019, p. 111). Positive early experiences during 'sensitive' periods of development are crucial to create well-adjusted adult dogs able to cope in their environment. There are currently six sensitive periods of early canine development that have been identified (Serpell et al., 2016), as noted in Figure 8.6. At different stages in this development, the nature and range of experiences a dog needs vary.

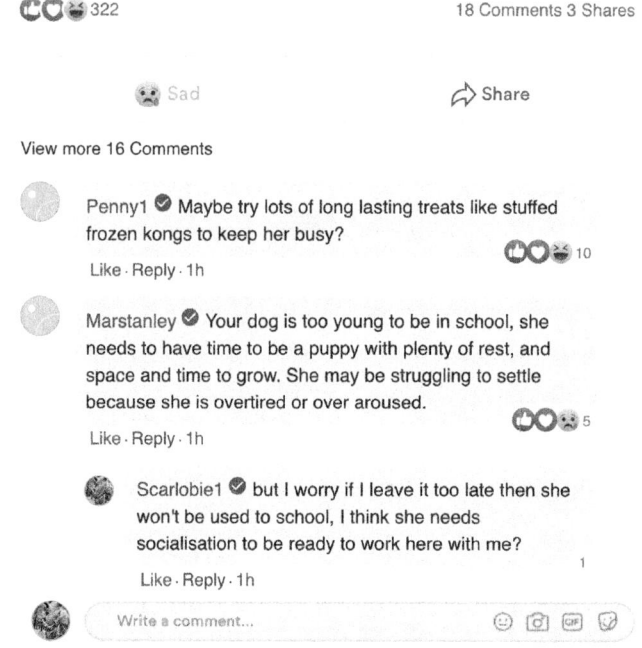

Scarlobie 1 Sunshine High School
Yesterday at 4:45am · 🌐

Any suggestions of activities I can do around the school with my 4 month puppy? She is in therapy dog training but with minimal contact with the children at the moment.
She's fine in the mornings and is settled in her crate for most of the time, with a break in the middle of morning. I take her home for lunch where she has a good run around in garden and a change of scenery. But she doesn't really settle for the rest of afternoon and seems bored. She is in school this young to get used to the environment and she is doing so so well. I just need to occupy her in the afternoon a bit.

❤️👍😢 322   18 Comments 3 Shares

           😢 Sad   ↪ Share

View more 16 Comments

        Penny1 ✅ Maybe try lots of long lasting treats like stuffed
        frozen kongs to keep her busy?
                                                  ❤️👍😆 10
        Like · Reply · 1h

        Marstanley ✅ Your dog is too young to be in school, she
        needs to have time to be a puppy with plenty of rest, and
        space and time to grow. She may be struggling to settle
        because she is overtired or over aroused.
                                                  ❤️👍😢 5
        Like · Reply · 1h

              Scarlobie1 ✅ but I worry if I leave it too late then she
              won't be used to school, I think she needs
              socialisation to be ready to work here with me?
                                                          1
              Like · Reply · 1h

        Write a comment...   ☺ 📷 GIF 🎴

FIGURE 8.5 Social media message: puppies.

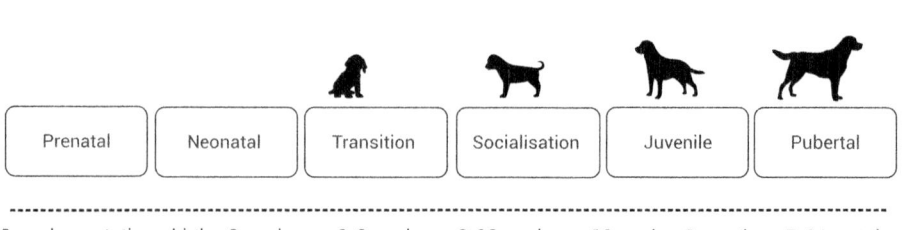

| Prenatal | Neonatal | Transition | Socialisation | Juvenile | Pubertal |

9 weeks gestation   birth - 2 weeks   2-3 weeks   3-12 weeks   12 weeks- 6 months   7-24 months

FIGURE 8.6 Sensitive periods of early canine development.

Rottier (2023) aligns the stages of development in a young puppy's life to key principles we should consider when raising them to be happy and healthy, and ready to thrive in their lives as they grow older. These echo our own principles for effective pedagogy. They are respect, safety, enjoyment, acceptance, training, and relationships, and together they provide positive foundations for the puppy. From birth, Rottier suggests that puppies should have experiences that are based upon these principles and would include opportunities for her litters of Shetland Sheepdogs to walk on different textures such as towels, mats, and rugs; hear different sounds; play with different toys; meet different people; and so on. All these experiences should be carefully managed, planned, and taken at a pace that the puppy feels comfortable. As the puppy grows, and becomes increasingly mobile and is vaccinated, these experiences can extend beyond the immediate home. Mann (2019) provides an extensive list of stimuli a puppy could have carefully managed exposure to, including a variety of people, vehicles, animals, smells, textures, weather, and heights.

Knowing if the puppy has had such experiences is relevant to those selecting a new puppy for life as a school dog. Has the puppy been raised in an environment that has fostered these early experiences? Certainly, the recent COVID-19 pandemic has been reported to raise concerns over dog behaviours because of reduced levels of puppy socialisation. For example, Brand et al. (2022) found that 'Pandemic Puppies' were less likely to have attended puppy training classes or received exposure to people from outside the home before 16 weeks of age, and concerns were raised about their subsequent adult behaviours because of this.

However, there are debates around the process of socialisation and the impact early experiences can have on a puppy's development. Just like any type of learning, socialisation is an ongoing process rather than a series of events to 'tick off' on a sheet. Wormald et al. (2016) found no protective advantage of earlier or more frequent public exposure on the development of aggression as adult dogs. They reported that every week an owner waited to expose their puppy to public areas, the more reduced the odds were that the puppy would show aggressive behaviour towards unfamiliar dogs when older. This study demonstrates that what happens during socialisation experiences needs to be understood by owners and handlers. Indeed, Wormald et al. suggest simple introductions, such as exposures to unfamiliar dogs in a public park, may have more effects on future behaviour and a dog's ability to cope with stress, when compared to more controlled, structured introductions during events like puppy classes. Similarly, Blackwell et al. (2013) suggest that early exposure to frightening noises was associated with fear of those noises as adults. These studies suggest that negative experiences with noises or other dogs may contribute to adverse reactions to these stimuli in later life, highlighting the need for positive interactions with potentially aversive stimuli in early life. Otherwise, there is a danger that puppies will be flooded with overwhelming sensory experiences. However, this research only identifies correlations and not causations, again highlighting the need for more robust, longitudinal studies.

What is important is that we recognise the puppy's agency in the process of socialisation. If we show respect and understanding, we should allow the puppy as much choice as possible. They need to be able to approach new situations or stimuli in their own time, with their owner there to make the experience as positive as possible. This may be challenging in the school environment, where there can be pressing demands on teacher's time and unpredictability in terms of events. Chapter 9 considers this in more detail, giving practical advice about managing socialisation.

PUBLIC PERCEPTIONS AND 'DANGEROUS DOGS'

The most successful interventions will have support from all stakeholders, including members of the public and local community. But people's perceptions are shaped by many factors, such as dogs in movies and literature, perceptions of service animals and personal experiences. Being mindful of any preconceptions, individuals may have of dog breeds to ensure that any undue anxiety or stress is avoided is important. Preconceptions about a breed may arise from an individual's personal experience. However, research suggests that there are some general commonly held perceptions. For instance, the coat colour of a dog can have an impact of perceptions of them. Black, brown, and brindle dogs are more likely to be abandoned, and fawn, black and tan, grey, and red dogs, if lost, have a better chance of being reclaimed. Furthermore, stray black dogs typically spend longer in shelters than dogs with other coloured coats (Voslarova et al., 2019).

The media plays a role in shaping public opinion in relation to specific breeds, yet media reports are often inaccurate and subjective. Any dog, whatever the breed, may react instinctively under certain circumstances, and there are many individual differences between dogs of the same breed. Nonetheless, certain breeds are perceived as more likely to be aggressive, with ongoing debate around banning the American XL Bully in the UK. Current legislation in the United Kingdom bans the breeding, sale, purchase, exchange, and promotion of the following dogs:

1 American Pitbull Terrier
2 Dogo Argentino
3 Fila Brasileiro (Brazilian Mastiff)
4 Tosa Inu

These breeds must be muzzled and kept on a leash in public places, be registered, have insurance, be neutered, and have a microchip. Legislation varies in other countries. For example, in New Zealand, 'He kurī whakamataku mōrearea' (menacing and dangerous dogs) can be classified by either breed or behaviour. These dogs must be muzzled in public except when in a vehicle or cage, neutered and microchipped. Five breeds are automatically classified as menacing, no matter how they behave individually:

1 American Pit Bull Terrier
2 Brazilian Fila
3 Japanese Tosa
4 Dogo Argentino
5 Perro de Presa Canario.

Public perceptions of dog breeds are heavily influenced by the media. Podberscek (1994), reviewed UK newspaper articles both before and after the implementation of the UK Dangerous Dogs Act of 1991 and suggested that the media could negatively influence the public perception of specific dog breeds without adequate, accurate information. One American study by Kogan et al. (2022) found that participants rated Pit Bulls as the breed rated most likely to bite, followed by Rottweilers, German Shepherds, Chihuahuas, and Doberman Pinschers. Breeds such as Chow Chows, Huskies, Akitas, and Belgian Malinois were rated as low bite risk breeds. However, this was not in line with perceptions of veterinarians, who rated Chow Chows, Chihuahuas, German Shepherds, Rottweilers, Akitas, and Belgian Malinois as high risk of biting. Other breeds rated as minimal risk by participants such as Dalmatians and Cocker Spaniels were viewed as higher risk by veterinarians (Kogan et al., 2019).

Hammond et al. (2022) found no evidence that the legislated breeds as a group were differentiated from the non-legislated breeds because of the behavioural traits related to the risk of aggressive behaviour. But people may interpret behaviours differently depending on the breed of dog acting in that way. Certain breeds, such as the Dobermann and English Bull Terrier, are more likely to be perceived as dangerous when lunging and barking than, for example, a Golden Retriever, regardless of the underlying emotional state that is driving the behaviour (Clarke et al., 2016). However, whilst there are differences between specific breeds of dogs in some of the traits that might affect the risk of aggressive behaviour, this is not consistently related to the legislative status of these breeds. For example, Oxley et al. (2018) report that Border Collies are amongst the breeds involved in bite incidents most frequently in the United Kingdom (although this may reflect their popularity), but they do not fall into the 'Dangerous Dog' breed categories.

One study points out that the owner has a significant influence on how a dog behaves. Indeed, many individual dogs of banned or legislated breed types may act aggressively not because of their intrinsic higher than average aggressive tendency, but because they more frequently have owners who mistreat them and/or specifically train them to act aggressively. This may lead to a correlation between 'dangerous breeds' and aggressive behaviour that may be independent of the natural aggressive tendencies in these dogs. It is also possible that certain dog breeds elicit more negative attention than others when they're acting as service dogs (Link & Wice, 2021).

Different organisations who train and provide volunteer school dog teams may have different perspectives. For example, Burns By Your Side in south Wales, who train dogs to read with children, take the position that it is the individual dog's personality that is the deciding factor. Amber Roach (the Project Officer) points out:

> In terms of breeds, we don't ban any breeds from the scheme (if they are legal). We strongly encourage bull type and larger type breeds on the scheme to break the stigma surrounding them. We currently have a beautiful German Shepherd in training, and a Staffordshire bull terrier x boxer has just passed through the last round of training! It's all down to individual temperament on initial assessment and how we feel they're progressing over the course of the 16 weeks training.

Conversely, in Owego (New York), one school's legal team would not ensure any dog that was a Great Dane, pit bull, or German Shepherd.

There may also be historical and cultural reasons for differences in how some breeds are perceived to consider. During World War II, dogs such as German Shepherds and wolfhounds were employed in Nazi concentration camps. Reports suggest that their exact purpose varied from camp to camp, but that in some cases dogs were trained to specifically attack exhausted prisoners, where 'one word or gesture from the SS and the dogs will tear the prisoner apart' (Beón in Hediger, 2013, p. 109). The use of dogs as a tool for oppression is not restricted to times of conflict. For example, Stewart argues that dogs such as bloodhounds and German Shepherds have long been used to oppress Black citizens:

> The use of dogs as tools of oppression against African Americans has its roots in slavery and persists today in everyday life and police interactions. Due to such harmful practices, African Americans are not only disproportionately terrorized by officers with dogs ... the use of dogs in oppressive acts is a critical layer of racial bias in the United States that has consistently built injustices that impede social and legal progress.
>
> (Stewart, 2020, p. 183)

This is echoed by Swistara (2021), who states that police dogs are disproportionally set loose on people of colour, and sniffer dogs are used on black motorists more often than white drivers.

THE CASE FOR THE CROSSBREED

So far in this chapter, we have considered how breed traits may impact dog suitability for classroom work. It is of course important to recognise that many dogs involved in schools are not pedigrees with traceable ancestors but fall into the category of 'mixed' or unknown breeding. In a recent survey of teachers involving dogs in their practice, Lewis and Oostendorp-Godfrey (2021) found that as well over 40 breeds of pedigree dogs mentioned by teachers, there were a wide range of crossbreeds in schools, from labradoodles and cockerpoos to those with unknown parentage.

This is unsurprising. There has been a rise in so-called designer crossbreeds in recent years, defined as the hybrid offspring that result from intentionally breeding dogs belonging to different breeds. Fuelled by the popularity of the labradoodle (Labrador × poodle) and the cockerpoo (cocker spaniel × poodle), there are now many such breeds, such as bernedoodles (Bernese Mountain Dog × poodle), sprockers (springer spaniel × cocker spaniel), puggles (pugs × beagles), and jugs (Jack Russell Terriers × pugs).

However, there is a myth that these dogs will be hardier, healthier, and a perfect blend of characteristics from each of their parents. For example, a survey of 2,191 owners of doodles and non-doodle dogs found that, when selecting their dogs, doodle owners were more influenced than non-doodle owners by their dog's appearance and by the perception that doodles are good with children and are generally healthy. Although doodle owners reported being highly satisfied with their dogs, more than twice as many doodle owners than owners of the other groups of dogs reported that their dog's maintenance requirements, such as their need for regular grooming, were more intensive than they had expected (Hladky-Krage et al., 2022).

Mixed breeds are not necessarily healthier. For instance, crossing the Labrador and a standard poodle to breed a litter of labradoodles can have a detrimental impact on the health and welfare of the offspring since both breeds are susceptible to similar genetic disorders, such as hip dysplasia and diseases of the eyes and joints (Farrell et al., 2015). Another common misconception is that cross bred dogs have better temperaments than their parent breeds. However, in a survey completed by

5,141 dog owners, labradoodles were not found to display any significant differences in 14 behavioural categories compared to poodles or Labradors. One exception to this was the goldendoodle, which scored significantly higher than their parent breeds in problematic behaviours, including dog-directed aggression, dog-directed fear, and stranger-directed fear (Shouldice et al., 2019).

These factors mean that it is essential to consider the suitability of any school dog from several perspectives, not least considering the perceptions that a particular breed may carry amongst members of the school community. This also means that a suitable school dog may come in many different shapes and sizes and will have a personality all their own. The key is to carefully match dog, child, intended activity, and environment to ensure that all fit well together.

PART 2: ASSESSING A DOG'S SUITABILITY FOR SCHOOL-BASED ACTIVITIES

So far, this chapter has explored the great variety of type that dogs come in, and the influence that this can have on a dog's suitability for involvement in educational contexts based on breed traits, appearance, and possible preconceptions and perceptions. However, it is crucial to note that all dogs are individuals, and so we need to go beyond generalisations to ensure that every dog is well-suited to the tasks they are asked to undertake. There are certain behaviours and personality traits that dogs working in educational contexts need if they are to thrive. Sarah Ellis is a highly experienced dog trainer, who has been instrumental in developing and coordinating the canine assessment and volunteer training for an educational canine assisted therapy scheme in west Wales. She looks for key qualities in a dog who is going to go into educational contexts (Figure 8.7).

These general qualities are very important to ensure that a dog is comfortable interacting with people in a school context, and that the dog behaves appropriately when meeting and greeting people. These also suggest that the dog demonstrates a sociable nature and is confident and curious about exploring new places and meeting new people. A dog who is relaxed and happy at home may respond very differently in the unfamiliar context of a busy school environment.

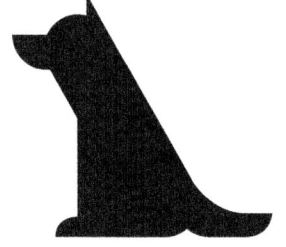

- Polite body language
- Willing to be touched all over body
- Enjoys being stroked
- Does not jump up
- Walks calmly on the lead
- Confident but not overbearing
- Calm and happy demeanour

FIGURE 8.7 Key qualities when choosing a dog to go into schools.
Adapted from Lewis and Grigg (2021, p. 176).

One international study of over 600 educational practitioners revealed that dogs are expected to work very flexibly in schools. For example, the specific environment where interventions take place varied greatly, 153 (48.6%) took place within the general classroom, 125 (39.7%) within the school grounds, and 116 (36.8%) in a quiet area other than the school library. Other areas included corridors and the offices of head teachers, counsellors, halls, and designated areas set aside for nurture groups or teaching children with special educational needs (classified under 'other'). Some respondents reported that space was used flexibly. In three cases, there was no fixed location as the dog followed the owner or therapist. The survey also indicated that many dogs are expected to work with varying numbers of people, and often for considerable amounts of time. Whilst many responses indicated that dogs typically work with individual children (45%), one in ten responses indicated that the dog worked with whole classes (Lewis et al., 2022). Therefore, for many school dogs, a typical day will involve spending time with multiple people in multiple environments.

Given these expectations, it is essential to consider each individual dog's suitability in detail, thinking through the nature of the interactions they will be likely to engage in. This goes beyond general breed type and traits to look closely at individual dogs in depth. Van Fleet and Faa-Thompson (2017) present an observation scale that can be used to look closely at an individual dog's characteristics (Table 8.3). This is the 'Animal Appropriateness Scale', which has four broad domains: physical/sensory functioning; social functioning; adaptability and psychological functioning. Each domain has several items, which are scored on a 5-point rubric after observation. These scores help make decisions around an individual's suitability for working in specific contexts.

These scores can then be considered against the 'job description' for the role to help determine an individual dog's suitability, although, as with any rating scale, care must be taken to ensure that all those using it are doing so consistently regarding judgement. It is also important to ensure that observations are made several times and also that the dog is observed in contexts where they will be working.

TABLE 8.3 Animal appropriateness scale.

Physical/sensory functioning items include	Social functioning items include
• Energy level	• Friendliness/sociability
• Vision, hearing, olfaction	• Interest/engagement
• Arousal	• Playfulness
• Stamina	• Cooperation
• Tolerance, e.g., to movement, sound, touch	
Adaptability items include	**Psychological functioning items include**
• Ability to learn	• Confidence
• Curiosity	• Independence
• Flexibility	• Freedom from behavioural problems
• Persistence	• Soundness/stability
• Impulse control	

Adapted from Van Fleet and Faa-Thompson (2017, p. 122).

Another way to consider the suitability of a dog for a specific role is to use Suzanne Clothier's 'CARAT' tool.[2] This looks specifically at the traits an individual dog has regardless of age, breed, or gender. These include looking at how socially tolerant the dog is, how resilient they are under stressful situations, and the levels of physical energy a dog has. Whilst many behaviour scoring systems describe overall behaviours, CARAT does not group together many different traits. Instead, CARAT differentiates at a finer level, for example, the scale allows the observer to note differences between a dog who distracted but distracted for different reasons. For instance, a dog in the school playground who is stressed and demonstrating avoidance sniffing compared to a dog who is confident but visually distracted by birds. In another rating system, they may have the same distraction score. This may enable a nuanced evaluation of a dog's suitability for specific contexts.

CONCLUSION

This chapter highlights the importance of considering a wide range of factors when selecting a dog so that their presence in school is mutually rewarding for both children and the dog. These include consideration of the individual dog's temperament and their physical characteristics, and how these relate to the environmental conditions and the needs of individual children. Whether a particular breed, or a puppy should be chosen is a point for much debate. Ultimately, the choice will be an individual one, but this should be an informed choice that considers what is best for all partners. Therefore, what is not contentious is the need to undertake careful research and preparation so that those involved are knowledgeable about both individual children and individual dogs, and to ensure that all are suitable for the intended activities and classroom contexts where they will meet.

NOTES

1   We do not discuss ear cropping or tail docking here. Both are illegal in the UK unless performed by a vet for medical reasons and are referred to as 'mutilation' under the Animal Welfare Act 2006.

2   https://suzanneclothier.com/carat/

REFERENCES

Arvelius, P., Asp, H. E., Fikse, W. F., Strandberg, E., & Nilsson, K. (2014). Genetic analysis of a temperament test as a tool to select against everyday life fearfulness in rough collie. *Journal of Animal Science*, 92(11), 4843–4855. https://doi.org/10.2527/jas.2014-8169

Brand, C. L., O'Neill, D. G., Belshaw, Z., Pegram, C. L., Stevens, K. B., & Packer, R. M. A. (2022). Pandemic puppies: Demographic characteristics, health and early life experiences of puppies acquired during the 2020 phase of the COVID-19 pandemic in the UK. *Animals*, 12, 629.

Burnett, E., Brand, C. L., O'Neill, D. G., Pegram, C. L., Belshaw, Z., Stevens, K. B., & Packer, R. M. A. (2022). How much is that doodle in the window? Exploring motivations and behaviours of UK owners acquiring designer crossbreed dogs (2019–2020). *Canine Medicine and Genetics*, 9(8). https://doi.org/10.1186/s40575-022-00120-x

Clothier, S. (2002). *Deepening our relationships with dogs*. Grand Central Publishing.

Doodle Trust. (n.d.). *Doodles and the allergy myth.* https://www.doodletrust.com/education/doodle-the-allergy-myth/

Farrell, L. L., Schoenebeck, J. J., Wiener, P., Clements, D. N., & Summers, K. M. (2015). The challenges of pedigree dog health: Approaches to combating inherited disease. *Canine Genetics and Epidemiology, 2*(3). https://doi.org/10.1186/s40575-015-0014-9

Fratkin, J. L., & Baker, S. C. (2013). The role of coat color and ear shape on the perception of personality in dogs. *Anthrozoös, 26*(1), 125–133. https://doi.org/10.2752/175303713X13534238631632

Frederick, E. (2019). Huans haven't just altered what dogs look like - we've altered the very structure of their brains. https://www.science.org/content/article/humans-haven-t-just-changed-what-dogs-look-we-ve-altered-very-structure-their-brains?utm_campaign=SciMag&utm_source=Facebook&utm_medium=ownedSocial&fbclid=IwAR0jV4WhDtLymrJ-gU7TQitWERn25CEE_llOSTQV1kihUfZmEKLZyqiR6E

Frederickson, M., & Howie, A. R. (2000). Methods, standards, guidelines, and considerations in selecting animals for animal-assisted therapy: Part B: Guidelines and standards for animal selection in animal-assisted activity and therapy programs. In A. H. Fine (Ed.), *Handbook on animal-assisted therapy: Theoretical foundations and guidelines for practice* (pp. 99–114). Academic Press.

Hamilton, L. (2022). *Canine types and abilities.* [PowerPoint Slides]. University of Denver.

Hammond, A., Rowland, T., Mills, D. S., & Pilot, M. (2022). Comparison of behavioural tendencies between "dangerous dogs" and other domestic dog breeds – Evolutionary context and practical implications. *Evolutionary Applications, 15*(11), 1806–1819. https://doi.org/10.1111/eva.13479

Hediger, R. (Ed.). (2013). *Animals and war studies of Europe and North America.* Brill.

Horowitz, A. (2009). Disambiguating the 'guilty look'; Salient prompts to a familiar dog behaviour. *Behavioural Processes, 81*(3), 447. https://doi.org/10.1016/j.beproc.2009.03.014

International Association of Human-Animal Interaction Organisations (IAHAIO). (2018). *The IAHAIO definitions for animal assisted intervention and guidelines for wellness of animals involved in AAI.* https://iahaio.org/wp/wp-content/uploads/2021/01/iahaio-white-paper-2018-english.pdf

Kogan, L. R., Packman, W., Erdman, P., Currin-McCulloch, J., & Bussolari, C. (2022). US adults' perceptions of dog breed bans, dog aggression and breed-specific laws. *International Journal of Environmental Research and Public Health, 19*(16). https://doi.org/10.3390/ijerph191610138

Lewis, H. (2022). *Thinking of a school dog?* Presentation at Osiris World Education Summit (online).

Lewis, H., Grigg, R., & Knight, C. (2022). An international survey of animals in schools: Exploring what sorts of schools involve what sorts of animals, and educators' rationales for these practices. *People and Animals: The International Journal of Research and Practice, 5*(1), Article 15. https://docs.lib.purdue.edu/paij/vol5/iss1/15

Lewis, H., & Oostendorp-Godfrey, J. (2021). Taking the Lead: innovations in classroom practices involving dogs. Society for Companion Animal Studies Annual Conference Paper.

Link, J., & Wice, M. (2021). Best in Show: Public Perceptions of Different Dog Breeds as Service Dogs. *Human-Animal Interaction Bulletin.* https://www.cabidigitallibrary.org/doi/10.1079/hai.2021.0005

MacLean, E. L., Snyder-Mackler, N., VonHoldt, B. M., & Serpell, J. A. (2019). Highly heritable and functionally relevant breed differences in dog behaviour. *Proceedings of the Royal Society B, 286*(1912). https://doi.org/10.1098/rspb.2019.0716

Mann, S. (2019). *Easy peasy, puppy squeezy.* Blink Publishing.

Mervosh, S. (2019). Do floppy-eared dogs look friendlier? The T.S.A. thinks so, 10 January, *New York Times.* https://www.nytimes.com/2019/01/10/science/tsa-dog-ears-floppy.html

Nicholas, C. E., Wegienka, G. R., Havstad, S. L., Zoratti, E. M., Ownby, D. R., & Johnson, C. C. (2011). Dog allergen levels in homes with hypoallergenic compared with nonhypoallergenic dogs. *American Journal of Rhinology & Allergy, 25*(4), 252–256. https://doi.org/10.2500/ajra.2011.25.3606

Oxley, J. A., Christley, R., & Westgarth, C. (2018). Contexts and consequences of dog bite incidents. *Journal of Veterinary Behavior, 23*, 33–39. https://doi.org/10.1016/j.jveb.2017.10.005

Rottier, M. (2023). Puppy Socialization and Animal Assisted Play Therapy™. *Presentation at the 3rd Annual International Institute of Animal Assisted Play Therapy conference,* online.

Smalley, S. (2009). A designer dog's life. *Newsweek*, 52–55.

Stewart, S. (2020). Man's best friend? How dogs have been used to oppress African Americans. *Michigan Journal of Race and Law*, 25(2), 183. https://doi.org/10.36643/mjrl.25.2.man

Swistara, M. (2021). Mutual liberation: The use and abuse of non-human animals by the carceral state and the shared roots of oppression. *University of Miami Race & Social Justice Law Review*, 12(2), 312–349.

Van Fleet, R., & Faa-Thompson, T. (2017). *Animal assisted play therapy*. Professional Resource Press.

Voslarova, E., Zak, J., Vecerek, V., & Bedanova, I. (2019). Coat color of shelter dogs and its role in dog adoption. *Society & Animals*, 27(1), 25–35. https://doi.org/10.1163/15685306-12341491

Watson, K. (2022). *Good autism practice for teachers*. Critical Publishing.

Westgart, C. (2021). *The Happy Dog Owner*. Wellbeck Publishing.

Wormald, D., Lawrence, A. J., Carter, G., & Fisher, A. D. (2016). Physiological stress coping and anxiety in greyhounds displaying inter-dog aggression. *Applied Animal Behaviour Science*, 180, 93–99.

CHAPTER 9

IMPLEMENTATION

This chapter focuses on practical issues associated with implementing happy, humane dog-assisted interventions. It is structured in four parts. The first discusses the fundamental ethical question of whether it is right to bring a dog or any animal into school. The second considers matters of health and safety, including guidance around conducting appropriate risk assessment to ensure children's and animal welfare needs are met, and about how to prepare stakeholders for the arrival of a dog. The third suggests possible approaches to planning the day-to-day interactions between dogs and children so that they can happen in a playful manner. And finally, the chapter discusses difficult issues such as the loss of a dog, the impact this may have on children and how this can be managed.

PART 1: IS IT ETHICAL TO HAVE ANIMALS IN SCHOOLS?

There are several considerations to be made when bringing any animal into a classroom because of the commitment and responsibilities that this brings. Lewis and Grigg (2021) outline practical considerations such as life expectancy, costs, welfare needs, as well as considering which is the most suitable species for any individual context. Ng et al. (2019) notes that any animal-assisted activity places certain demands on the animal partners. These demands can impact negatively on the welfare of the animal. For example, when learning about life cycles, many schools decide to hatch chicks in an incubator. However, to do this successfully is not simple. Mother hens typically turn their eggs up to 30 times a day to avoid the chick sticking to the walls of the shell. At the end of the school day, or over the weekend if the incubator is left in school, this can be impossible to manage. Eggs can hatch on weekends when no one is in school to check on the health of the newborn chick. Furthermore, being born in an incubator deprives the baby of a key part of their natural life – bonding with their mother. In nature, these bonds are formed before the chick is born. Two to three days before they are ready to hatch, they start peeping to notify their mother and siblings. This builds communication amongst the baby birds, and between the baby birds and their mother. In a school-chick hatching project, there is no opportunity for these natural relationships to develop between baby and parent. Additionally, projects involving hatching in schools often do not plan what will happen to the chicks at the end of the process. In many cases, the birds return to the farm where they were bred with their fates unknown (British Hen Welfare Trust, n.d.).

In terms of a school dog programme, a dog has little choice over when they will be there, how long they will be there for, where they will work, and who they

DOI: 10.4324/9781003257073-13

will meet. Opportunities for the dog themselves to exercise their own free will, for example, in choosing who to interact with, may be limited. This creates some ethical dilemmas to consider and address before embarking on an animal-assisted programme.

For instance, real-life hatching projects can be replaced with many resources such as books, videos, computer programmes, and plastic models. An understanding of the natural life of birds can be encouraged by quietly observing birds in the school grounds. Visits to parks, farms, or gardens can allow children's first-hand experiences of seeing birds engaging in natural behaviours such as socialising, dust-bathing, sunbathing, and feeding. Every year in the United States alone, over 3 million frogs are dissected in science classrooms. The organisation People for the Ethical Treatment of Animals (PETA) has worked with a manufacturer of realistic, synthetic models to develop a new simulated whole-body frog model called a Syn-Frog™. This can replace the use of frog cadavers completely in classrooms around the world. And in terms of spending time with dogs, there are several studies that report on the impact on children involving stuffed toys, robotic dogs, or online dogs (e.g., Steel, 2023).

MacNamara and MacLean (2017) suggest one approach that settings should take to ensure that the animal is well-suited to the intervention is to draw up a job description, thinking about the goal of including an animal, session logistics, and optimal animal characteristics (behaviours/physical, etc.) before selecting a suitable animal – or indeed deciding that the context may not be right for an animal. By reflecting on the job description, it may be easier to identify a suitable dog – or it may become apparent that there are alternative approaches that are more ethical.

For example, although I (HL) have involved my three dogs in CAE activity, all three are very different and each suits different situations. Table 9.1 summarises key characteristics of these dogs and how this might influence the CAEs that they become involved in.

Bearing this in mind, each dog is involved in practice in different ways. For instance, if a session was to be on a one-to-one basis with a student who was not very familiar with working with dogs, Scarlet would probably be best suited to the interaction. This is because she is smaller, physically less intimidating and her overall body language is calm. She would be very responsive in a situation where an individual wanted to play a puzzle type game with her. For a group of more dog-confident individuals, Carlo is a very responsive dog to interact with and would happily allow new people to stroke him or play fetch with his favourite squirrel toy. If the session involved presenting to a larger group of students in a lecture style setting, or students who liked to 'walk and talk' Obie would be well suited. He enjoys a quick sniff to familiarise himself with the setting but then is quite happy to spend some time watching the audience, but equally enjoys a slow, sniffy walk around campus. Although Carlo would also enjoy a walk around campus, the many squirrels which live there would be distracting for him, and he would be on high alert. This is less relaxing for all concerned. Knowing the dog and the environment well helps make informed decisions.

TABLE 9.1 Considering the preferences of individual dogs

Dog	Characteristics	Suitable for
Carlo 7-year-old Italian Spinone Neutered male 35 kg Wiry coat and beard	• Comfortable interacting with strangers • Enjoys being stroked and will spend time with individuals or groups by choice • Enjoys playing with toys • Food motivated • Nervous in clinical situations • Plays with soft toys and balls • Strong on lead	• Large and small group sessions • 1:1 with dog confident individuals • Environments that are calm and relaxed • Relaxing sessions where the participants want to stroke the dog • Play based sessions
Obie 18-month-old Otterhound Neutered male 42 kg Wiry coat and (often wet) beard	• Highly food motivated • Comfortable interacting with strangers, • Enjoys attention from an audience but independent • Can be distracted by scent • Plays with puzzle toys • Generally laid back but does not like elevators	• Large and small group sessions • 1:1 with dog confident individuals • Training sessions using food rewards • Scent detection activities
Scarlet 10-year-old cockerpoo Neutered female 15 kg Fleecy coat	• Enjoys 1:1 attention from familiar people • Highly responsive to training or puzzle games • Prefers to remain close to handler • Does not pull on lead • Does not like new dogs	• Small group sessions • 1:1 sessions with less dog confident pupils • Activities with handler and child • Walks around school

Sentience and Umwelt

An important consideration to make is how the interaction that takes place between dog and people will make the participants feel. Oftentimes in school, emphasis is placed on how the pupil will benefit (e.g., Lewis et al., 2022), but for happy, healthy and humane relationships the dog's emotions must also be considered. Bekoff and Pierce (2019) alert us to two ways to do this, one is by reducing the number of stresses a dog encounters, and the second is to increase the enrichments that they have. This means we must start to view the world from the dog's perspective to understand how they experience it.

Animal emotions and sentience refer to the capacity of animals to experience emotions and consciousness. Studies have shown that certain animals, such as dogs, horses, and primates, can experience a range of emotions, including joy, fear, anger, and love. The extent to which different species experience emotions and consciousness is still a topic of scientific debate. However, this means that we must recognise the fact that the life of every single individual is important (Bekoff, 2022).

We also need to remember that a dog will experience and relate to the world in a very different way to the way we experience it. This is described as the dog's 'Umwelt' (from the German, meaning 'environment'; von Uexkell, 1934 in Tedeschi & Jenkins, 2019, p. 303). Understanding a dog's Umwelt acknowledges that they will perceive the school environment and experiences within this differently to us, and we need to respect this and be aware of the possible implications of this. For example, dogs experience their world through more highly attuned senses than humans do. A dog's olfactory cortex, which deals with smell, is 40 times larger than a human's, meaning a typical dog's nose is at least a hundred thousand times more sensitive than our own (Bekoff, 2018). I notice in my own dogs that if one has been out of the house without the others, when they return home, they are sniffed thoroughly by the other two. This olfactory information must enable my pack to reacquaint with each other and gather valuable information about what has been going on whilst they have been apart. It is hard to comprehend therefore how the myriad of smells in a busy school environment will be perceived by a visiting dog.

Horowitz (2009) also reminds us that dogs do not perceive objects in the same way we do. What a person thinks an object is for may not match what the dog understands the function to be. For example, whilst I (HL) perceive the function of an oven glove as a handy piece of equipment to save my fingers from being burnt, Obie perceives this same object to be something exciting to chew, carry, and play with. Whilst we may perceive a barking dog as annoying, or a dog who wants to sniff the headteacher's groin as rude, the dogs are simply using their natural communication systems to make sense of the world (Bekoff & Pierce, 2019).

So, if we think about a school dog's typical day, we need to consider what may be challenging for them. For example, the dog's journey to school may be very different to their normal routine, and they may perceive the experiences they have on the way to school very differently to how their handler might. These will include several multi-sensory situations, and unfamiliar people and contexts. Figure 9.1 highlights some of these, from the clanging of the school gate to the sights and smells of the playground, or the sounds of the photocopier or school bell, to the texture of slippery school floors. The dog may deal well with each of these confidently as singular events, but when they encounter all in a short space of time this may be overwhelming.

To think through my own (HL) practice with my dogs, I carefully consider the experiences they are likely to have, and how they may perceive these before I undertake any activity. To do this I go beyond thinking through who they will meet, to also ensure I consider when, how, and where they will meet them. For example, I plan my day so that I arrive and set up the room to include a familiar blanket, water bowl, and toy that will help reassure the dog as soon as they enter the room. I ensure that I plan so that the dogs can visit the room before any of my students arrive. I book parking close to the venue so that there is less chance of unfamiliar experiences e.g., a loud delivery lorry overwhelming them on the way to the class. Knowing that Carlo is nervous in situations that remind him of a veterinarian's clinic (e.g., very bright lights, slippery floors, clanging crate doors), or that Obie does not like elevators would influence where I choose to run a CAE activity with them. I manage the way that students and dogs enter the room and ensure that greetings and interactions are carefully managed. I also ensure that the experiences feel positive and playful, and that reassurance and rewards are available. Thinking through how to successfully introduce a dog to the environment is crucial.

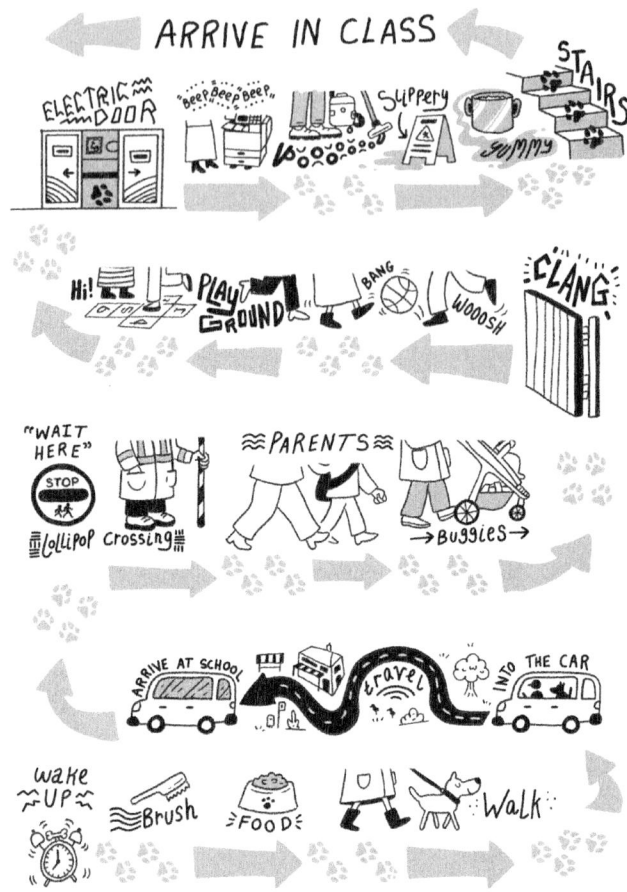

FIGURE 9.1 Considering the journey to school through the dogs' senses.
Reprinted by permission of Tom Bradraw.

Socialisation and Localisation

As discussed in Chapter 8, the age at which a dog should be brought into school is much debated and there is currently a gap in research in this area. Ideally more research would explore how to successfully introduce a dog so that their well-being is carefully observed and protected. Socialisation does not mean just exposing a young puppy to as many different things as possible in their early life. We need to remember that exposure can create negative as well as positive associations. Puppies may easily become overwhelmed and sensitised negatively to environmental stimuli, especially if there are bad associations with the first experience of something new. In a multisensory school environment, there are many potential challenges for a young puppy to cope with.

The localised noise, smells, textures, and sights that abound in any school may be overwhelming for any dog. It is difficult to overcome experiences that produce strong negative emotional responses. Dogs do not readily habituate to scary

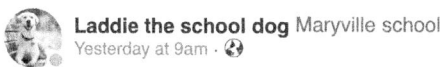

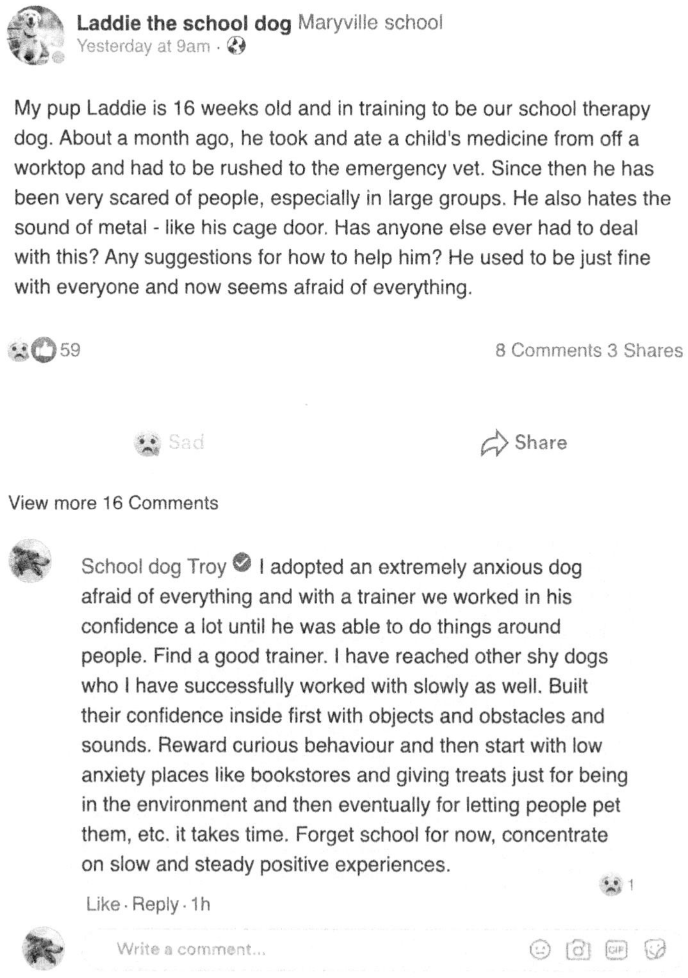

Laddie the school dog Maryville school
Yesterday at 9am ·

My pup Laddie is 16 weeks old and in training to be our school therapy dog. About a month ago, he took and ate a child's medicine from off a worktop and had to be rushed to the emergency vet. Since then he has been very scared of people, especially in large groups. He also hates the sound of metal - like his cage door. Has anyone else ever had to deal with this? Any suggestions for how to help him? He used to be just fine with everyone and now seems afraid of everything.

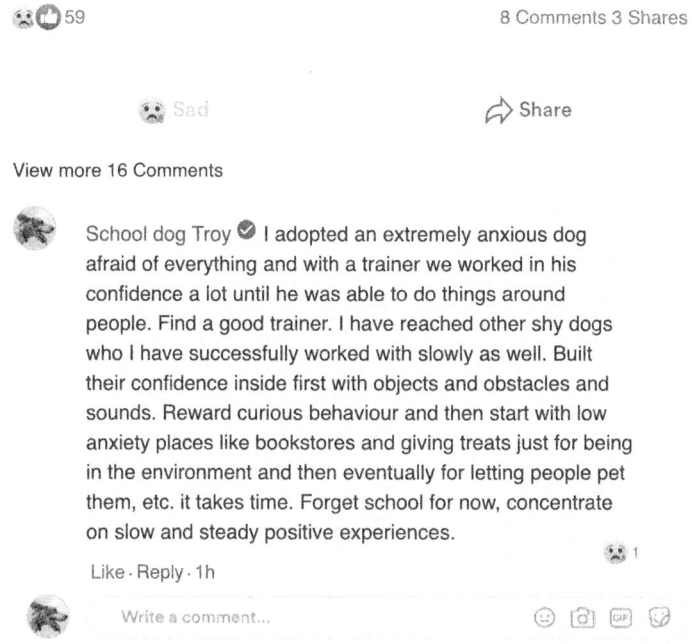

😢❤ 59   8 Comments 3 Shares

😢 Sad   ⤷ Share

View more 16 Comments

School dog Troy ✅ I adopted an extremely anxious dog afraid of everything and with a trainer we worked in his confidence a lot until he was able to do things around people. Find a good trainer. I have reached other shy dogs who I have successfully worked with slowly as well. Built their confidence inside first with objects and obstacles and sounds. Reward curious behaviour and then start with low anxiety places like bookstores and giving treats just for being in the environment and then eventually for letting people pet them, etc. it takes time. Forget school for now, concentrate on slow and steady positive experiences.

😢 1

Like · Reply · 1h

Write a comment...   ☺ �📷 GIF 🎁

FIGURE 9.2 Social media message: Fear in dogs.

situations. Instead, undesirable flight or fight responses become ingrained (Martin & Martin, 2016), as Figure 9.2 exemplifies.

Although in this case the teacher had the best of intentions, this experience overwhelmed the young dog. It may take some time before Laddie feels confident enough to return to a school environment.

It is important to be clear about the differences between 'socialisation' and 'localisation' to better understand how to introduce a dog successfully. Although often used synonymously in literature these terms may represent different developmental processes (McEvoy et al., 2022). Martin and Martin (2016) suggest that socialisation is 'the process of learning to communicate and relate with humans, members of the same species, and other animals', whereas 'localization is the process of learning to be attached to specific environments'. Socialisation and localisation are not simply about access to many varied experiences; first and fore-most, these processes are about making these experiences pleasant, fun and devel-opmentally appropriate.

For example, a class of undergraduate education students at Swansea University helped identify potential areas of the university campus that might cause Scarlet, Carlo, and Obie anxiety or surprise when they visit. Firstly, the students observed each dog in a familiar environment (one at a time) and found out more about their background, experiences, and personalities. They then worked in small groups around the campus to identify locations they thought would be unfamiliar to the dogs. In each of these locations, they planned activities that they felt would help the dog feel confident and supported in these spaces. For instance, one pair of students identified the electronic entrance doors as being ones that might cause Obie con-cern. They felt that the sudden sound and movement might scare him. They sug-gested a slow approach, with plenty of positive verbal encouragement and rewards would help him manage this new situation successfully. They observed Obie carefully as he came towards the door, noticing:

> Obie firstly observed humans entering and leaving through the automatic doors. Obie was alert but more interested in trying to sniff and interact with the humans who were watching. He went through the door calmly and was rewarded on the other side.

Other students in the group also noticed that having people on either side of the doors to provide treats may have helped Obie feel relaxed, and I noted that just before going through the doors he did a quick check in with me – glancing quickly up at me, just for a split second. This may have been for reassurance, but it would have been easy to miss if I had not been totally focused on him. At that moment, I was able to give him verbal encouragement. This is part of the reason that I would only ever work with one dog at a time, as I need to be able to focus fully on them as individuals.

The students identified other local areas for Obie to experience for the first time, including stairs, drain covers, and new floor surfaces. For each of these, they suggested ways to support him to have a positive experience, such as loose lead walk-ing, high quality treats, and lots of positive verbal encouragement. Obie faced these new situations calmly and in a relaxed manner, he was inquisitive but calm through-out. This was totally different from his experience at a large dog show when he was 8 months old. There, the large, echoing hall, the sounds, sights, and scents of many unfamiliar dogs, the bright lights, and the slippery flooring were quite overwhelming for him. In that situation, his body language was much less relaxed, and he showed some signs of anxiety. For Obie, a career in the show ring would not be in his best interest, but as a visitor in lectures, he seems well-suited.

It is important to ensure that the dog is ready for each new experience. Obie's first visit to campus did not come until he was 12 months old, and then this was a short and carefully planned event. The session was designed to be positive – there were plenty of high value treats and favourite toys available, Obie had choices throughout the session, and he engaged with the students as and when he chose. As a result, his body language was relaxed and interested throughout. This meant that the teaching in that session had to adapt, students understood that there would be some flexibility in how and when we discussed certain content. For example, part of the way through discussing one piece of research we paused the discussion to watch as Obie became fascinated by the magpie on the windowsill. This provided a valuable opportunity to look at body language. However, balancing his needs and those of the students is a constant process, just as it is for teachers who bring a dog into their classrooms.

The key question to ask is perhaps then not what age the dog should be brought in from, but rather whether the school can provide positive, varied, and context-specific experiences alongside the age-appropriate care needed for any individual dog. Crucial to this is whether there is deep understanding amongst staff, children, and the wider school community of the developmental needs of the dog, whatever age they are.

Beyond the physical environment, any teacher deciding to bring a dog into their classroom must be aware of the possibility that involvement in CAE can have implications for the dog's own emotional well-being. For example, research suggests that dogs can empathise with human emotions. Karl and Huber (2017) argue that the relationship between dogs and humans enables dogs to communicate with us emotionally, by responding adaptively to our expressions of emotion. Similarly, dogs in a study by Albuquerque et al. (2018) showed more lip-licking (stress signals) when showing faces of humans in distress than humans not in distress. In one study on the effectiveness of AAT on children with multiple disabilities, the therapy dog Cody demonstrated symptoms of stress like excessive panting and tiredness, which led to the study being terminated early (Heimlich, 2001). Thus, if our planned interventions are intended to support children who may be anxious, upset, or emotionally vulnerable, we must be aware that this may unintentionally impact the umwelt of the dog themselves.

Another ethical point to consider relates to how we view the dog, as this may impact on how we interact with them. Pierce (2016) suggests that any animal's status in the family or community can shift and change. Relationships are complex and can become strained, so when a dog is added into an already pressured classroom context, teachers can find this difficult, and maintaining a positive, calm relationship with a dog may be challenging. Since dogs pick up on our stress signals so effectively, this may impact on their well-being. Furthermore, there is evidence to suggest that talking in a pleasant, friendly voice to dogs creates a positive atmosphere, encourages more desirable behaviours, and can help make training sessions more effective (Coren, 2023). If the classroom context is one where there is more disciplinary style interaction taking place, the dog may find this difficult to cope with.

Behaving Ethically: Asking the Dog If They Would Like to Join in

If we are to promote happy, healthy, and humane interactions between children and dogs, we must ensure that all participants can consent to take part. Seeking such consent from all involved is an ongoing process that goes beyond an assessment of a dog's temperament or a child's agreement at the start of the project. We must recognise that the right to withdraw from an activity may be sudden, brief, and transient. Teachers are generally well versed in their children's rights, but we need to ensure we also listen to the dog. Clothier (2014) talks about six elemental questions that we should ask of our dogs before any interactions. These questions reaffirm that this is a relationship, built on trust and respect, and the ability to interpret carefully what our dogs are telling us (Figure 9.3).

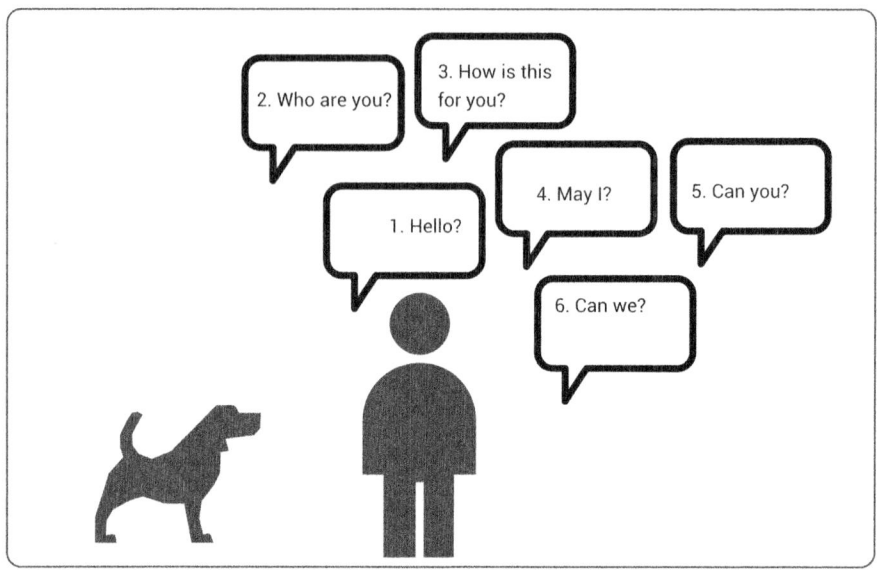

FIGURE 9.3 Six elemental questions.
Based on Clothier (2014).

The first question, 'Hello?', asks the dog whether she would like to interact with anyone today. This may vary from day to day, moment to moment. The important thing for teachers to plan for is if the dog does not consent what will happen to the children. Having a back-up plan is essential. The second question, 'Who are you?', encourages us to reflect on who our dog is – their likes, dislikes, etc. so that we can ensure they are well matched to the interactions taking place. Knowing what motivates a dog is important. The third question, 'How is this for you?', reminds us to observe the dog carefully throughout the session to ensure that they are happy to participate. Understanding the individual dog here is very important as they will have individual behaviours to indicate their mood. The fourth question, 'May I?', ensures that we observe the dog's preferences and respect them if they do not want to participate. The fifth question, 'Can you?', focuses on the dog's ability to undertake an activity or interaction – where ability refers to physical, intellectual, and emotional characteristics. And the final question, 'Can we?', reminds us that throughout our interventions, we must ensure that decisions made are mutual and respect all participants. By asking these questions before beginning any CAE, and observing the dog's responses, teachers can ensure that the needs of the individual dog, on any chosen day, and in any chosen activity, are recognised and respected.

PART 2: WHAT IS A SAFE INTERACTION?

All schools should carry out a detailed risk assessment before bringing a dog into the environment. This needs to cover practical and health-related matters such as allergies, phobias, or waste disposal arrangements. For visiting school dogs, the external organisation will typically have a risk assessment or guidance that can be tailored to the specific needs of the school. For schools having a permanent school dog, a specific risk assessment needs to be developed.

A good risk assessment is not just undertaken to protect children from harm but also serve to protect everyone in the school setting, such as teachers and teaching staff, supply teachers, kitchen staff, administrative staff, visitors, and of course the dogs themselves. Risk assessments also support vulnerable children and staff.

Schools should record findings of the assessment by identifying:

- hazards, for example, allergies, tripping, hygiene;
- how someone may be harmed, for example, allergic reaction, scratches, or bruises;
- what the school has put in place to control and reduce risk, for example, inform parents and carers, restrict dogs to certain areas, assess dogs' behaviour carefully, ensure dogs and handlers are easily identifiable (such as with a bandana or logo on harness, Photo 9.1).

There are many templates on-line to help guide the development of a school dog risk assessment.[1] Schools also frequently share their examples of risk assessment on-line. These can be valuable starting points. However, it is important to ensure

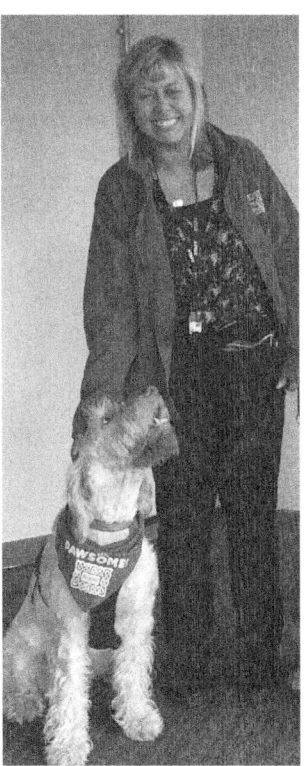

PHOTO 9.1 Helen and Carlo the dog in their volunteer uniforms.

Reprinted by permission of Vanessa Thomas.

that the risk assessment is created specifically for each unique context, and that the needs and welfare of the dog are included in the assessment (Appendix A1). For example, there may be a risk to the dog if the children he is working with are prone to unpredictable behaviours. How the intervention is planned to mitigate against these eventualities is important to consider.

Accidents can happen. As well as having human first aid contingencies in place, having a member of staff trained in canine first aid, and having a canine first aid kit (containing, e.g., saline pods, dressings, bandages, disposable gloves, tweezers, sterile gauze) on hand is something to also consider.

Schools should also examine what insurance is available to them. Again, visiting dogs are likely to be covered via the organisation's arrangements, but schools with their own dog will need to explore their options. This is important. Lewis and Oostendorp-Godfrey (2023) found that unexpected incidents such as a dog barking or growling at a child, toileting in the class or jumping up had happened in a number of cases. For example, one teacher reported that their dog:

> ... slipped the lead and one student who is quite fearful for the dogs ran away because he was scared. What the dog thinks is 'great you're running', and because the child is screaming the dog was jumping up in excitement. We had to hold the child and get the dog. And he did scratch his arm, not out of malice, just because he's jumping up because there's a kid running and screaming.

Ongoing discussion with parents, carers, and the wider community is also important. There may be health-related, psychological, cultural, or religious sensitivities to consider before bringing a dog into the school. Clear and accessible communication with stakeholders will help ensure that the needs of all pupils and their families are considered. A typical letter to parents and carers will explain the rationale for bringing a dog into school, information about the dog themselves, who they work with, when they will be on site, how to meet and greet the dog, and how to raise any concerns (Appendix A2). A simple information sheet for pupils to introduce them to the dog, including information about them (e.g., name, age, breed, favourite treat, favourite walk/toy/trick, etc.) is useful (Appendix A3). In the case of a visiting dog, a simple fact sheet about the school and appropriate information about the pupils they will work with is helpful for the handler.

Once the dog starts to attend school, signs to show where the dog is working, or when he is resting should be visible (Appendix A4). Many schools will encourage the community to see the dog as a member of the school team, often having a notice board for the dog, or an entry in the school Yearbook (Appendix A5).

It is also important to continue to monitor the interactions that take place. This can be done in several ways. Martino's website[2] recommends that we follow certain principles when planning an intervention with animals and by following these we can build a rapport with dogs, get to know their personalities, and develop an understanding of how the environment and individual animals interact. These principles can be adapted to a school context, as illustrated in Table 9.2.

To ensure that we are creating interactions and interventions that are happy and humane, we must consider the dog as a partner. To understand what a dog is trying to tell us, Horowitz (2010, p. 21) reminds us that '... we must ask the dog what he wants. You only need to know how to translate his answer'. To do this, all participants must learn to read their dog's body language, and act according to what they are

TABLE 9.2 Principles for planning a dog-assisted intervention

Principle	Action	Application to school environment
Pausing to notice all conditions	Stop and observe	• Awareness of environmental conditions. • Awareness of both child and dog body language and communication.
Recognising that all have needs	Appreciate individuals and their needs	• Ensure interactions are bespoke to each individual child and dog • Ensure that child and dog are well matched.
Advocate for everyone	Set up conditions for success	• Ensure a balance between needs of dogs and children. • Speak up for children, handlers and dogs as appropriate, and ensure they consent to participate throughout.
Celebrate often	Name and notice the successes	• Know what motivates individuals and use this to reward success regularly • Notice the small steps
Get curious	Understand what each dog is likely to be interested in Ask questions about the interactions that are taking place	• Create a learning environment that is engaging for all
Observe labels and language	Question whether we are communicating effectively as a partnership	• Are we communicating effectively as a partnership

telling us. Pelar (2013) suggests looking at a dog's communication based on a traffic light system:

- Green – enjoyment. Things are going well. All partners are comfortable. Continue observing, but no need to intervene;
- Amber – tolerance. There is a level of tension or disengagement in the interaction. There may be things that can be done to improve the situation, or the interaction should end;
- Red – enough. Intervene immediately. The participants should be given time apart, and future interactions monitored carefully.

To be able to use the traffic light system effectively, all participants need to observe carefully. Whilst many human participants may be able to verbalise how they are feeling, the signs that dogs give us are subtle and nuanced. Dogs use all their bodies to convey emotions, and we must look closely at the signals they are giving us and interpret them carefully (Figure 9.4).

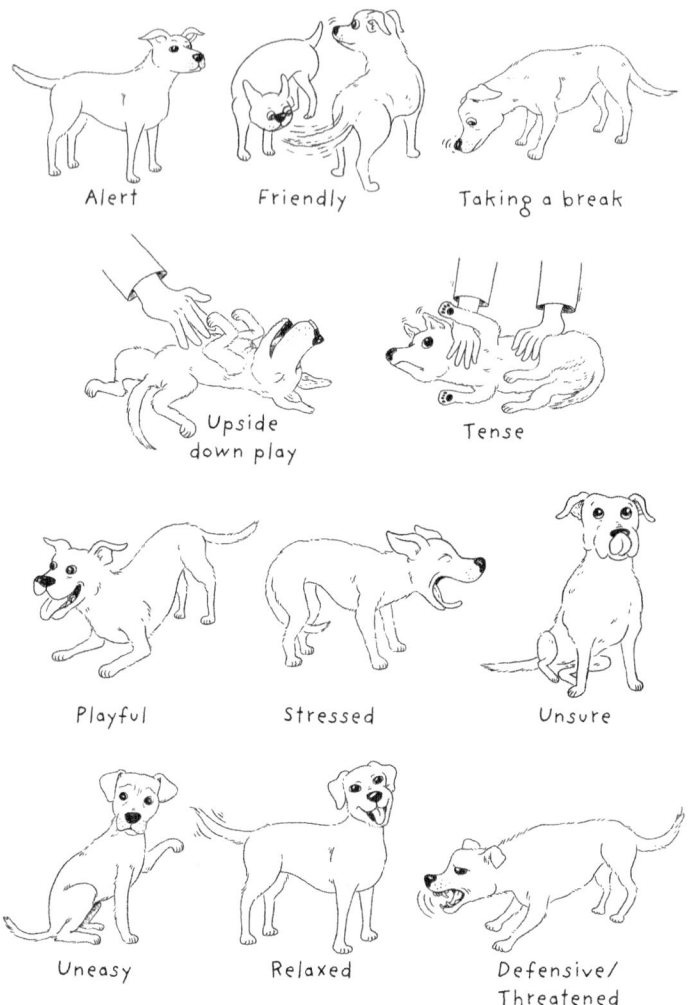

FIGURE 9.4 Interpreting dog signals.

Reprinted by permission of Tom Bradraw.

There is a tendency to make generalisations; for example, I often hear people say that a dog must be feeling happy because their tail is wagging. Dogs use their tails to convey many messages. A dog holding their tail horizontally may be feeling relaxed, whereas a low tail may be signalling feelings of anxiety. A tentative, narrow wag suggests a dog may be less sure of the situation compared to a wide, broad sweep of the tail (e.g., Lewis & Grigg, 2021). Furthermore, evidence suggests that the direction of the tail wag also conveys information. Dogs looking at positive stimuli (e.g., the owner) wagged more to the right than dogs looking at negative stimuli (e.g., an unfamiliar, unfriendly dog), whose tails moved more to the left (Siniscalchi et al., 2018).

Therefore, helping children understand more about dog body language, safe greetings, and consent is vital if interventions are going to be happy and safe.

Children need to recognise stress signals in the dogs they interact with and understand how to behave if they see these. Misunderstandings are common amongst children, and this can lead to significant risk. For example, in one study, Meints et al. (2010) found that 69% of 4-year-olds interpreted aggressive dog's faces as smiling and happy. This is understandable. When people smile, we typically show our teeth – when a dog shows his teeth, they are usually telling us they want space. However, we must acknowledge the individual in this. My own (HL) Irish setter Stanley would greet us with bared teeth, but this was accompanied by a low, gently sweeping tail and soft body language. He was smiling to welcome us home.

Thus, these interpretations will be based on our knowledge of the individual dog, as well as the context and environment that they are in. For example, as shown in Figure 9.4, a dog may roll on her back because she wants more petting or because she feels tense or anxious.

Typically, a dog who is feeling increasingly uncomfortable will move through a series of behaviours to try and inform us how they feel. These may start with lip licking, paw lifting, or averted gaze, but may escalate to growling, barking, or snapping if a dog feels particularly threatened or uneasy. Shepherd (2002) describes this as a ladder of aggression. At each level, the dog is trying to signal his feelings. If these signals are ignored, the dog may climb a step on this ladder, showing more stressful behaviour.

For instance, in Figure 9.5, the dog is looking tense and uncomfortable. Her lead is tight and therefore she has no escape route. Her ears are back, her brow is furrowed, she is leaning away, and the whites of her eyes (a whale eye) are showing.

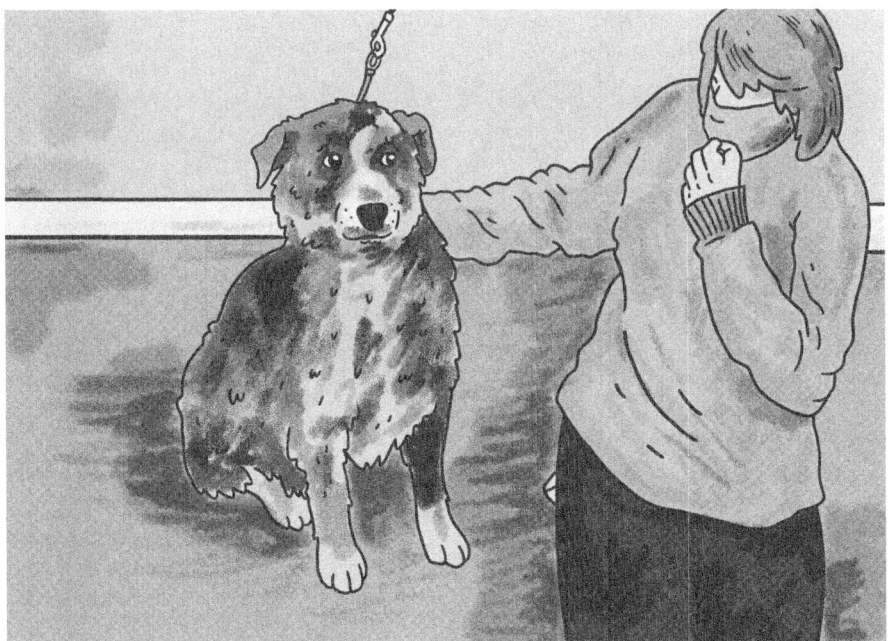

FIGURE 9.5 A dog showing uncomfortable body language.

Reprinted by permission of Tom Bradraw.

She may be concerned by the mask on the human, or there may be other circumstances making her feel anxious. This is an amber traffic light interaction that could become more serious if the adult does not respond appropriately (e.g., leave the space; avoid touch; loosen the lead).

Including reference to canine communication, and how all stakeholders are made aware of this (and act accordingly) is important to include in any risk assessment documentation, and in whole school preparation activity.

How Can Teachers and Children Evaluate Interactions?

Children need an opportunity to explore canine body language in a variety of safe ways. Before the dog begins coming into school, it is advisable to run 'meet and greet' events and hold information sessions, such as assemblies where key messages can be shared. There is no doubt that when a dog first arrives, excitement (or in some cases anxiety) levels will rise. Managing children's expectations regarding appropriate behaviour, what to expect, and key facts about the dog will be useful preparation.

For example, whilst observing real dogs is very useful, the children could start by looking at images and discussing what they see. From there, moving to watch dogs in real life carefully can be engaging and useful in advance of the dog arriving. Dogs certainly watch us very closely. Indeed, Duranton and Gaunet (2018, p. 347) found that dogs

> … synchronize their behaviors with that of humans in a variety of situations, and the degree of behavioral synchronization is dependent upon the degree of affiliation between the interacting partners.

I (HL) watch dogs wherever and whenever I see them. Today, I passed two Labradors, one Staffordshire Bull Terrier ('Staffie'), three doodles, a greyhound, and a little black ball of fluff on my journey to work. I cannot help but notice their body language, and I watch how they interact with other people, dogs and the environment. I often observe how closely they watch their owners too. They are highly attuned to our body language. The little black dog I passed today trotted along the street alongside the person walking him. Every few feet, he would quickly glance up at the person for a split second. These check-ins might have been for reassurance, or out curiosity (unfortunately, his person was looking at their phone, so missed these opportunities for relationship-building interactions). Observation is a skill that needs to be learnt. Dog body language is subtle, fleeting, and nuanced. It takes practice to learn to interpret what the dogs are telling us.

Teachers as well as children therefore need to have structured opportunities to observe dogs carefully. This may start with looking at images or films of dogs, and talking about what is seen. Marikris De-Leon, a postgraduate student at Swansea University, analysed video segments of children and dogs interacting. She reflected on the value of taking time to look in detail at interactions, and the potential benefits of video as a tool. She suggested that video is powerful for several reasons. Video captures human and dogs' visual (e.g., facial and bodily gestures) and auditory behaviour. Replaying the video allows teachers to focus on key elements of the interaction, and to examine these in more depth. Micro expressions that are not easy to see during a lesson may be captured, whereas in live observations, observing may be quite difficult and it is easy to miss details. Marikris does warn however that:

> While videos may work adequately to provide audiovisual information, it should be noted that they do not show tactile and olfactory elements, and the audiovisual factors they present are limited by the angle or movement of the camera and the acoustic range of the microphone. Videos do not capture all factors that may distract participants or influence their behaviour. Complementary observer notes may contribute to a better understanding of the immediate environment. In terms of cognitive factors as well as participant wellbeing and emotions, videos capture only audiovisual behavioural indicators so it may be useful to supplement them with self-assessments and other measures, if necessary.

Another potentially useful tool for teachers, support staff (and older learners) to use when observing interactions between humans and dogs is the Human-Animal Interaction Scale, or HAIS (Fournier et al., 2016). The HAIS is a 24-item self-reported scale developed to assess human–animal interaction. The scale was designed to 'describe and quantify behavior performed by human and nonhuman animals during an episode of interaction' (Machová et al., 2020). This breaks down behaviours of the human (e.g., talking to the animal, grooming the animal, holding the animal) alongside the behaviours of the animal themselves (e.g., making friendly sounds, accepting food, sniffing the human). Lydia Morgan and Bethany Hill, two students at Swansea University, used the HAIS when observing school dogs and identified strengths and potential limitations of this as a tool, as well as some interesting features (Table 9.3).

Using a tool like the HAIS means that there are objective measures in place to consider the interactions taking place. It is possible of course that there are other

TABLE 9.3 Student researchers' reflection on using HAIS

Positives	Minuses	Interesting
• Clear way to code the behaviours of children and dogs. • Categories are clearly defined and easy to understand. • Easy to record the reciprocity/mutuality of the child-dog interaction because of the broadly equivalent actions for each. • Can use HAIS in a lot of environments which is helpful in a busy school context. • Can capture evidence of where the interactions between dog/child work best.	• Difficult to use with more than one dog and child (e.g., meet & greet at school gates, walking around the school). • Must interpret why the behaviours are happening • No room to record mediating influence of the handler (in this case, the teacher), who was present • Could be a distraction for the participants if they were not used to being observed	• The actions coded on the HAIS could be easily supplemented by a comments box for recording verbal communication by the child towards the dog during a session. • Not all behaviours included on the HAIS would be observed in a school setting (e.g., grooming and feeding would be less likely to take place). • Can also observe how the staff interact with the dog and what approach they use, and the impact of this.

interactions occurring beyond observable behaviours, but as a starting point to consider CAE, there is merit in adopting such approaches. Chapter 10 explores capturing data and evaluating CAE in more depth.

PART 3: SCHOOL DOGS: PRACTICAL IDEAS FOR HAPPY, HEALTHY AND HUMANE INTERACTIONS

Training Your Dog

Whilst dogs are generally very willing to fit in with our lifestyles and live closely with us, some training is usually required so that they can do this comfortably (Hollin, 2021). There are many approaches that can be taken, and these have developed over time so that ideas such as dominance/pack theory have been discredited due to better understandings of how dogs learn best (Van Fleet & Faa-Thompson, 2017). Positive, force-free training methods use rewards such as treats, praise, and play to encourage desired behaviours. These methods aim to build a positive relationship between the dog and the trainer and to reinforce desired behaviours. This is not about developing a dog who behaves like a robot, but rather to provide the dog with 'a toolbox of skills, understanding and communication techniques that allow them to calmly navigate their surroundings' (Bekoff & Pierce, 2019, p. 39).

Aversive training methods, on the other hand, use punishment or discomfort to discourage undesired behaviours. This may include physical punishment, such as hitting or pulling on a lead, or psychological punishment, such as scolding or shouting. To develop happy, healthy relationships, positive training methods are desirable as they do not damage the relationship between the dog and the trainer. Punishment and negative approaches can lead to a lack of trust, or even fear, anxiety, and aggression.

As humans, many of the behaviours we automatically teach our dogs – such as 'sit' or 'lay down' are not necessarily beneficial for the dog. In fact, for some breeds, they may even be uncomfortable or unpleasant. For instance, some greyhounds find sitting uncomfortable due to their anatomy. Furthermore, it is important that training allows safe interactions, but does not create dogs who behave like automatons. It is important to ensure that they keep their individuality and can enjoy their experiences in schools. Each dog is different, so it is always important that we take the time to get to know the dogs as individuals. Training sessions also work best if they are short and based on playfulness. Several five-minute sessions a day would maintain a dog's interest better than a single longer period (Van Fleet & Faa-Thompson, 2017). Training is an on-going process rather than a one-off event, and continues throughout the dog's life.

Katie Gardner and Amber Roach are dog trainers for Burns By Your Side, the reading with dogs' scheme run by The John Burns Foundation in Kidwelly, South Wales. In the following section, they share their ideas on ways to train dogs positively, and to build playful activities into interactions.

The Basics: Marking and Rewarding Behaviour

Marking and rewarding is a way of helping a dog to build an association between a sound and a positive reward to aid the training process, which is known as secondary reinforcement. Once the dog realises that whenever they hear a particular marker sound, it is followed by a positive reward, they begin to recognise which behaviours are rewarding for them, and the frequency with which they display these behaviours will increase in anticipation of that reward.

A marker word should be a unique sound with which the dog has no existing association. The best types of words are short and sharp such as 'Yes!' or 'Good!', as they are unlikely to hear this word said in any other context than having done something right. It is vital that any time the dog hears this word, they are rewarded. Words such as 'Good Boy' are not so effective because the dog is likely to hear this phrase said numerous times a day by numerous people and in numerous contexts, thus decreasing the effectiveness of the mark and reward contract. Some choose to use a clicker which has a similar effect, being a short and unique noise that is only heard in the context of the desired behaviour being demonstrated.

Before beginning training the dog, it is important to 'load' the marker word or clicker to begin to build the positive association. Say the word or click the clicker and treat the dog immediately. Do not ask the dog for anything during this exercise; this is just allowing them to begin to associate that sound with a reward. Repeat this at least ten times before asking anything else of the dog.

Luring

Many behaviours we ask of our dogs are not necessarily naturally rewarding behaviours that they would use in a non-human-oriented world. Luring, encouraged by tempting with tasty treats, encourages the dog into the positions we desire, allowing them to focus on making positive, rewarding choices so that over time these behaviours become meaningful and will be offered more frequently. There is no point in us asking them to perform certain behaviours using cue words before we have taught them what those words relate to. Therefore, Katie and Amber suggest that we should not 'name a behaviour until they know it'.

To make the most of luring, they suggest holding a treat like a magnet to the dog's nose and allow them to follow the hand back and forth. After a couple of movements, mark and reward the dog for following the treat magnet. Repeat this a few times so that the dog gets used to the luring process and realises they will be rewarded for following the hand. This process can be built up to train more complex behaviours, and ultimately the motions made with the hand will become signals for various behaviours.

Luring is a positive, rewarding experience for the dog, and prevents the temptation to push, pull, or force dogs into position. Positive training methods will give the dog the confidence to make desirable choices as well as allowing your relationship to flourish.

Six Essential Behaviours for a School Dog

We want to ensure that a school dog's personality can shine through CAE activity. We want them to make us smile and for them to enjoy themselves. Nonetheless, there are some key behaviours that are important building blocks for happy and safe interactions in the classroom. Every dog will respond differently to training, so it is important to remember that what follows are general pointers. When training, it is important to bear in mind who the dog is because personality, breed, and experience will have shaped them. As Denise Fenzi reminds us 'train the dog in front of you' (2016, p. 7). These six behaviours are those identified by Katie, Amber, and the authors. Specific dogs working in specific school contexts may of course need other essential behaviours – such as polite greetings with other dogs if they are in a multiple dog school.

1. Leave It

This is an essential behaviour for keeping the dog safe (Figure 9.6). They may come across things in school which are dangerous or generally unpleasant which we do not want them to pick up or eat. For example, a bar of chocolate from a lunch box, or a box of raisins on the tuck trolley, both of which are poisonous to dogs. It is important when we are asking the dog to 'leave it' that they never get what it is you are asking them to leave – we do not want them to assume they will eventually get it! This behaviour is also not best used for asking a dog to drop what they have already picked up.

2. Swap and Drop

This is for when the dog has picked up something which you need them to give up (Figure 9.7), for example, a child's pencil case or ball, or their socks or brand-new trainers. When asking a dog to drop something which they deem valuable, it is

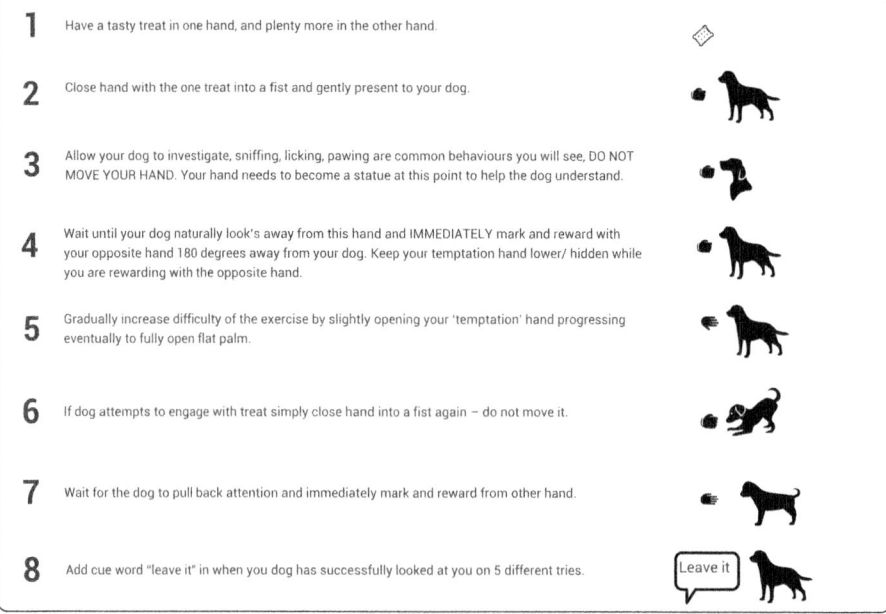

1 Have a tasty treat in one hand, and plenty more in the other hand.

2 Close hand with the one treat into a fist and gently present to your dog.

3 Allow your dog to investigate, sniffing, licking, pawing are common behaviours you will see, DO NOT MOVE YOUR HAND. Your hand needs to become a statue at this point to help the dog understand.

4 Wait until your dog naturally look's away from this hand and IMMEDIATELY mark and reward with your opposite hand 180 degrees away from your dog. Keep your temptation hand lower/ hidden while you are rewarding with the opposite hand.

5 Gradually increase difficulty of the exercise by slightly opening your 'temptation' hand progressing eventually to fully open flat palm.

6 If dog attempts to engage with treat simply close hand into a fist again – do not move it.

7 Wait for the dog to pull back attention and immediately mark and reward from other hand.

8 Add cue word "leave it" in when you dog has successfully looked at you on 5 different tries.

FIGURE 9.6 Taught behaviours for 'Leave It'.

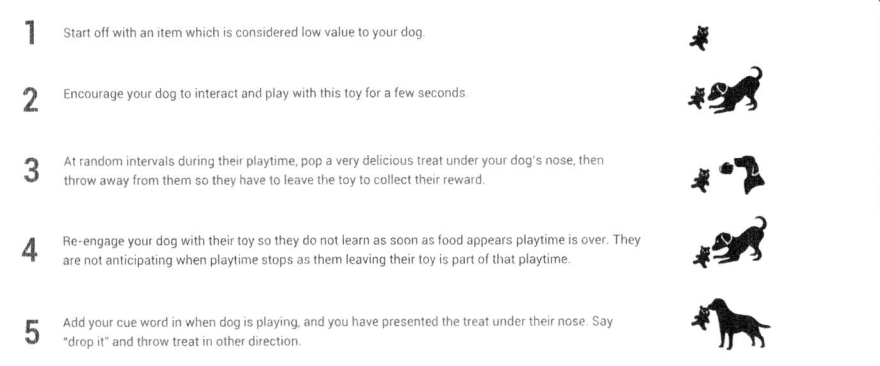

FIGURE 9.7 Taught behaviours for 'Swap and drop'.

important to offer them a better alternative. If they are asked to give up something and they get nothing in return, resource guarding issues may arise. It is still good to offer rewards for this behaviour even once well established to keep it at the forefront of their minds and to guarantee they realise that 'giving something up' isn't a bad thing as they get something equally (or more) valuable in return.

3. Recall

Having a good recall with the dog is imperative if they are to be able to have the freedom to play safely off-lead (Figure 9.8) or should they ever find themselves in a situation where a child or adult drops the lead in the school. Whatever the distraction,

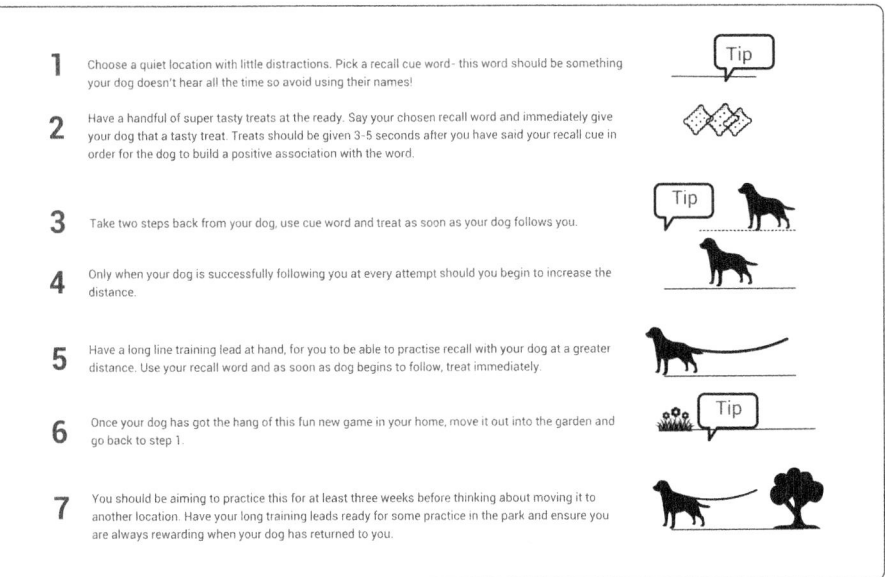

FIGURE 9.8 Taught behaviours for 'Recall'.

having reliable recall provides peace of mind. Recall must always be practiced at home before taking the dog to school.

4. Settle

This is a useful behaviour to ensure the dog can enjoy some down time (Figure 9.9). The behaviour of settling can be used as it is, or eventually build on it to help with sending the dog to their bed or crate. Settled behaviour is fantastic when encouraging a dog to rest, or if events in the classroom mean that you need to intervene unexpectedly in a situation with the children. It is essential for the dog to have a very positive relationship with their bed area.

5. and 6. Wait and Stay

These behaviours are useful in multiple contexts, for safety and to make life a little easier. 'Wait' is a mobile behaviour (Figure 9.10). We want the dog to wait where they are until called to join us or walk with us, for example, waiting at the roadside until we want them to cross or waiting at the bottom of the stairs before we call them up. This is helpful in a school context, for example if waiting whilst a child goes through a door first. This contrasts with 'stay', where we may want the dog to stay where they are until we get to them. It is useful to train these as two distinct behaviours for clarity. Training begins in a similar way for both behaviours. It is important to remember that if you want your dog to return to you after waiting, call them back with one cue. However, if you want your dog to stay where they are until you return to them, make sure you do not offer that reward until you get back to them.

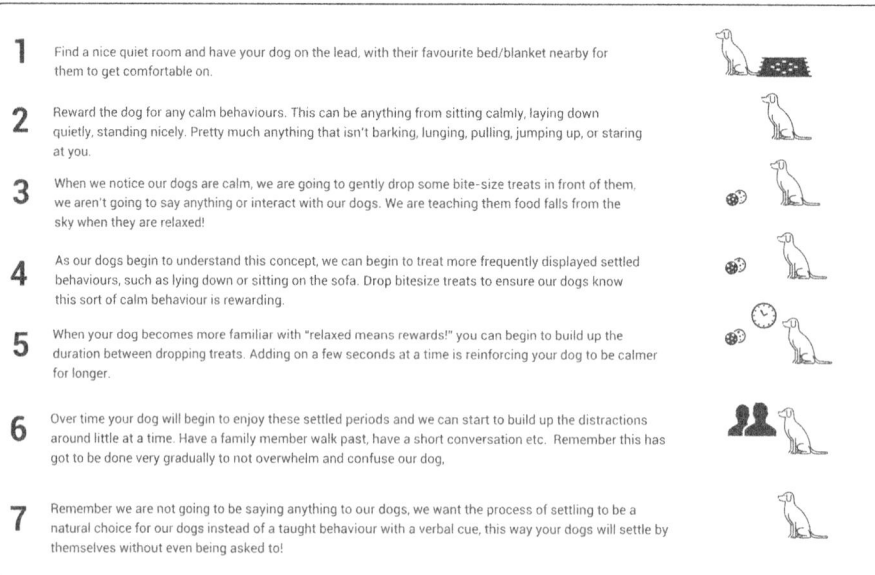

1 Find a nice quiet room and have your dog on the lead, with their favourite bed/blanket nearby for them to get comfortable on.

2 Reward the dog for any calm behaviours. This can be anything from sitting calmly, laying down quietly, standing nicely. Pretty much anything that isn't barking, lunging, pulling, jumping up, or staring at you.

3 When we notice our dogs are calm, we are going to gently drop some bite-size treats in front of them, we aren't going to say anything or interact with our dogs. We are teaching them food falls from the sky when they are relaxed!

4 As our dogs begin to understand this concept, we can begin to treat more frequently displayed settled behaviours, such as lying down or sitting on the sofa. Drop bitesize treats to ensure our dogs know this sort of calm behaviour is rewarding.

5 When your dog becomes more familiar with "relaxed means rewards!" you can begin to build up the duration between dropping treats. Adding on a few seconds at a time is reinforcing your dog to be calmer for longer.

6 Over time your dog will begin to enjoy these settled periods and we can start to build up the distractions around little at a time. Have a family member walk past, have a short conversation etc. Remember this has got to be done very gradually to not overwhelm and confuse our dog.

7 Remember we are not going to be saying anything to our dogs, we want the process of settling to be a natural choice for our dogs instead of a taught behaviour with a verbal cue, this way your dogs will settle by themselves without even being asked to!

FIGURE 9.9 Taught behaviours for 'Settle'.

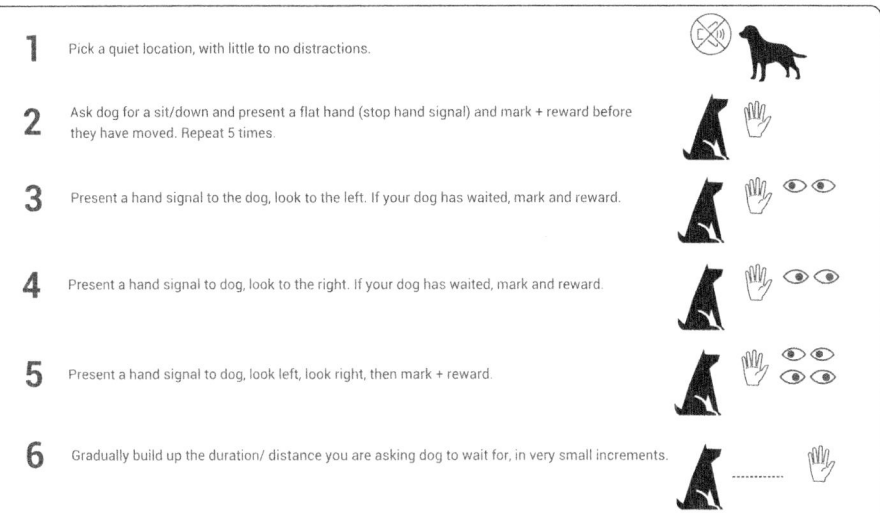

FIGURE 9.10 Taught behaviours for 'Wait/Stay'.

The Power of Play

Whilst training can be done in a playful and rewarding manner, play as an activity by itself is something different and powerful. Play is a natural part of behaviour repertoires of many species and is typically something children and young animals do frequently. Play brings a range of benefits. For example, play releases neurochemicals in the brain which makes play desirable as it helps an individual feel good (e.g., Bekoff, 2018). Play also supports social development, physical development, and cognitive development in both non-human and human infants. As such, it truly is 'the language of childhood' (Van Fleet & Faa-Thompson, 2017, p. 45). But play is not only for youngsters, and like many humans, many dogs remain playful throughout their lives. McConnell (2002, p. 88) describes this tendency to continue to play as adults as 'paedomorphic', and suggests that dogs and humans are amongst the few species to truly demonstrate this capacity into adulthood.

Playful behaviour happens when an animal or person is relaxed and comfortable. Burghardt (2005) identifies five criteria for play activities: play is voluntary, pleasurable, self-rewarding, different from related serious behaviour system, and initiated in benign situations. In short, play is essential for happy, healthy dogs (Glazebrook, 2021), and happy, healthy children.

Dogs will play with other dogs, with people, with other species or by themselves (Bekoff & Pierce, 2019). When dogs play with other dogs, there are rules that they follow, for example, they take turns, self-inhibit, and invite others to play via a 'play bow', as seen in Image 9.10 below which is a type of social contract (Bekoff, 2018). How dogs play with one another is also influenced by how well the dogs know one another, and how frequently they have had opportunities to play in the past. This shows the importance of building understanding, trusting relationships over time.

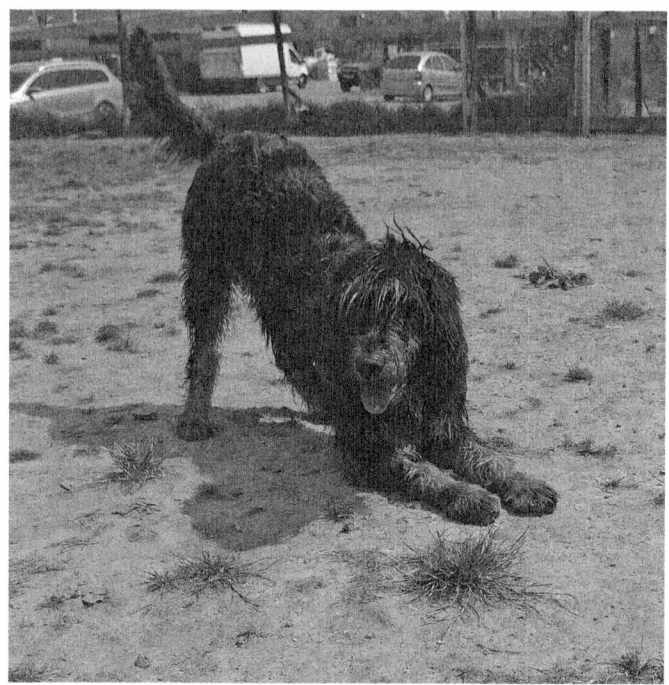

PHOTO 9.2 Obie signals he would like to play by 'play bowing'.

The play relies on a variety of body language and verbal cues and signals. But dogs can also play with other species, which is why they are potentially so well suited to playful learning experiences in schools, if we take time to learn how they are inviting us into the interaction (Photo 9.2).

Practical Ideas for Playful Interaction

Whilst there are times when an interaction between child and dog may take the form of a relaxed, low energy activity (e.g., reading to a gently snoozing dog), if play is so beneficial and intrinsically motivating for both humans and dogs, then incorporating some playful activities into sessions could be valuable for all. Playtime helps child, handler, and dog build a closer bond through teamwork and communication. Some games are a great way to teach the dog and new skills and can help develop impulse control.

Therefore, knowing what excited and enthuses your dog is important. If we know what motivates them, we can develop training and rewards that build on this. Once we know what they enjoy, it is helpful to have a variety of activities that we can use in the school setting to enrich their experiences. Furthermore, knowing the dog well may help decide which games are less suitable. Many herding breeds such as collies will become quickly fixated when playing fetch games, perhaps barking constantly and, jumping up in their eagerness. In this case, scent work or puzzle games might be a better option. There are numerous toys available for dogs, from bacon-flavoured bubbles to cuddly toys in their own image. However, dogs are happy to play with very simple resources. Appendix B includes a series of simple games that children can play with dogs in school, based on ideas from Katie Gardner and Amber Roach, Dog Trainers and Project Officers at Burns By Your Side, Wales. These include ideas for dogs who love to sniff, rip, paw, fetch, and solve problems.

PART 4: WHEN SCHOOL DOGS LEAVE US: ANTICIPATORY LOSS AND GRIEF

There will be times when a CAE will need to end, and this might be for a range of reasons. The planned intervention may reach the end of its timeline, the child may leave the school, or the intended result be achieved. In the case of a visiting dog, the volunteer may leave the organisation or move away. There may be situations where the dog may not enjoy school anymore or might become too old or sick to continue. And sadly, in some cases the dog or handler may die. Indeed, when we compare a human and a dog's lifespan, it becomes painfully apparent that any dog will only be with us for part of our lives. This is difficult to deal with for those of us who love our dogs and can become an additional challenge when the dog is involved in the life of a school, and how to tell children needs to be carefully thought through (Peralta and Fine (2021)). Schneider (2005) describes these as the three goodbyes. They are the decision-making good-bye, the working relationship good-bye, and the good-bye of death. Whatever the goodbye, ending the relationship between a child and a dog (or handler) can be sad and understandably difficult.

Wherever possible, planning and preparation for the transition are crucial. Van Fleet and Faa-Thompson (2017) recommend simple, honest explanations, allowing children time to ask questions. For instance, if the child is going to be leaving the school, planning a celebration to mark the event may help signal the end of this part of their school lives. As well as missing the dog, they may have questions about whether the dog will miss them or whether she will be ok without seeing them. Having mementoes to take with them such as photographs or opportunities to maintain some contact via social media may be an option.

Planning carefully for transition can take many forms. In one primary school that I (HL) worked with, at the end of the school year teachers were very aware that several of the children who had been working with the visiting school dog were feeling sad about the end of the programme. They discussed this with the handler who arranged to visit the local library on a Saturday morning so that the children had the opportunity to maintain contact with the dog. In another secondary school, one young person, Carrie, had worked three times a week with the resident school dog Wilbur. She had formed a close relationship and the teachers had seen improvements in her (previously troubled) behaviour. However, the CAE programme was only scheduled to run for a 12-week period before a new student would have the opportunity. As the twelfth week drew nearer, Carrie's behaviour began to deteriorate. She became withdrawn and was prone to violent outbursts. Her teacher explored this with her, and it soon became apparent that Carrie was upset because she felt that she had a close bond with Wilbur and was feeling upset and jealous about him working with anyone else. The school helped Carrie to develop a series of tasks to support the next child get to know Wilbur, where she could take the lead as the expert in his life, allowing her to develop a sense of self-esteem and also maintain some contact with him. This helped manage the transition period.

Another transition will come if the dog (or indeed handler) reaches an age where they need to retire. It may be possible to phase out involvement over time. Knowing when the time is right will depend on the dog themselves. Roz Rimes (see Chapter 7 for more about Roz's work) knew when her dog Flash was ready for retirement:

> I knew that Flash was ready to retire when, after a visit to a student who lives with complex trauma, he started to shake on the way home in the car. I thought that he had injured his back and took him straight to the Vet. She examined him and found nothing wrong. When it came time for the next trip in the car to see the student Flash started to shake again. I realised he was no longer taking pleasure in these visits. I knew it was time for Flash to enjoy semi-retirement. He continues to enjoy his monthly visits to the University of Melbourne Student Village where the high, playful energy of the mostly international students fills his wellbeing cup. He approaches different ones in turn with a full body wag, his body language communicates that he is having fun and after a snooze on the way home he's back to his playful self.

For Roz, this was a manageable situation as succession planning was something she thought of well in advance. She began 'Live with Zest', with Labradoodle Flash, but welcomed new dog Rafa to the team when Flash was eight years old. This was so that when Flash retired, Rafa would be ready to take over. Recognising that one dog cannot simply replace another, Roz still felt that this was important since many of the young people she works with may have experienced a sense of loss during their life. As they then develop a relationship with the dog, they need time to adjust to the transition that takes place when a dog leaves.

In preparing the young people for the transition to retirement from Flash to Rafa, Roz introduced Rafa in conversation to pique curiosity. She then began to show photos and video footage to enable the young people to start to develop an emotional relationship with Rafa prior to the initial physical introduction. Once Rafa was old enough, he and Flash were working interchangeably, with Flash being gradually withdrawn from the programme. This promoted a smooth transition for the young person.

Roz continues to provide 'news flashes' about Flash enjoying his retirement for her clients, letting them know that he is continuing to run in the park and enjoy his well-earned daytime naps. This approach, where children can see that the dog is happy may be beneficial for them. In other cases, a retired dog may revisit the school for special occasions or may make an appearance via an app or online video call.

However, sometimes the goodbyes are more final. Children and the wider community need support when they face the death of a school dog, whether this be unexpected and sudden, something that has been anticipated as the dog has a diagnosed illness, or ages naturally. If this is sudden, the natural grief that will be felt needs to be acknowledged and processed.

Preparing for loss is never easy, and neither is watching our precious dogs age. As dogs age, just like people they may experience loss of senses, trouble with digestion, muscle loss, incontinence, or even dementia. Certain breeds of dog have shorter life expectancy than others (Figure 9.11), and this is something that might be worth considering when selecting a dog for CAE. Children's story books can be a helpful way to explore feelings of sadness and grief with children.

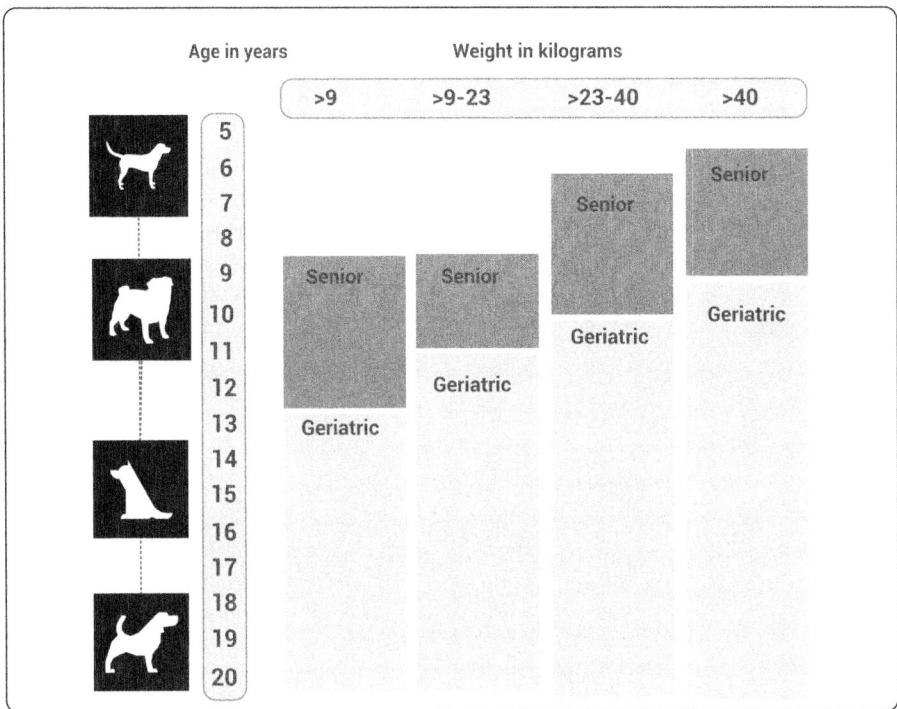

FIGURE 9.11 Life expectancy of dogs related to their weight.

Adapted from Westgarth (2021).

Teachers who involve a dog in their practice will naturally find serious illness or loss of the dog a devastating time. We love our dogs and grieve for them when they die. Individuals may also feel a sense of loss in terms of no longer being able to involve an animal in their practice. This may be amplified by worries over how to support children cope with the situation (Figure 9.12).

How children and young people deal with the loss of a school dog depends on their age, experiences, and levels of attachment to the dog. One study by Schmidt et al. (2020) explored how children of different ages use 'continuing bonds' (CB) to manage their emotions following the loss of a pet. These bonds include fond memories, lessons learned from their deceased pet, belongings/possessions used to feel closer to the deceased pet, continuing connection, being drawn to places associated with the deceased pet, thoughts of being reunited with pet, intrusive memories, reminiscing with others about the deceased pet, creating memorials/shrines or attending special events in memory of the deceased pet, dreams including the pet, talking to deceased pet, and having the deceased pet influence everyday choices and preferences (everyday choices). The researchers found that bonds that promoted greater internalisation, or symbolic representation of the relationship between the bereaved and the deceased, following the loss (e.g., fond memories, reminiscing) may be more beneficial for children. This study also highlights the role of a child's age, attachment to the pet, and level of grief in determining the types of coping/CB used.

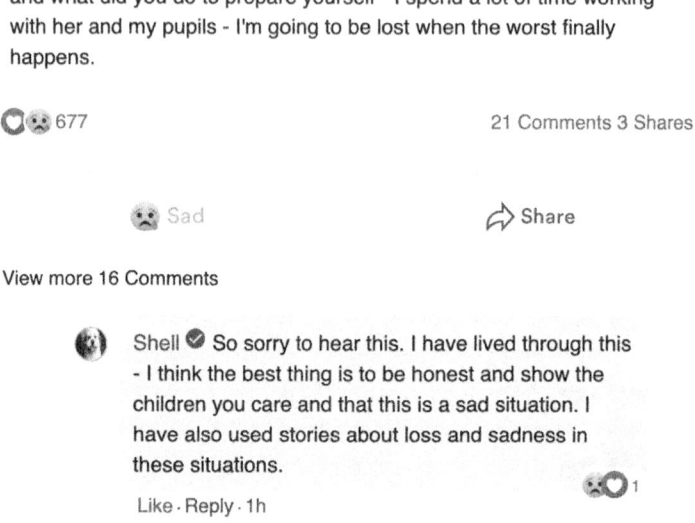

FIGURE 9.12 Social media post relating to school dog bereavement.

In the case of serious illness or aging, children and teachers may experience feelings of anticipatory grief, which is a natural reaction that occurs before the loss of a pet. This can impact negatively on emotions. Animal Hospice and Palliative Care providers such as veterinarians support people experiencing anticipatory grief relating to a pet through:

- recognition and awareness;
- acknowledging, normalizing, and validating feelings;
- providing education;
- redirecting focus – on what they can control = empowering;
- fostering hope – creating a bucket list;
- preparing for pet death – making a plan, alleviating fears;
- encouraging clients in seeking support;
- developing coping strategies;
- referring to a pet loss specialist or mental health professional.

These ideas may be useful for teachers in schools in the situation of needing to prepare or support pupils when the loss of a school dog is experiences or anticipated.[3]

Finally, as we acknowledge the sentience of dogs, we must also recognise that they themselves may experience grief. Many animals display grief at the loss or absence of a close friend or loved one (e.g., Bekoff, 2000). For example, McConnell (2002) talks of Goldie the dog, who, after the death of the family's young son would wait at the door for him. After several hours, Goldie would lie down and refuse walks or food. This behaviour continued for several months. Although this is an area needing more research, it is likely that some dogs will experience grief at the loss of a loved one, be they human or non-human. This may be demonstrated in changes to behaviour such as hiding, a change in appetite, sudden signs of aggression or irritability, and anxious reactions to their normal routine. Recognising this and allowing the dog time to heal is also important.

CONCLUSION

We conclude that it is ethically appropriate to bring a dog into school, provided we consider the experience through their eyes and meet the preconditions discussed in Chapter 3. To ensure that interactions with dogs are safe and meaningful, it is key for children and adults to be taught how to interpret canine communication. It is also important for children and dogs to derive enjoyment from such interactions, and this can be promoted through playful learning experiences. At times, unfortunately, schools will face the difficult task of explaining the loss of a dog. We have discussed various ways in which such loss, either through death, retirement, or other reasons, can be best managed. An essential element of effective CAE is reflecting continually on whether children and dogs are benefiting from their time together. Hence, the final chapter considers how schools can research and evaluate the impact of dog-assisted interventions.

NOTES

1   https://schoolleaders.thekeysupport.com/administration-and-management/risk/premises-risk-assessments/dogs-in-school/
2   https://pawsandreward.com/connectionprinciples/
3   Dickie, E. (n.d.). The Grief Journey that starts before the loss: Anticipatory Grief. https://www.aplb.org/anticipatory-grief/

REFERENCES

Albuquerque, N., Guo, K., Wilkinson, A., Resende, B., & Mills, D. S. (2018). Mouth-licking by dogs as a response to emotional stimuli. *Behavioural Processes*, *146*, 42–45.

Bekoff, M. (2018). Secrets of the snout: A dog's nose is a work of art. *Psychology Today*, 6 April.

Bekoff, M. (2022). Time to stop pretending we don't know other animals are sentient beings. *Animal Sentience*, *31*(2). https://doi.org/10.51291/2377-7478.1699

Bekoff, M., & Pierce, J. (2019). *Unleashing your dog: A field guide to giving your canine companion the Best life possible*. New World Library.

Burghardt, G. (2005). *The genesis of animal play: Testing the limits*. Massachusetts Institute of Technology.

Clothier, S. (2014). Presentation for the Reflected Relationship seminar. 23 September, St Johnsville.

Coren, S. (2023). Talk nicely when training dogs: It makes a difference. *Psychology Today*. 22 March, https://www.psychologytoday.com/gb/blog/canine-corner/202303/talk-nicely-when-training-dogs-it-makes-a-difference

Duranton, C., & Gaunet, F. (2018). Behavioral synchronization and affiliation: Dogs exhibit human-like skills. *Learning Behaviour*, 46, 364–373. https://doi.org/10.3758/s13420-018-0323-4

Fenzi, D. (2016). *Train the dog in front of you*. Fenzi Dog Sports Academy Publishing.

Fine, A. H. (2020).

Fournier, A., Berry, T., Letson, E., & Chanen, R. (2016). The human–animal interaction scale: Development and evaluation. *Anthrozoös*, 29(3), 455–467. https://doi.org/10.1080/08927936.2016.1181372

Glazebrook, L. (2021). *The book your dog wishes you would read*. Orion Spring.

Heimlich, K. (2001). Animal-assisted therapy and the severely disabled child: A quantitative study. *Journal of Rehabilitation*, 67(4), 48–54. https://www.proquest.com/scholarly-journals/animal-assisted-therapy-severely-disabled-child/docview/236288875/se-2

Horowitz, A. (2010). *Inside of a Dog: What Dogs See, Smell, and Know*. Scribner Book Company.

Karl, S., & Huber, L. (2017). Empathy in dogs: With a little help from a friend – A mixed blessing. *Animal Sentience*, 14(13), 1–4.

Lewis, H., and Oostendorp-Godfrey, J. (2023). Research Exploring Interactions Between Children, Dogs, and Handlers in School Settings. *Proceedings of the 2023 Animal Assisted Play Therapy Conference* [online].

Lewis, H., & Grigg, R. (2021). *Tails from the classroom. Learning and teaching through animal-assisted interventions*. Crown House.

Lewis, H., Grigg, R., & Knight, C. (2022). An international survey of animals in schools: Exploring what sorts of schools involve what sorts of animals, and educators' rationales for these practices. *People and Animals: The International Journal of Research and Practice*, 5(1), Article 15. https://docs.lib.purdue.edu/paij/vol5/iss1/15

Machová, K., Juríčková, V., Nekovářová, T., & Svobodová, I. (2020). Validation of the human-animal interaction scale (HAIS). *International Journal of Environmental Research and Public Health*, 17(20), 7485. https://doi.org/10.3390/ijerph17207485

MacNamara, M., & MacLean, E. (2017). Selecting animals for education environments. In N. R. Gee, A. H. Fine, & P. McCardle (Eds.), *How animals help students learn* (pp. 182–196). Routledge.

Martin, K., & Martin, D. (2016) Canine socialization: More than meets the eye *American Veterinarian*, 1(3). https://www.dvm360.com/view/canine-socialization-more-than-meets-the-eye

McEvoy, V., Espinosa, U.B., Crump, A., & Arnott, G. (2022). Canine Socialisation: A Narrative Systematic Review. *Animals*. 12(21):2895. https://doi.org/10.3390/ani12212895.

McConnell, P. B. (2002). *The other end of the leash: Why we do what we do around dogs*. Ballantine Books.

Meints, K., Syrnyk, C., & De Keuster, T. (2010). Why do children get bitten in the face? *Injury Prevention*, 16(Suppl. 1), A172–A173.

Ng, Z., Morse, L., Albright, J., Viera, A., & Souza, M. (2019). Describing the use of animals in animal-assisted intervention research. *Journal of Applied Animal Welfare Science*, 22(4), 364–376.

Pelar, C. (2013). *Living with Kids and Dogs...Without Losing your Mind*. Dream Dog Productions.

Peralta, J., & Fine, A. (2021). The welfare of Animals in Animal-Assisted Interventions: Foundations and Best Practice Methods. Springer. to refs here and main refs.

Pierce, J. (2016). *Run, spot, run*. University of Chicago Press.

Schmidt, M., Naylor, P., Cohen, D., Gomez, R., Moses, J. Jr, Rappoport, M., & Packman, W. (2020). Pet loss and continuing bonds in children and adolescents. *Death Studies*, 44(5), 278–284. https://doi.org/10.1080/07481187.2018.1541942

Schneider, K. S. (2005). Practice report: The winding valley of grief: When a dog guide retires or dies. *Journal of Visual Impairment & Blindness*, 99(6), 368–370.

Shepherd, K. (2002). Development of behaviour, social behaviour and communication in dogs. *BSAVA Manual of Canine and Feline Behavioural Medicine*, 8–20.

Siniscalchi, M., d'Ingeo, S., Minunno, M., & Quaranta, A. (2018). Communication in dogs. *Animals*, *8*(8), 131. https://doi.org/10.3390/ani8080131

Steel, J. (2023). Reading to Dogs in schools: A controlled feasibility study of an online Reading to Dogs intervention. *International Journal of Educational Research*, *117*, 102117, https://doi.org/10.1016/j.ijer.2022.102117.

Tedeschi, P., & Jenkins, M.A. (2019). *Transforming Trauma: Resilience and Healing Through Our Connections With Animals Connections With Animals*. Purdue University Press.

Van Fleet, R., & Faa-Thompson, T. (2017). *Animal assisted play therapy*. Professional Resource Press.

von Uexküll, J. (1934). A stroll through the worlds of animals and men: A picture book of invisible worlds. *Semiotica*, 89–4, 1992, 319–391.

Westgarth, C. (2021). *The Happy Dog Owner*. Wellbeck Publishing.

CHAPTER 10

RESEARCHING AND EVALUATING IMPACT

Over recent decades the concept of impact has gained considerable attention in education as policymakers and schools themselves want to know whether interventions are worthwhile. This chapter focuses on what impact means in relation to CAE. It describes the various ways in which researchers aim to collect data and evaluate the outcomes of such interventions.

THE MEANING OF IMPACT

The word impact is derived from Latin (*impactus*) and, as a verb, it originally meant the effect of pressing one thing against another. In education, this means understanding the impact of interventions primarily on children and young people, as potentially the most significant beneficiaries. As Chapter 2 noted, most of the literature has focused on how dog-assisted interventions have impacted children's reading, the ways in which dogs have been used to support children with specific social or communication difficulties, and more generally how they have contributed towards improved aspects of children's well-being. In our survey of more than 600 educators in 23 countries, we found that the overriding reason for involving animals in educational settings is the perception that they make an important contribution to children's well-being (Lewis et al., 2022).

Less attention has been given to how dog-assisted interventions impact teachers' own well-being, their approaches to pedagogy, or the wider school ethos. Similarly, we have little evidence of the impact such programmes have on dog handlers and the wider community, nor the feelings of children who are *not* selected to participate in such programmes (Figure 10.1).

THEORY OF CHANGE

Any intervention in education should be accompanied by a clearly articulated rationale. Many organisations use a Theory of Change (TOC) to explain why they are introducing an intervention, what change (impact) they anticipate, and how this will happen (activities). A full TOC also includes the assumptions underpinning the intervention and the factors (enablers) needed to be present or absent for the goal to be achieved (Figure 10.2). Often, a logic model accompanies a TOC, setting out more narrowly what needs to be done to implement the change.

A TOC is typically represented as a flow chart or diagram, showing a causal chain of outcomes from an initial needs assessment to realising the long-term goal. The process begins by identifying key stakeholders and their needs. In the case of a Reading to Dogs programme, pupils, parents, dogs, dog handlers, and teachers are all key stakeholders. But to illustrate the process, let us consider the children as the primary stakeholder. Suppose a school identifies a group of six children who are struggling

DOI: 10.4324/9781003257073-14

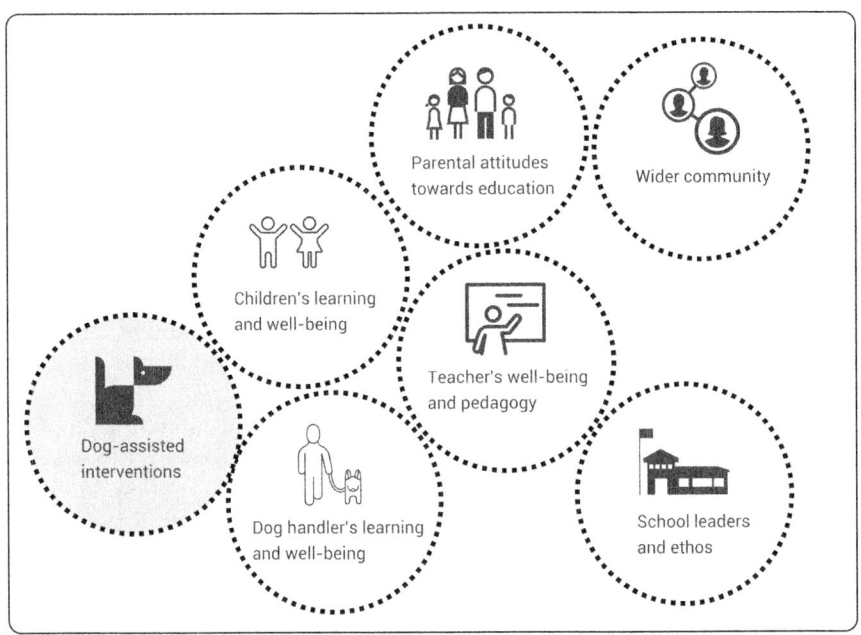

FIGURE 10.1 Dog-assisted interventions and potential impact on different audiences.

to read and who are well behind where they should be in terms of their reading development. Teachers might prioritise ways of increasing children's reading motivation, confidence, and enjoyment, which are commonly seen as predictors of reading attainment. The long-term changes could be for children to read for pleasure, to engage in reading daily, and to become competent readers at a level appropriate to their age.

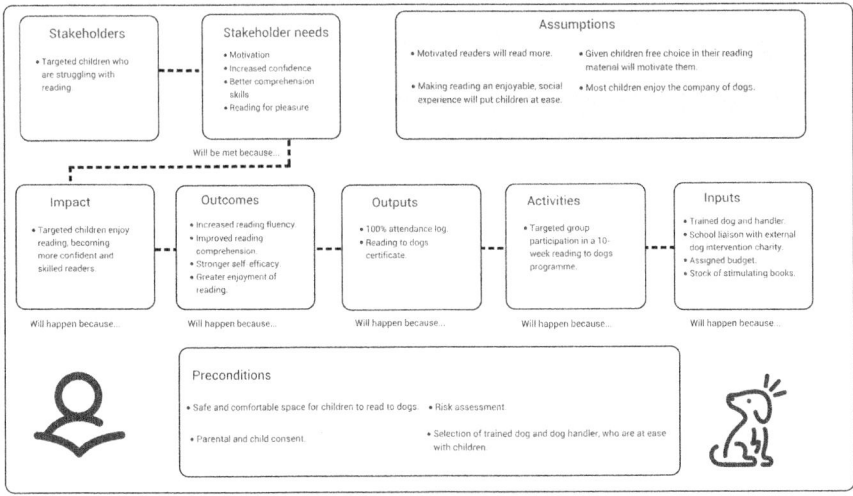

FIGURE 10.2 Theory of change for reading to dogs programme.

Working backwards from these end results, the school can show visually what needs to be done through a sequential change of events. The long-term goal depends upon achieving short-term behavioural changes (outcomes). For example, an increase in the group's enthusiasm for reading, extended attention spans, a richer range of vocabulary, higher level of self-confidence, reduced anxiety, or a greater inclination to share their views about reading.

Whereas outcomes are concerned with behavioural changes in pupils' knowledge, skills, and attitudes, outputs are tangible, countable things. The outputs from a Reading to Dogs programme might be a simple reading certificate awarded to participants or a log of what each child has read during the session, including such details as the date, title of the text, number of pages read, any reading strategies observed, reading time, and frequency of dog.

Outputs arise directly from the activities. The pattern for Reading to Dogs programmes might be as follows: An individual or small group of children read to a dog for say 30 or so minutes in the presence of the dog handler. Where research is being conducted, then the activities of the researcher can also constitute outputs such as a running observational record, reflective diary, or an audio or visual recording. Videotape analysis, for example, can focus on signs indicating children's nervousness such as throat clearing, coughing, jiggling the foot or leg, and playing with or fiddling with objects (London, 2021).

Before activities can begin, certain preconditions should be met as noted in Chapter 3. From a researcher's perspective, the overriding consideration is to ensure that any research is conducted ethically and in line with appropriate guidelines (e.g., APA, 2017; BERA, 2018). This means exercising responsibilities to the participants, for example in gaining assent, being transparent, and ensuring they have a right to withdraw. Information sheets and parental consent forms are standard practice (Figure 10.3 and 10.4). They include such details as the purpose of the research, what is expected of any volunteers, and what happens to the data.

Such consideration should apply equally to dogs as well as humans, which means that researchers need to prepare carefully to ensure that they do not put excessive demands on the dogs, for example, in terms of time indoors without a break. It is also important to ensure that children are taught to recognise signals from dogs that indicate that they are uncomfortable or in some form of distress. In such circumstances, research activity should end at any point that the participants appear to be suffering. It is standard practice to anonymise data and ensure that it is not traceable back to the school, although there are occasions when teachers and schools as participants want to be named, for example, to raise awareness of their research profiles.

Procedural aspects are important to ensure that any intervention is implemented as intended and that the well-being of all is kept to the fore. Attention to detail matters. For instance, thought should be given to when best to introduce a dog and its handler into school or when a researcher should visit. Most reputable dog-assisted programmes ensure that their dog handler visits the school without the dog to plan and agree upon logistical issues, conduct a risk assessment, and agree with the teacher the programme objectives. From the perspective of a visiting researcher, there is also much to be said for a preliminary visit to learn about the school context and explain to the children in age-appropriate ways what the researcher will be doing (e.g., 'I will be looking at how the dog responds to you'). This is also a good opportunity to address any concerns and set out rules for interacting with dogs.

Pen Llech Primary School
School Dog Information Sheet

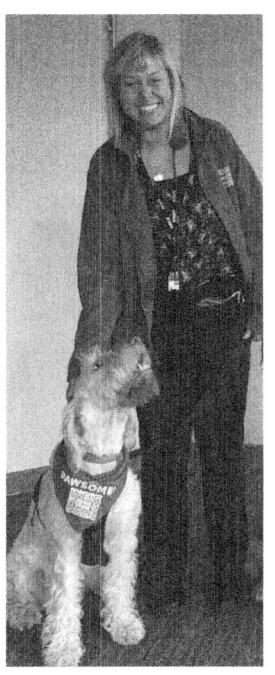

In July 2023 the Governors of Pen Llech Primary School approved the involvement of school dogs for the purpose of supporting children's learning and well-being. All dogs must be trained and fully vaccinated.

School dogs are known to bring many benefits, particularly in the area of well-being. For example, they provide emotional support, reduce anxiety, and make reading enjoyable. They are also known to help children socialise, take responsibilities and show compassion for others.

Our first dog is Carlo, a two-year-old Spinone. He has a sociable, docile, and a very patient nature. He enjoys playing with squeaky toys and loves biscuits.

The designated contact for this project is Mrs Lewis, who is an experienced dog handler. She will teach the children how to interact safely with dogs. Mrs Lewis is happy to discuss any particular questions or concerns. She can be contacted on 01234 456789.

Carlo will visit Pen Llech Primary School every Monday and Wednesday in the Autumn Term. He will be in school between 9.15 and 11am, and will be based in the Well-being space.

He will work with some selected individual pupils, or small groups for up to 20 minutes at a time. He will also attend some assemblies and wallk in the playground during morning break. He will always be with Mrs Lewis.

There will be an introductory meeting for all parents on Monday 8th September at 3.30pm in the hall. Please come along to find out more about this project, and to meet Carlo.

Last Updated: September 2023.

FIGURE 10.3 Example of Parents' Information Form.

It should be possible with a well-designed TOC to trace a connection back from the long-term goal to the short-term outcomes, outputs, activities, preconditions, and the inputs that are needed at the outset. Inputs for dog assisted interventions obviously include the programme itself delivered by a suitably trained dog and its handler, a dedicated space, and targeted pupils.

School Dog Consent Form

Pen Llech Primary School
September 2023

Dear Parent/Guardian

We will soon welcome Carlo, a specially trained dog, as part of our school community.

Carlo is a two-year-old Spinone, an Italian breed known for their sociable, docile, and patient nature. He has received all necessary vaccinations and training.

School dogs are known to bring many benefits, particularly in the area of well-being. For example, they provide emotional support, reduce anxiety, and help make reading enjoyable. Our School Information Sheet provides more details.

Carlo will always be accompanied by Mrs Lewis, who is an experienced dog handler. She will also teach the children how to interact safely with dogs. Mrs Lewis is happy to discuss any particular questions or concerns. She can be contacted on 01234 456789.

If you would prefer that your child does not interact with Carlo, please sign and return the slip below to the school. Please also inform Mrs Lewis if your child has any known allergies or animal phobias.

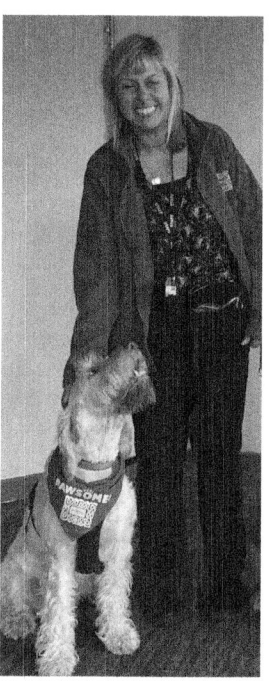

I prefer that...[insert child's name]
does not participate in the school dog programme.

Signed: Date:

FIGURE 10.4 Example of a Parents' Consent Form.

In conducting research into the efficacy of a dog-assisted intervention, the researcher should establish selection or inclusion criteria for the sample. For example, Friedrich (2019) identified nine special education needs teachers (and one child study team member from the local district) in her doctoral study exploring the role of AAIs in supporting the communication skills of children with autism.

The teachers were required to have implemented AAI programmes in their class-rooms for a minimum of one day a week or one day every two weeks. Criteria should also apply to children who agree to participate in research. In all cases, for instance, no child should be included who has a known allergy to the coat of dogs or fears dogs.

A TOC can help visualise what an intervention is aiming to achieve and guide its subsequent evaluation. It originated as a form of programme evaluation within complex community initiatives where it was easy to lose track of the small changes needed to accomplish bigger goals. Similarly, in the busy environment of schools, it can be difficult to isolate the factors that make a significant difference to children's learning, which is why evaluative research is so important. This is particularly so in the case of dog-assisted interventions which attract considerable media hype.

CAUSES AND CORRELATIONS

'Reading to a dog leads to more improvement than reading to a person', so declared a headline in a popular psychology magazine (Coren, 2022). Media headlines often represent simple cause-and-effect arguments, which satisfy readers who do not have the time or inclination to engage in nuanced academic debate. Such reporting also reflects how the concept of cause-and-effect is rooted in society. The word 'because' is one of the most frequently used in the English language and shapes how we think about the world.

Yet, few experienced educational researchers use the concept of causation faced with interpreting the complex realities of classroom life. They prefer terms such as 'independent variable', 'treatment variable', or 'antecedent' (Punch, 2009). Often, in terms of changes in children's behaviour, there is more than one cause at work in any single effect, just as there may be more than one effect from a single cause. As Cohen et al. (2011, p. 55) point out, 'causation in the human sciences is much more tentative and may be probabilistic rather than deterministic.' Stern et al. (2012) offer a useful reminder that most interventions prove to be 'contributory causes', which work in tandem with other 'helping factors' such as related programmes and pol-icies, alongside cultural and social forces. They point out that the key question to keep in mind is: 'Did the intervention make a difference'? rather than 'Did the inter-vention work'? because this allows space to consider the impact of the intervention and other factors.

Many studies report correlations or associations between dog-assisted interven-tions and children's learning. A correlation is simply an association between two variables. Causes and correlations should not be confused. When thirteenth-century Prince Llewlyn the Great returned home to find his baby son missing and Gelert his favourite hound dripping with blood, he naturally connected the two events. In a rage, Llewelyn slayed his dog, but his conclusion that Gelert had caused the death of his son was wrong. There was a correlation, however. Gelert had saved the baby by killing an intruding wolf, whose body Llewelyn later found alongside his son, alive and well under an upturned cradle.

Correlations are concerned with mutual relations. Whenever one variable changes, the other is likely to also change. For example, Uccheddu et al. (2019) report that children's attendance was significantly higher (100%) on days when they read to dogs compared to 'no-dog' days (75%). But, of course, this is not the same as claiming that the dogs' presence in school was the cause of the children's improved attendance. Other factors not discussed by the authors may have accounted for differences in attendance, such as wider school incentives, home appointments, or illness. In fact, it was only during the final two days of the 10-day programme that the difference in attendance was statistically significant. Moreover, although the children in the study were randomly assigned to the experimental ($n = 5$) and control ($n = 4$) groups, the total sample size was very small ($n = 9$). This meant that one child's absence from the control group equated to 25% of the total attendance. The bottom line is that the children's attendance may have been high with or without the presence of dogs.

To say with confidence that a dog's presence is associated with improvements in any aspect of a child's learning or well-being requires three conditions to be met. First, the researcher needs to prove that a correlation exists between the dog (predictor) and the outcome (e.g., improved attendance, reading fluency, reduced anxiety, increased self-confidence). Second, the introduction of the animal must precede the outcome. And finally, there can be no plausible alternative explanation for the outcome.

Connor and Herzog (2017) suggest how to meet these three conditions. First, researchers need to ask questions that are answerable. They cite two simple examples: 'Does the presence of service dogs reduce school absences for the target student'? and 'does the number of classroom disruptions change when the dog is present'? These kinds of questions can be answered through pre-and post-test data using measures such as the number of days absent, notwithstanding earlier comments about attendance, and the total minutes of disruptive behaviour observed. Second, a longitudinal design needs to be adopted so that the predictor precedes the outcome and that repeated observations of the same variables can be secured. Most longitudinal studies usually last at least a year (in some cases several decades) although there is no reason why these cannot be conducted over a shorter period. And the third condition is met when the research methodology ensures that no other more plausible explanations exist for the causal inference. Counterfactual thinking helps here. The counterfactual position is to ask whether something would have happened without the intervention, which is why experimental researchers use randomisation and control groups who are not exposed to the intervention.

RANDOMISED CONTROL TRIALS (RCTS) AND QUASI-EXPERIMENTAL STUDIES

The gold standard of scientific research is the use of randomised control trials (RCTs). These involve the random assignment of individuals to one of two groups: one (the experimental group) receives the intervention that is being tested and a control group receives a conventional treatment (Figure 10.5). Hence children participating in an AAI would form the experimental group and their peers join a control group. Over recent decades, steps have been taken to introduce RCTS into educational settings (Hutchinson & Styles, 2010; Styles & Torgerson, 2018). Most other approaches are seen as susceptible to selection bias, which means that it is difficult to say whether the outcomes are due to the dog-assisted intervention or the selection characteristics.

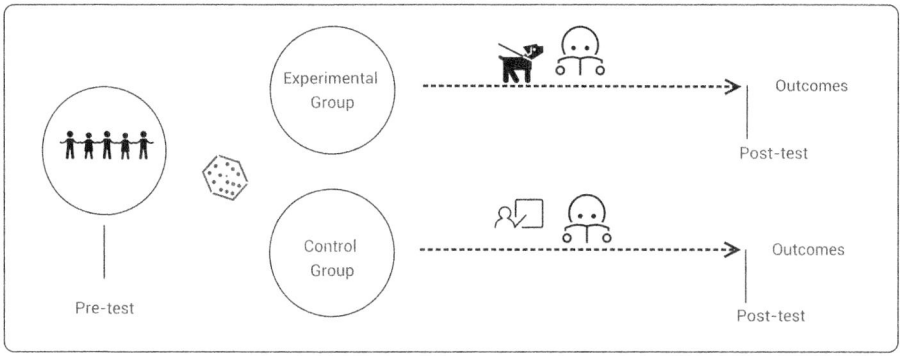

FIGURE 10.5 The design of a randomised control trial.

Pre-tests are recommended before randomisation because if it occurs after randomisation, then knowledge of the group may influence the pre-test scores. The post-test represents the outcome measure and reveals whether the intervention has had a significant impact or not on children's achievement or well-being. Such tests should be administered under the same examination conditions, with the children's answers anonymised to alleviate markers' conscious or unconscious bias.

Of course, schools are not scientific laboratories, and much of the research which takes place inside classrooms is descriptive rather than experimental by nature. In any event, the appropriateness of RCTs in evaluating the impact of AAIs has been questioned (Signal et al., 2017). RCTs deal with large sample sizes whereas AAIs are typically associated with individuals or small groups. Critics raise what they perceive as ethical issues associated with RCTs in education (e.g., 'Should not all children be exposed to potential benefits?'), while highlighting the excessive demands in terms of time and expense. Hutchinson and Styles (2010) counter this pointing out that in educational research, we rarely know something works in advance and invite readers to 'contrast randomisation with the cost (both monetary and educationally) of rolling out an untested intervention' (Hutchinson & Styles, 2010, p. 5).

Given the debate around RCTs, quasi-experimental design is often used as a kind of compromise (Figure 10.6). The aim remains to draw causal inferences about

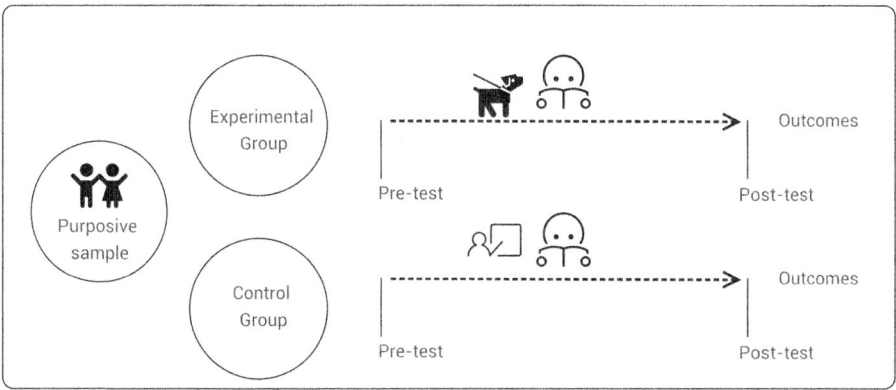

FIGURE 10.6 A quasi-experimental design.

change over time using post-tests, but without the random assignment of subjects necessary for true experimentation. This means that the treatment and control groups may not be comparable at baseline. Quasi-experimental design has featured in a wide range of contexts, including the role of AAIs in supporting children who have experienced sexual abuse (Signal et al., 2017), young offenders given the opportunity to train a dog (Duindam et al., 2021), and attempts to reduce the anxiety of hospitalised children through the visit of a therapy dog and a trained handler (Hinic et al., 2019).

Quasi-experimental studies often involve purposive sampling. As the name suggests, purposive sampling is a matter of choosing participants whose characteristics suit a specific purpose and likely to produce the most relevant and complete data. For example, schools which use Reading to Dogs programmes typically select children who they think might benefit from such an intervention to boost their reading confidence or skills. Purposive sampling is deliberately selective and biased towards meeting the researcher's needs and makes no claim for representing the wider population.

In such quasi-experimental research design, it is essential to be clear about the conditions. A researcher in the treatment ('dog') and control ('non dog') groups should follow the same basic protocols. In one research study, the same researcher brought the children to the reading spaces, observed and documented the interactions between the children and dog, offered praise irrespective of their reading performance, and returned them back to the classroom (Wohlfarth et al., 2014). In the treatment group, the dog handler only introduced the dog to the children whereas in the control group, she sat close to each child on a shared floor cushion, invited the child to read the text to her, and verbally praised the reading performance. The researcher observed behaviour by using a stopwatch to time the children's attentiveness to the dog handler in the control group (measured by face-to-face encounters) and their body contact (e.g., petting) with the dog in the treatment group.

The authors used a cross-over design. This meant that the 24 children were randomly assigned to two groups (12 each). Group 1 first read the text to the dog and, in another session, a second text to the dog handler (without the dog). The conditions were swapped for Group 2, who read the first text to the dog handler and the second text to the dog (Figure 10.7). The texts were validated for comparability by language teachers who judged their qualitative (e.g., level of meaning) and quantitative

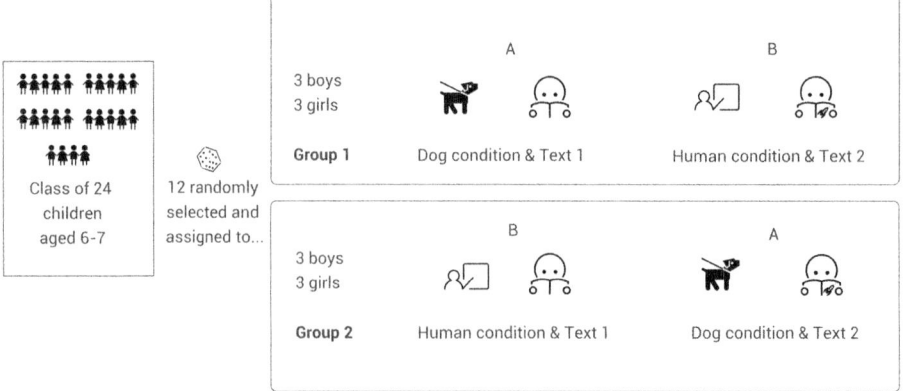

FIGURE 10.7 An example of a cross-over research design (Wohlfarth et al., 2014, p. 64).

features (e.g., number of words), while a separate group of children read the text so the researchers could assess minimum reading time. The assessment showed that both texts were similar in terms of the required reading skills.

Approaches to Research

Attitudes, beliefs, values, previous experiences, and assumptions all shape how an individual approaches research. There are four main worldviews or paradigms that characterise the assumptions we hold about the nature of reality. First, positivism describes the traditional scientific view that objective knowledge can be exactly determined through reason, logic and careful observation rather than intuition. Those who adopt this view prefer an experimental approach to researching dog-assisted interventions. For example, if their focus is measuring impact on children's reading attainment, they will establish a baseline using standardised tests and employ control groups. In contrast, there are researchers who are more interested in interactions, say between teachers and children, or children and dogs. They do not see research as a matter of uncovering indisputable facts. Rather, they recognise that participants provide them with subjective interpretations, which they then reinterpret in the research process. An interpretivist view emphasises the individual experience of reading to dogs, which differs from one participant to the other. Interviews and case studies are seen as more appropriate means of finding out the rich details of what individuals feel and think about dogs. Interpretivists are interested in telling stories and the purists among them reject the notion of exploratory inquiries too concerned with reaching generalised conclusions. As Gilbert (2008) points out, the distinctions between positivists and interpretivists are more of a caricature because many researchers take a more nuanced view and are willing to see the value in a variety of research.

Hence, the appeal of the paradigm of pragmatism, which moves away from binaries (e.g., objective vs. subjective) to accept the evolving nature of reality. Pragmatists adopt a mix of methods to suit whatever research project they are pursuing rather than be weighed down by philosophical concerns. A fourth paradigm sees the world through a critical realist lens and questions the conventional knowledge, assumptions, and underlying structures that have the potential to produce inequalities, social oppression, and alienation. Critical theory is particularly concerned with concepts of gender, race, class, and power and how these operate in the world. Adopting a critical realist perspective would thus mean exploring the relationships between 'real' objects (e.g., the child, dog, teacher, and dog handler) and contextual factors (e.g., the dog behaviours and the school setting) to identify forces that shape how children and dogs behave. Many Reading to Dogs programmes are carefully designed but like all interventions, their implementation is mediated by individuals who bring their own experiences and subjectivity to the context. Critical theory also recognises the importance of dogs as key actors in the social world. Pawson et al. (2005) offer a useful mantra to keep in mind, 'What works, for whom, and in what circumstances?'

METHODS OF COLLECTING DATA

There are various methods that can be used to gather data to inform an evaluation of dog-assisted interventions. The choice depends upon factors such as the project objectives, time, and other resources available and who and what is being evaluated. A researcher may want to find out the impact of the intervention in terms of 'hard' measurable outcomes such as children's reading scores, their levels of physical exertion, or physiological changes. For example, assessments of children's physical well-being while interacting with a dog are likely to require the use of timed exercises and measures of cardiovascular activity at different points – typically, before, during and after the activities. To measure something a researcher needs to know what has changed numerically over time.

BASELINE DATA

Baseline data describe what is known about the current situation before the start of the intervention, for example, pupils' attainment in reading, their attendance record, psychological or emotional state, social skills, and confidence levels. In programmes which involve reading to dogs, for instance, it is important to establish the children's reading attainment levels and attitudes to reading using standardised tests such as Neale Analysis of Reading Ability (NARA), or Elementary Reading Attitudes Scale (ERAS). Case studies (e.g., Fisher & Cozens, 2014), which have done so have shown gains in the scores of children who participated in a reading to dogs' scheme. But there are few studies which have established a baseline for reading performance of both those children who participated in a reading to dogs' programme and a control group who did not (see Hall et al., 2016). Post-tests are also needed for comparison of data, and to show what progress has been made during the intervention.

Some researchers have measured children's physiological responses (blood pressure) when they were with a dog and engaging in reading and when they were resting, compared to when they were not with a dog and reading and resting. Friedmann et al. (1983) pioneered such research and found that children's blood pressure was reduced while reading to a dog and when they were resting. However, Hall et al.'s (2016) review of the recent literature, which features physiological indicators, shows a lack of agreement over whether dogs have a calming or excitatory effect on children, or no effect.

Baseline data are not exclusively numerical (quantitative) in nature. It can be qualitative or a combination of both. The key point is that whatever data is collected, it must be appropriate for measuring changes with respect to the goals of the intervention. Qualitative baseline data might include semi-structured interviews with the teacher or children ahead of the dog arriving in school to gauge their knowledge of and interest in dogs, and attitudes towards the intervention.

OBSERVATIONS

Many studies gather data as it happens through observations, which is more than just looking. Observation allows for the systematic capture of 'live' data from naturally occurring situations (Cohen et al., 2017). This means that the researcher does not need to rely on second-hand accounts and can use observation as a means of validating what people might say they do. Dog handlers and teachers may say that the children enjoyed interacting with the dog, or that the dog settled easily during a session, and observations may or may not provide data that concurs with these views.

In terms of what to observe during dog-assisted interventions, there are facts that can be immediately noted such as the number of participants, the location, the time, and the duration. There are also events that can be recorded, such as the number of times a child pets or stares at the dog, the duration of their eye contact, or the amount of talk by adults. And then there are qualities or behaviours that can be observed; for example, the degree of friendliness exhibited by the dog handler, the body language of the child or children when the dog first enters the room, or the turn-taking exhibited by children if observing a group.

The observer's role and degree of participation can vary from being completely independent, almost unnoticed by the children being observed, to being completely involved as a participant, adopting an 'insider' view and working alongside the children. Teachers as observers may find that they naturally adopt a mid-way position in which they contribute comments occasionally. The challenge from a research perspective is ensuring that the subjects or situations are not manipulated by the observer. Schedules or checklists can help identify focal points and chart anticipated incidence or frequencies of behaviour. Such structured observations enable the researcher to gather numerical data in a systematic manner.

But observers bring their own bias and beliefs to the experience, which can compromise the reliability of the observation. Unless observers are highly trained, the likelihood is that they will focus on different things and particularly those that they want to see. Two observers may interpret the same observed behaviour differently, such as a dog wagging its tail as a child brushes its coat. Moreover, it is difficult for observations to capture feelings of affection or anxiety associated with dog-assisted interventions. This calls for other techniques such as interviews with participants.

Another drawback associated with observations is that the act of observation inevitably distorts the phenomenon. If subjects know that they are being observed, their behaviour will be different to when they are not observed. This could be countered by conducting covert observations, but this raises separate ethical issues around consent. Gilbert (2008) compares such actions to a doctor carrying out an experiment on patients without their agreement. Where an observer is positioned and the choice of observer (e.g., whether they are familiar with the subjects) can also influence the nature of the observation. Despite these reservations, observations can prove very insightful particularly if there is a clear focus. For example, whether the dog's presence is calming or exciting, if the dog's mood changes, how children talk to the dog, the kind of social interaction that the dog facilitates, or whether the act of touching a dog affects a child's reading.

STRUCTURED INTERVIEWS AND FOCUS GROUPS

Structured interviews can vary in format and the degree of formality. Most researchers create questions to guide the discussion. Schedules typically include prompts arranged in sections. For example, if interviewing school leaders about their reading to dogs programmes, section topics might cover logistical issues (e.g., when the programme started, how many children have participated, how children are selected), why the programme was adopted, the management of the programme, perceived benefits and challenges, and the nature of the interactions (e.g., role of the adult and tasks).

Focus groups are discussions with individuals (4–10) who meet together either in-person or online, to express their views on particular subjects defined by the researcher. The discussion is guided either by the researcher acting as a facilitator or an independent moderator whose level of involvement can vary, depending upon their own experience, the objectives, group composition, and stage of the project. If the researcher is intent on gaining the views of the participants on precise topics, then the style of facilitation may warrant a high degree of direction and structure to retain focus. On the other hand, a more open-ended and self-managed discussion might be appropriate if the researchers want participants to develop their own views on a subject, perhaps in areas that have not previously been discussed. In such cases, the facilitator's role might be limited to introducing the subject, keeping the conversation flowing and ensuring that all have the opportunity to have a say.

Teachers are familiar with conducted group discussions with their pupils. In relating to dog-assisted interventions, sometimes these discussions are most insightful when children are asked broad questions such as 'How do you feel when you hear that a dog is coming to visit?'

SURVEYS AND QUESTIONNAIRES

Surveys and questionnaires are also widely used to describe and interpret the impact of dog-assisted interventions. Surveys describe the content, method, and means of analysis (e.g., use of computer software), whereas questionnaires relate only to the questions respondents are asked to answer. Surveys vary in format, characteristics, complexity, and how they are administered. The data generated typically enable researchers to manipulate variables to derive frequencies (e.g., 'How many times does a child pet a dog during a session?'), detect patterns (e.g., 'Does this vary depending on the breed of dog?'), and ascertain whether exist correlations exists between gender and responses (e.g., 'How do boys and girls compare in their view of dog-assisted interventions?'). Attention needs to be given to the sample if the intention is to draw conclusions on wider applicability. More generally, it is worth bearing in mind that respondents to dog surveys predominantly hold positive perception of dogs which limits generalisation.

Survey design begins with understanding its purpose and targeted audience. For example, Morrow (2009) wanted to know what school counsellors thought about AAIs in their practice. Her purpose was to help aspiring practitioners create an implementation plan that addresses the challenges and promotes the reported benefits of AAIs. To collect responses, she used the Pet Attitude Scale Modified (PAS-M), which measures attitudes towards animals and distributed this online to a sample of 220 public school counsellors. The mode of distributing surveys should be considered. In-person and telephone surveys can be time-consuming but allow the facilitator to answer any questions on the spot. Online surveys are convenient, low cost, and save time since data are automatically collated with programmes such as Microsoft Forms, Google Forms, and SurveyMonkey®. Recent examples of online surveys include exploring the impact of COVID-19 on the delivery of AAIs, albeit in health settings (Shoesmith et al., 2022), and an examination of UK primary teachers views of reading to dogs in schools, gathered via a survey distributed to online teaching forums (Steel et al., 2021).

Of course, online surveys carry the basic assumption that respondents have access to the Internet, while there is also a danger of survey fatigue and the lack of an interview to probe and clarify responses can lead to less reliable data. Nonetheless, it is common for academic researchers to use digital survey management tools such as Qualtrics survey software or SPSS (originally, Statistical Package for the Social Sciences). Prospective participants are typically directed to a link to complete the survey where they are first presented with a Participant Information Sheet and consent form.

The type, wording, order, and structure of questions are important. Surveys including anonymous ones typically begin with a section to complete on the characteristics of the respondents. For teachers, this might include their length of teaching experience and role, while basic information about dogs might cover their breed, age and size. Most questionnaires feature a mix of closed and open-ended questions. Closed questions are best used when alternative replies are known and can elicit people's beliefs about a topic (e.g., 'Do you agree that puppies should not feature in AAIs?'). Ranking scales for closed questions can help ascertain the level of importance for particular items, such as the reasons for bringing dogs into school. Open-ended questions are best suited when the objective is to find out why people believe what they do and to explore more complex subjects (e.g., the relationship between the well-being of the child and dog).

Occasionally researchers use vignettes as a means of teasing out what participants think about a topic. For example, one study exploring UK parental perceptions of canine-assisted activities in school posed the following vignette as part of its online survey:

> Your child is in a low mood as well as trouble making friends. The school suggests they spend weekly lunch breaks walking, playing and learning tricks with a trained AAT dog with an adult watching. This is intended to help their social skills, self-esteem, mood, and reduce anxiety.
>
> (Fynn & Runacres, 2022).

In this scenario, parents were then asked to rank their level of agreement (from strongly disagree to strongly agree) with statements such as the following:

- I find this treatment to be an acceptable way of dealing with the given problem;
- I believe the child will experience discomfort during the treatment;
- I believe it would be acceptable to use this treatment with individuals who cannot choose treatments for themselves (Fynn & Runacres, 2022).

The value of such vignettes is that they afford an authentic context for respondents to relate to, although there are limitations. The authors acknowledge several, including the wording of the vignettes and even the placement of a photograph of the researcher and her dog on the first page of the survey. This may have influenced which participants went on to complete the survey by appealing more to dog lovers. Moreover, in this study, almost half the sample owned a pet dog, which was more than double the reported percentage (24%) of UK households with a child and pet dog (PFMA, 2019). There is a danger of posing hypothetical scenarios along the lines of 'What would you do if …?' because what people say they might do is not always a reliable guide to their actual future behaviour (Gilbert, 2008). That said, hypothetical questions and problem-based scenarios can prove a useful means of stimulating debate between participants, especially in the context of group discussions.

Sometimes survey designers modify their surveys, for example to make them more reliable. For example, Munsell et al. (2004) found inconsistencies in the format of the original Pet Attitude Scale (PAS). Some of the questions were directed towards individuals who already had pets, whereas only one question had a qualifier for those who did not own pets. Hence a revised scale was drawn up (PAS-M) with reworded items, e.g., 'My pet means more to me than any of my friends' became 'My pet means more to me than any of my friends (or would if I had one)', although this additional tag could still be misread (is the 'one' referring to a pet or a friend?). Sometimes researchers pilot a questionnaire for the purpose of improving the overall quality of the survey. Gilbert (2008) recommends that in a proposed survey of 2,000 respondents, a pilot sample should include between 10 and 20, and this initial group must have similar characteristics to those of target population. Teachers might opt to run a questionnaire by a colleague or academic friend to check the questions are relevant, clearly and sensitively worded while avoiding pitfalls such as double-barrelled and leading questions.

As a check for internal consistency among respondents, surveys often include statements, the responses to which do not contribute to the overall score. For example, on the Stirling Children's Wellbeing Scale, the statements 'I have always told the truth', 'I like everyone I have met', and 'I always share my sweets' form a social desirability sub-scale. Overall scores of 14/15 (5 is the maximum for each statement) here means that the participants' well-being scores should be treated with caution. Grajfoner et al. (2017) used three scales while comparing the mood and well-being of university students before, during, and after interacting with a dog, a handler or both during a 20-minute session.

The general well-being surveys in Table 10.1 and those relating to AAIs in Table 10.2 have been chosen for convenience based on those we are familiar with, rather than the number of studies using these surveys or the rigorous methodology underpinning them. However, they do illustrate the kinds of surveys available, and the nature of items featured.

TABLE 10.1 Examples of scales used to measure aspects of well-being

Instrument and source	Focus and sample statements/questions	Age
The Warwick-Edinburgh Mental Wellbeing Scales (WEMWBS) https://warwick.ac.uk/fac/ sci/med/research/platform/ wemwbs/using/faq/	It assesses the change in mental well-being of individuals along a five-point scale. However, the survey is not designed to measure depression, but low scores do relate to depression. [None of the time – rarely – some of the time – often – all of the time] • 'I've been feeling relaxed'. • 'I've been dealing with problems well'. • 'I've been feeling close to other people'.	13–74

(Continued)

TABLE 10.1 (Continued)

Instrument and source	Focus and sample statements/questions	Age
Stirling Children's Wellbeing Scale Liddle and Carter (2014)	Measure emotional and psychological well-being along a five-point scale. [Never – not much of the time – some of the time – quite a lot of the time – all of the time] • 'I think good things will happen in my life'. • 'I always share my sweets'. • 'I feel I am good at some things'.	8–15
UWIST Mood Adjective Checklist (UMACL) Matthews et al. (1990)	A scale using factor hypothesis and associated adjectives: e.g., Hedonic: pleased, cheerful, optimistic, happy, gloomy, sad, sorry Anger: impatient, annoyed, angry, irritated, grouchy Tense: stirred up, fearful, anxious, tense, stressed, nervous Energetic: active, paler, bright, idle, sleepy, dull, tired, passive N.b. these are only examples of adjectives for each category	17–62
Myself as a Learner Scale (MALS) Burden (2014)	Young people's perceptions of themselves as learners and problem-solvers, based on responses to 20 questions along a five-point scale e.g., [definitely true (a) – a bit true (b) – not sure (c) – not very true (d) – definitely not true (e)] 'I know how to be a good learner'. 'I know how to solve the problems that I meet'. 'Learning is difficult'.	8–16
Pupil Attitudes to Self and School® (PASS) https://www.gl-assessment.co.uk/	Assesses how students feel about school and themselves as a learner, including connectedness, self-efficacy, and motivation using a 20-minute survey.	4–16+
Positive and Negative Affect Schedule for Children (PANAS-C) Ebesutani et al. (2012)	Assesses the frequency of positive and negative emotions in children, with the scale being shortened to suit needs, e.g., five points Question stem: 'Thinking about yourself and how you normally feel, to what extent do you generally feel …' positive affect (joyful, cheerful, happy, lively, proud) negative affect (miserable, mad, afraid, scared, sad)	6–18

TABLE 10.2 Examples of scales used to measure human-canine relationships

Instrument and source	Focus and sample statements/questions	Target age
Pet Attitude Scale (PAS) Templer et al. (1981) Pet Attitude Scale Modified (PAS-M) Munsell et al. (2004)	Measures attitudes towards pets using 18 items along a seven-point scale [Strongly disagree – moderately disagree – slightly disagree – unsure – slightly agree – moderately agree – strongly agree] I would like to have a pet in my home I feel that pets should always be kept outside I love pets	
Companion Animal Bonding Scale (CABS) Poresky et al. (1987)	Measures attachment to a dog using eight items along a five-point scale, both retrospectively (as a child) and as an adult. [Always – generally often – rarely – never] How often were you responsible for your companion animal's care? How often did you clean up after your companion animal? How often did you hold, stroke, or pet your companion animal?	16+
Child-Companion Animal Attachment Scale Endenburg et al. (2014)	Based on an adapted version of CABS, a nine-item measure of the attachment of Dutch children to their companion animals. How often do you hug [name of pet] per day?	3–13
Lexington Attachment to Pets Scale (LAPS) Johnson et al. (1992) and Zaparanick (2008)	Originally a telephonic survey in which respondents were asked to say whether they agree or disagree with very brief statements about their favourite pet. Later developed as an e-survey. [Strongly agree – somewhat agree – somewhat disagree – strongly disagree] General attachment, e.g., my pet understand me. People Substituting, e.g., my pet means more to me than any of my friends. Animal rights/welfare, e.g., pets deserve as much respect as humans do.	18+

MIXED METHODS RESEARCH

It is common for researchers to use a mixed methods approach. For example, one of our teacher researchers (Nicholas, 2021) wanted to know the benefits and limitations of a Reading to Dogs scheme, as perceived by ten of her Year 1 pupils (as participants), their parents, the teacher, and the headteacher. Her methodology involved a control group of five children who continued to read to staff only while the intervention group of five children read to a dog accompanied by a trained handler. All the pupil participants were of the same level of reading attainment and were allocated to groups based on random selection. Each session was held on the same afternoon each week for the same period. Diagnostic Reading Accuracy and comprehension assessments (DRA) were conducted at the start and end of the programme. To ascertain attitudes to learning, the teacher-researcher used the 'Myself as a Learner' (MALS) scale. Pupils were also asked pre and post initiative to complete a questionnaire regarding their views on reading and of themselves as learners. She captured qualitative data by keeping a diary of her experiences, through confidential, semi-structured interviews with pupils and teachers and by video-recording the reading sessions. By combining quantitative (numerical) and qualitative (textual) sources, her aim was to build up a more rounded picture of how the participants perceived the Reading to Dogs programme.

EVALUATING IMPACT

The implementation of any intervention can be analysed in multidimensional terms. Humphrey et al. (2016) identify eight dimensions, which we have adapted to form a simple framework to evaluate the impact of dog-assisted interventions (Table 10.3).

TABLE 10.3 Implementation dimensions and prompts for canine-assisted education

Dimension	Application
Fidelity/adherence treatment model	To what extent did the teacher and/or dog handler follow the intervention protocols? For example, follow any training guidance for dog handlers such as frequency of rests for dogs.
Dosage	How much of the intended intervention has been delivered and/or received? For example, in a programme of six 1-hour sessions over six weeks, how many were delivered? and how many were received by each individual child?
Quality	How well were different components of an intervention delivered? E.g., risk assessment, location, selected children, nature of activity.
Reach	How many children participated and for how long? Who else does or might benefit?
Responsiveness	How well did the child/children engage with the dog(s)? How well did the dog respond to the children and environment?
Programme differentiation	How different is this intervention to other, existing practice? E.g., reading to a dog compared to reading to a teacher.
Monitoring of control/comparison groups	What is taking place (in a trial context) in the absence of the intervention? For example, How do the feelings of children reading to a dog and toy dog compare?
Adaptation	Determination of the 'counterfactual' the nature and extent of changes made to the intervention, and how these elements interact

Based on Humphrey et al. (2016).

First, fidelity or 'delivery as intended' describes the extent to which implementers (e.g., teachers and dog handlers) adhere to any guidance provided, such as allowing children to choose which book to read with a dog or handwashing protocols. Second, the concept of dosage typically refers to the timed amount of an intervention, such as the number of reading sessions provided and the actual take-up among individuals. Children may miss certain sessions because of illness or if they were required to complete other work.

Fidelity and dosage are concerned with what and how much is delivered, whereas the third dimension of quality is about *how well* an intervention was implemented. Matters of quality include how well the teacher or dog handler prepared for the session, their understanding of basic concepts such as respecting the sentience of a dog and catering for its welfare needs, and the skills they demonstrate in the implementation of the intervention. Fourth, responsiveness refers to the extent to which the children interact with the dogs and are engaged in the tasks. This involves focusing on how well the intervention appears to stimulate children's interest and hold their attention. Fifth, reach is about the proportion of an eligible population that took part in the programme. For example, if school leaders identified four vulnerable children on the registers who they thought might benefit from therapy dog sessions, how many in practice did so.

The concept of reach can also apply to the potential that exists to extend the intervention to others. Sixth, programme differentiation describes what makes the intervention special or different to existing practices. In any school context, the likelihood is that several interventions will be occurring at a given moment. And so, it is important to be clear over whether changes in children's behaviour, learning, or well-being can be associated with the dog-assisted intervention and not something else. Seventh, researchers recognise the importance of setting up conditions that allow comparisons to be made between children exposed to an intervention and those who are not.

Researchers consider the need for a control/comparison group to be essential in ensuring that any change in outcome is attributable to the intervention and does not simply occur naturally over time. However, unlike hospital settings, in school contexts, it is very difficult to arrange for an 'untreated' control group because children are exposed to so many different influences. Durlak (1995) dismisses the idea as a fantasy. For teachers, it is more pragmatic and in keeping with professional enquiry to focus on the progress of individual learners over time. This can be measured using pre- and post-intervention measures such as surveys and interviews. Adaptation is the final implementation dimension. It is concerned with the changes that are made to any intervention.

The significance of the change depends upon the extent of the deviation from the programme objectives. If, for example, a school uses a therapy dog to support a child who has recently suffered bereavement, then whether the child reads or talks to the dog is insignificant. If, on the other hand, a school uses a reading dog to boost the confidence and fluency of reluctant readers, then it would be a significant change if the child decided only to play with the dog and not read during the session. Significant changes can also involve removal of core components of any intervention, such as the replacement of a dog handler with an untrained teacher assistant or a sizeable reduction in the duration of a programme. Such a change could also be of a philosophical nature. For example, if an intervention is based on the idea that a child reads to a dog who is laying down calmly, but the dog does not appear to settle, the handler may switch to a more active task such as throwing a ball outside.

CONCLUSION

One of the themes in this book is the need for school leaders to take seriously the question of bringing dogs into school. All interventions warrant careful planning, monitoring, and evaluating, particularly when these involve nonhuman animals who have their own thoughts, feelings, and needs. Ongoing research is also important in CAE because there is so much more we need to know about dogs in school, for example, in areas such as the most appropriate pedagogy, what doesn't work well, dog well-being, and sustaining perceived gains beyond the life of the intervention. If schools succeed in promoting happy, healthy, and humane relationships between children and dogs, then they will have gone a long way to nurturing the kind of values and dispositions which children need to flourish in this complex world. We should never take for granted the affection, companionship, and other qualities dogs provide:

> To be loved by a dog is a great privilege, perhaps one of the finest in a human life. May we prove ourselves worthy of it.
>
> (Wynne, 2019, p. 287)

REFERENCES

American Psychological Association (APA). (2017). *Ethical principles of psychologists and code of conduct.* https://www.apa.org/ethics/code

British Educational Research Association (BERA). (2018). *Ethical guidelines for educational research.* BERA. https://www.bera.ac.uk/publication/ethical-guidelines-for-educational-research-2018.

Cohen, L., Manion, L., & Morrison, K. (2011). *Research methods in education* (7th ed.). Routledge.

Cohen, L., Manion, L., & Morrison, K. (2017). *Research methods in education* (8th ed.). Routledge.

Connor, C., & Herzog, H. (2017). Methods for bridging human-animal interactions and education research. In N. Gee, A. H. Fine, & P. McCardle (Eds.), *How animals help students learn* (pp. 141–156). Routledge.

Coren, S. (2022). Kids who read out loud to a dog see improved literacy. *Psychology Today.* 3 November, https://www.psychologytoday.com/gb/blog/canine-corner/202211/kids-who-read-out-loud-dog-see-improved-literacy

Duindam, H. M., Creemers, H. E., Hoeve, M., & Asscher, J. J. (2021). Who lets the dog in? Differential effects of a dog-training program for incarcerated adults. *Anthrozoös, 34*(6), 839–861. https://doi.org/10.1080/08927936.2021.1938405

Durlak, J. A. (1995). *School-based prevention programs for children and adolescents.* Sage Publications.

Endenburg, N., van Lith, H. A., & Kirpensteijn, J. (2014). *Child-companion animal attachment scale [Database record].* APA PsycTests.

Fisher, B., & Cozens, M. (2014). The BaRK (Building Reading Confidence for Kids) canine assisted reading program: One child's experience. *Literacy Learning, 22*(1), 70.

Friedrich, J. A. (2019). The Role of Animal-Assisted Interventions in Communication Skills of Children with Autism, Ph.D. thesis, Walden University. https://scholarworks.waldenu.edu/cgi/viewcontent.cgi?article=7482&context=dissertations

Fynn, W. I., & Runacres, J. (2022). Dogs at school: A quantitative analysis of parental perceptions of canine-assisted activities in schools mediated by child anxiety score and use case. *ICEP, 16*(4). https://doi.org/10.1186/s40723-022-00097-x

Gilbert, N. (2008). *Researching social life* (3rd ed.). Sage.

Grajfoner, D., Harte, E., Potter, L. M., & McGuigan, N. (2017). The effect of dog-assisted intervention on student well-being, mood, and anxiety. *International Journal of Environmental Research and Public Health, 14*(5), 483. https://doi.org/10.3390/ijerph14050483

Hall, S., Gee, N. R., & Mills, D. S. (2016). Children reading to dogs: A systematic review of the literature. *Public Library of Science ONE, 11*(2). https://doi.org/10.1371/journal.pone.0149759

Hinic, K., Kowalski, M. O., Holtzman, K., & Mobus, K. (2019). The effect of a pet therapy and comparison intervention on anxiety in hospitalized children. *Journal of Pediatric Nursing, 46,* 55–61.

Humphrey, N., Lendrum, A., Ashworth, E., Frearson, K., Buck, R., & Kerr, K. (2016). *Implementation and process evaluation (IPE) for interventions in education settings: A synthesis of the literature.* University of Manchester. https://educationendowmentfoundation.org.uk/public/files/Evaluation/Setting_up_an_Evaluation/IPE_Handbook.pdf

Hutchinson, D., & Styles, B. (2010). *A guide to running randomised controlled trials for educational researchers.* NFER.

Lewis, H., Grigg, R., & Knight, C. (2022). An international survey of animals in schools: Exploring what sorts of schools involve what sorts of animals, and educators' rationales for these practices. *People and Animals: The International Journal of Research and Practice, 5*(1), Article 15. https://docs.lib.purdue.edu/paij/vol5/iss1/15

London, K. (2021). What happens when kids read books with dogs. 14 July, *The Wildest.* https://www.thewildest.com/dog-lifestyle/reading-dogs-benefits-children

Munsell, K., Canfield, M., Templer, D., Tangan, K., & Arikawa, H. (2004). Modification of the pet attitude scale. *Society & Animals, 12*(2), 137–142.

Pet Food Manufacturers Association (PFMA). (2019). Families with pets 2019. https://www.ukpetfood.org/_assets/docs/annual-reports/PFMA-2019-Annual-Report.pdf

Punch, K. (2009). *Introduction to research methods in education.* Sage.

Shoesmith, E., Gibsone, S., & Ratschen, E. (2022). The impact of Covid-19 on animal-assisted interventions: Perceptions of UK animal-assisted intervention providers, *Journal of Public Health,* fdac126. https://doi.org/10.1093/pubmed/fdac126

Signal, T., Taylor, N., Prentice, K., McDade, M., & Burke, K. (2017). Going to the dogs: A quasi-experimental assessment of animal assisted therapy for children who have experienced abuse. *Applied Developmental Science, 21*(2), 81–93. https://doi.org/10.1080/10888691.2016.1165098

Steel, J., Williams, J. M., & McGeown, S. (2021). Reading to dogs in schools: An exploratory study of teacher perspectives. *Educational Research, 63*(3), 279–301. https://doi.org/10.1080/00131881.2021.1956989

Stern, E., Stame, N., Mayne, J., Forss, K., Davies, R., & Befani, B. (2012). Broadening the range of designs and methods for impact evaluations. *Department for International Development Working Paper.* https://assets.publishing.service.gov.uk/government/uploads/system/uploads/attachment_data/file/67427/design-method-impact-eval.pdf

Styles, B., & Torgerson, C. (2018). Randomised controlled trials (RCTs) in education research – Methodological debates, questions, challenges. *Educational Research, 60*(3), 255–264. https://doi.org/10.1080/00131881.2018.1500194

Uccheddu, S., Albertini, M., Pierantoni, L., Fantino, S., & Pirrone, F. (2019). The impacts of a reading-to-dog programme on attending and reading of nine children with autism spectrum disorders. *Animals, 9*(8), 491. https://doi.org/10.3390/ani9080491

Wohlfarth, R., Mutschler, B., Beetz, A., & Schleider, K. (2014). An investigation into the efficacy of therapy dogs on reading performance in 6-7-year-old children. *Human-Animal Interaction Bulletin, 2*(2), 60–73.

Wynne, C. (2019). *Dog is love.* Quercus.

APPENDIX A

USEFUL TEMPLATES

The following examples provide starting points for developing documentation relating to implementing a school dog initiative. These would need adapting depending on the individual children and dogs involved, and the school context.

Risk Assessment for School Dog: **Buddy**

Hazard/ Risk	Who is at Risk?	How can the hazards cause harm?	Are the following adequate control measures in place?	Y/N/ N/A
Zoonoses: Ticks, fleas, roundworms etc.	Staff Pupils Visitors	Disease/infections, e.g., toxocariasis (roundworm)	• Buddy treated monthly for worms and fleas. • Buddy has annual health check and booster injections. • Buddy groomed and checked weekly. • Buddy has a specific and separate toilet area behind the car park so away from children. • Buddy's waste to be bagged appropriately and disposed of in designated bins • Handwashing policy in place for everyone interacting with Buddy. • Wipes/ cleaning products available.	
Bites and scratches	Staff Pupils Visitors	Disease/infections/ pain	• Children taught how to interact with Buddy safely. • Children closely supervised. • Petting by invite from handler and consent from Buddy only. • Buddy trained not to jump up. • Buddy's claws clipped regularly.	
Phobias	Staff Pupils Visitors	Fear and anxiety Possible non-attendance	• Parents/carers/children asked to inform of any concern. • Only those who have given consent will interact. • Contact with Buddy is not compulsory. • Clear working areas for Buddy identified, and his timetable shared. • Buddy has a sign on the door when he is in a room.	

(Continued)

Hazard/ Risk	Who is at Risk?	How can the hazards cause harm?	Are the following adequate control measures in place?	Y/N/ N/A
Allergy	Staff Pupils Visitors	Allergic reaction, e.g., skin rashes, irritation to the eyes and nose, breathing difficulties	• Parents/carers/children asked to inform of any concern. • Only those who have given consent will interact. • Buddy groomed thoroughly before visits. • Buddy regularly professionally groomed. • A lint roller is to be used on clothing after contact with the Buddy. • Children wash hands immediately afterwards. • Clear working areas for Buddy identified, and his timetable shared. • Buddy has a sign on the door when he is in a room.	
Slips, trips and falls	Staff Pupils Visitors Buddy	Injury may be caused by new hazards, e.g., leads, bowls, blankets.	• Provision of floor matting to be available for Buddy if he is working in the hall. • Sessions to take place away from busy areas – without causing obstruction to walkways or emergency exits. • Ensure we don't cause trip hazard to any persons while session taking place (e.g., no bags, leads in walkways).	

(*Continued*)

Hazard/ Risk	Who is at Risk?	How can the hazards cause harm?	Are the following adequate control measures in place?	Y/N/ N/A
Buddy's well-being	Buddy	Buddy may be overwhelmed, anxious, or hurt.	• Buddy has a well-being assessment from external behaviourist twice a year in school. • Buddy has a clear timetable that ensures he is only in school for set periods of up to 2 hours, and on set days, no more than three per week. • His visit to school will always start before children arrive and with a walk around the grounds. • Quiet 'spot' for Buddy to go to rest when he chooses. • Jane (Buddy's owner) present with Buddy when he is in school. • Buddy typically kept on loose lead if not in session with child. • Whole school training on canine body language, canine consent and positive training. • Physical contact during sessions with children must be under full guidance of Jane. • Planning includes plentiful opportunities for Buddy to enjoy sessions, e.g., in the garden. • Buddy loves treats but must be monitored so that he is not given anything dangerous, e.g., chocolate, or too many treats. • Any child with unpredictable physical or emotional behaviours will be monitored closely during interactions and these will cease if Buddy appears concerned.	

Additional control

	Further control measures	**Action by whom**	**Action by when**	**Action completed**	**RRR***
Purpose	To take account of local/ individual circumstances including changes such as working practices, equipment, staffing levels.	To list the name of the person/ people who have been designated to conduct actions.	**To set timescales for the completion of the actions –** remember to prioritise them.	To record the actual date of completion for each action listed.	
	A newly qualified teacher is joining the staff in September. A new reading scheme is being piloted in Year 2.	Jane is responsible for Buddy while he is in school and her timetable reflects this. Leadership Team to ensure that all of the above practices are carried out.	As required	September 2023	L

Evaluative comments:

Residual Risk Rating (RRR)*		**Action required**
Very high (H)	Strong likelihood of fatality/serious injury occurring	The activity must not take place at all.
High (H)	Possibility of fatality/serious injury occurring	You must identify further controls to reduce the risk rating.
Medium (M)	Possibility of significant injury	If it is not possible to lower risk further, to consider the risk against the benefit. Monitor risk assessments at this rating regularly and closely.
Low (L)	Possibility of minor injury only	No further action required, but monitor throughout year in case this changes.

LETTER TO PARENTS, CARERS AND CHILDREN

Insert School logo, etc.

Dear Parents, Carers, and Children,

We have news of an exciting project that will begin
at _____ school in October.

_____(e.g., Ms Jane Jones and her dog Buddy)
have been working very hard so that Buddy can
become our own School Dog.

Buddy will be able to provide comfort, encourage positive behaviour, motivate
speech, and inspire us all to have fun in school. Having Buddy in school will
also help us all to understand how to respect and care for animals and be less
fearful and safe around unknown dogs.

Buddy will be in school on _____ (e.g., Monday, Wednesday, and
Friday mornings between 8.40 and 11 am). Buddy will be based in _____
(e.g., Ms Jones' office). He will also visit _____(e.g., the hall, library, school
garden, and Classes 2 and 6) while he is in school.

We hope to seek your support for this project and ask you to sign the consent form below. We also offer the option for you to include some additional
information if you wish so that we can help your child get the best out of the
scheme.

Please could you return the form to _____(school email address).

If you would like more information about Buddy and the project, please see
the school's website where Buddy has his own section.

Parent/Guardian consent slip

Does your child have an allergy to pets?   Yes/No

Is your child nervous around dogs?   Yes/No

I am **happy/not happy** (*delete as appropriate*) to consent to my child .... spending time with Buddy the school dog.

Parent signature...

Date...............................

Please return to Ms Jones

Additional Information (Optional)

Name of child ....

Does your child have any experience in being around dogs? Please summarise, i.e., dogs at home/ relatives/friends' houses, etc.

Is there anything you feel it would be useful for (e.g., Mrs. Jones) to know so that your child may get the best out of the sessions? For example, specific interest in dogs, hobbies, etc.

DOG'S GETTING TO KNOW YOU PROFILE

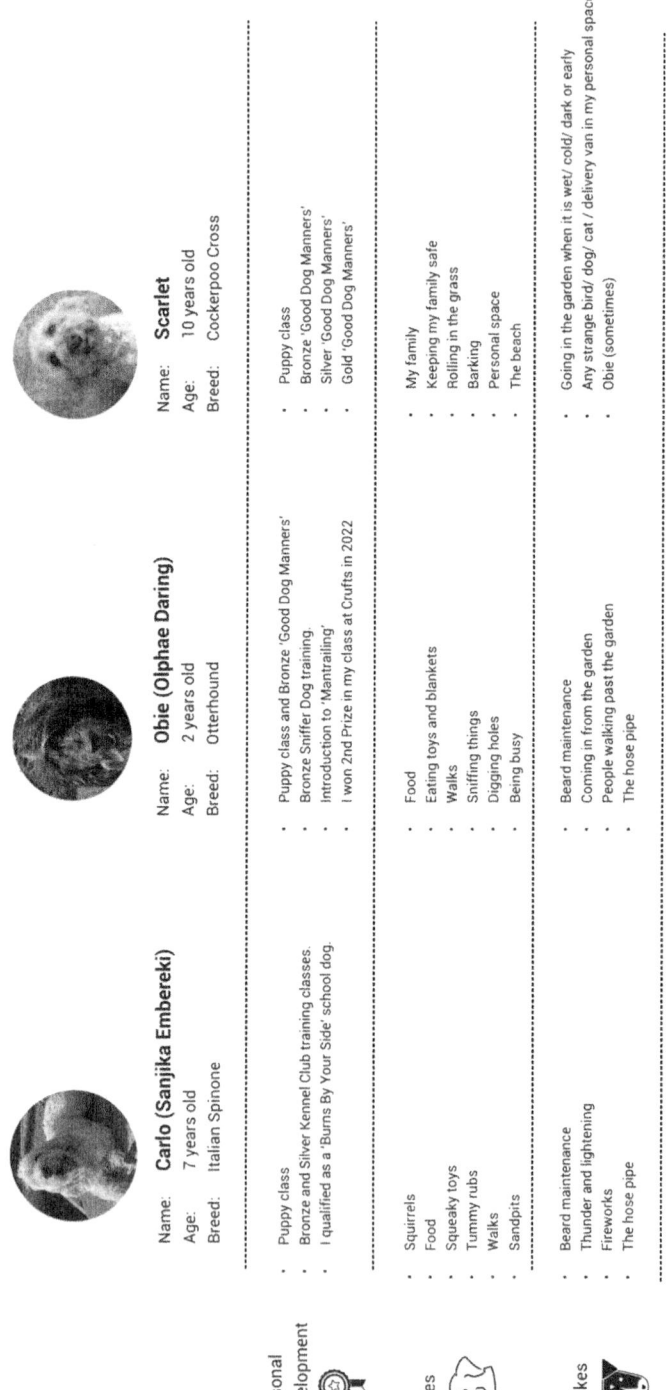

Name: Carlo (Sanjika Embereki)
Age: 7 years old
Breed: Italian Spinone

Name: Obie (Olphae Daring)
Age: 2 years old
Breed: Otterhound

Name: Scarlet
Age: 10 years old
Breed: Cockerpoo Cross

Personal development

Carlo:
- Puppy class
- Bronze and Silver Kennel Club training classes.
- I qualified as a 'Burns By Your Side' school dog.

Obie:
- Puppy class and Bronze 'Good Dog Manners'
- Bronze Sniffer Dog training.
- Introduction to 'Mantrailing'
- I won 2nd Prize in my class at Crufts in 2022

Scarlet:
- Puppy class
- Bronze 'Good Dog Manners'
- Silver 'Good Dog Manners'
- Gold 'Good Dog Manners'

Likes

Carlo:
- Squirrels
- Food
- Squeaky toys
- Tummy rubs
- Walks
- Sandpits

Obie:
- Food
- Eating toys and blankets
- Walks
- Sniffing things
- Digging holes
- Being busy

Scarlet:
- My family
- Keeping my family safe
- Rolling in the grass
- Barking
- Personal space
- The beach

Dislikes

Carlo:
- Beard maintenance
- Thunder and lightening
- Fireworks
- The hose pipe

Obie:
- Beard maintenance
- Coming in from the garden
- People walking past the garden
- The hose pipe

Scarlet:
- Going in the garden when it is wet/ cold/ dark or early
- Any strange bird/ dog/ cat / delivery van in my personal space
- Obie (sometimes)

APPENDIX B

STARTER ACTIVITIES FOR PLAYING GAMES WITH DOGS

With contributors Katie Howells and Amber Roach

The following ideas relate to games for dogs who like to sniff, retrieve, paw, rip, or problem-solve. Of course, many dogs would enjoy all these activities, but just like people they are likely to have preferences. Planning and preparing these activities can also be beneficial for children's independence and self-esteem, their fine and gross motor skills, communication, and creative and critical thinking skills. Furthermore, playing games together strengthens the relationship between child, dog, and potentially the handler.

Before starting, a useful behaviour to develop is 'Watch me'. This behaviour is an effective way to get the dog's attention before beginning any game. Start with a tasty treat. Show this to the dog, and then hold it out to the side. The dog will naturally look at the treat. Wait until they stop looking at it and make eye contact with you. Immediately mark and reward that behaviour – it may only be a fleeting glance, so timing is very important here. Keep practising until the dog starts making consistent eye contact and then introduce the 'Watch Me' command. Over time, as the dog begins to do this consistently, gradually increase the watch by a second at a time.

The following simple starter activities can use readily available items, so they are quick and easy to prepare. The activities can all become increasingly challenging once the dog masters the basics, although, just like children ensuring sessions finish with success and positive reinforcement is crucial.

1. DOGS WHO LOVE SNIFFING

Sniffing is important for all dogs, and it can give them the mental stimulation they need. But some dogs instinctively need to use their noses far more than others, for example, scent hounds such as otterhounds, and gundogs such as spaniels have been specifically bred to scent. These dogs have their noses to the ground almost constantly. They may love games such as those outlined in Figure B1.

1 Shoebox Hide and Seek

Collect a set of empty containers like shoeboxes or takeaway containers with a few holes in the top. Place the containers in a group on the floor and put some smelly treats in one. Then allow the dog to sniff all the containers to search for the hidden treasure. Mark and reward when they find the correct one. This can be extended to find boxes hidden in increasingly challenging places, or to find smaller and smaller boxes but build this slowly to ensure success. This activity is good for children's creative thinking and gross motor skills too.

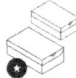

2 Snuffle Mat

These are textured mats, often with longer bits of material. Lay the mat out and scatter some kibble or other tasty treats such as small pieces of meat or cheese under the pieces of material. Let the dog sniff around until they have found each piece. Snuffle mats are widely available as readymade items online or in pet shops or can easily be made by cutting up some old material and threading/tying them through holes in an old towel (or doormat with holes). Preparing the snuffle mat is a good activity to develop fine motor skills in children.

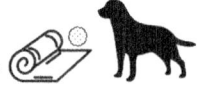

3 Find It

This is a game that helps build some impulse control. Start with a paper cup or empty tin (something light enough for the dog to knock over) and tasty treats. Ask the dog to wait and place a treat on top of the cup. Release the dog to get his treat. After a few times, place the treat in different places around the cup to get the dog used to the association between the cup and the food. Place the treat half under the rim of the cup, so it is still visible, and release the dog to fetch their treat. Place the treat fully under the cup and wait for the dog to find it. This may take them a while the first few times – this is all part of the game. Once the dog can manipulate the cup to get their treat out quickly every time, add in a cue word – "Find it!".

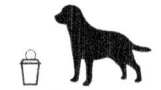

4 Scent bags

Make a 'scent bag' by tying something very smelly in a piece of cloth or small fabric bag (e.g., the ones that come with boxes of washing capsules). Blue cheese, liver, tripe or pate work well. Attach string to the bag so it can be pulled along the ground. Start with simple short trails before extending to a winding, zigzagging path. Leave a special surprise jackpot at the end of the trail for your dog to find, typically a small pot of soft cheese or peanut butter works well as the dog must lick this which takes a few seconds, building the satisfaction. Make sure the scent bag itself is out of the way, otherwise the dog may just focus on that.

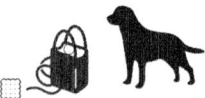

FIGURE B1 Games for dogs who love sniffing.

2.   DOGS WHO LOVE CHEWING, LICKING, AND RIPPING THINGS UP

Ripping up things (unfortunately sometimes mail, books, or boxes) is something many dogs do. This can be a sign of boredom, frustration, or anxiety when left alone, but for many dogs ripping behaviour is very satisfying. It provides plenty of mental stimulation and physical activity. Just like children who prefer playing with the empty box than the expensive toy, for many dogs the chance to shred, chew, and tear a box is very satisfying.

Many dogs will find licking an enriching activity. When a dog licks, it soothes and calms them, releasing endorphins and creating a sense of safety and calm. The bumps on a lick mat help to clean a dog's teeth, massage their gums, and promote salivation all of which can reduce tartar build-up and promote healthy oral hygiene. For dogs like these, the games depicted in Figure B2 may prove helpful.

1 **Destruction Box**

The simplest way to set this up is to keep aside some old boxes from deliveries and junk mail. Put a selection of items in the box, with a handful of kibble or smelly treats. Practice "wait" with the dog whilst preparing the box and set it aside for them. When ready, release the dog to search for the food in the box. They are free to rip up whatever they want in the box, and they get a reward at the end for finding the food. Predicting which items the dog will prefer, or how long they will take to find the treats might engage children. Adding different textures will provide even more mental stimulation for the dog. Try using kitchen roll, cardboard tubes, or egg boxes in the destruction box. This could be a good home-school connection, as parents may be willing to send in items from their recycling. Just be careful that all materials are safe.

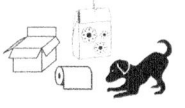

2 **Lick mat**

A lick mat is usually a flat silicon mat covered with small bumps and ridges to trap food and encourage licking. Children can develop fine motor skills as they spread different foods onto the mat for the dog. Lick mat recipes are a great way to add variety to a dog's diet, whilst also helping children gain a better understanding of healthy eating for dogs. Dry dog food or wet food can be put onto a lick mat. for example, by crumbling dry food, pouring on wet ingredients, or mashing up fruits. Children can test which recipes the dogs enjoy most or keep a record of how many licks a dog does in a certain amount of time.

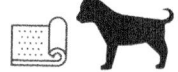

FIGURE B2 Games for dogs who love chewing, licking, and ripping things up.

3. DOGS WHO LOVE TO USE THEIR PAWS

Some dogs are keen to offer their paws, often to indicate that they would like attention. Just as most human favour using their right or left hand, many dogs show a preference for using one paw over the other. Finding out which paw a dog prefers to use could be an interesting enquiry project for children. Dogs may enjoy playing 'Which hand?' or Target Touches (Figure B3). However, it is worth being mindful that pawing behaviours for attention or food are generally not desirable in a CAE context, so these games need to be played judiciously.

1   High Five

Hold a treat for the dog in a closed fist and show the dog. As soon as they paw at the hand, give them the treat and either use a clicker to mark the action or say 'yes'. Continue doing this a few times before marking the action by saying 'high five'. Gradually move the hand so that the dog reaches for it, and over time try using an open hand and rewarding after the dog has touched this.

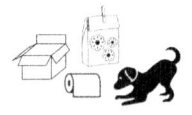

2   Which hand?

Ask the dog to stay in the sit position and allow them to watch as a treat is placed in one hand. Close hands into a downward facing fist and extend them out to the dog and ask, "which hand?" Once the dog touches or signals the correct hand praises them and gives them the treat. This game can be extended by moving hands behind your back for a few seconds before presenting them to the dog – they then need to also use their sniffing skills to find the correct hand.

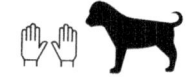

3   Paw target touches

Refresh the dog's skills at giving his paw, every time his paw touches your hand mark and reward with a tasty treat. Place a post-it note over your hand and ask the dog for paw. The dog may be a little unsure of the foreign object but give him time and when the paw touches the target, mark and reward. Practise step 2 at least 5 times to get the dog familiar with touching this new target. Move the target to the floor and ask the dog for paw. Move the target on to an object you'd like your dog to be able to touch e.g., a button or bell, every time your dog's paw contacts the button, mark and reward.

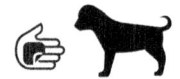

FIGURE B3 Games for dogs who love to use their paws.

4. DOGS WHO LIKE TO SOLVE PROBLEMS

Some dogs enjoy solving problems and puzzles and there are many to choose from. Food dispensing toys, for example, come in a variety of shapes and sizes, and provide challenge of differing levels. These might include tubes that a dog needs to knock to get food out of, or a puzzle box that the dog can learn to open. Whilst many are commercially available, there are simple activities that can be developed using resources such as paper cups (Figure B4).

1 The Shell Game (building on Find it)

Have three cups in front of the dog, place a treat under one cup and allow the dog to find the hidden treat. Increase the difficulty of this game by switching the cups around after hiding the treat.

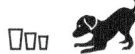

2 Hide and Seek

Have the dog sit in a stay position (or enlist help if the dog keeps following). Find a hiding spot. Call the dog. Praise them when they find you and use high quality treats. Increase the distances and complexity of hiding places over time to add excitement to the game.

3 The Muffin Tin Game

Use an empty muffin tin, for six (or 12) muffins. Take six (or 12) tennis balls. Put some of the dog's favourite treats into one or two of the muffin tin holes and cover them with tennis balls. Next, put tennis balls into all the other empty muffin tin holes. Give the "puzzle" to the dog and let them explore by moving the balls to find the treats hidden underneath.

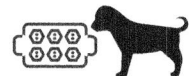

FIGURE B4 Games for dogs who like to solve problems.

5.   DOGS WHO LIKE TO FETCH AND CARRY

The word 'fetch' derives from Old English *facian*, which means 'grasp and bring near', just as dogs grasp things in their mouth before returning with them. Although breeds such as Golden Retrievers were specifically bred to retrieve prey to hunters without causing damage, not all dogs will naturally retrieve or know how to play fetch. But they can be taught to do so through games (Figure B5). These can also be rewarding for children to participate in.

1   Rope fetch

Tie between 2-5 knots into a length of rope. Bear in mind that the longer the length of rope, the heavier the rope will be to toss. Throw the rope at increasingly further distances and in different directions to test your dogs' agility and co-ordination

2   Squeaky toy throw

For dogs who love the noise, squeaky toys are very popular. Lightweight rubber versions are easy to throw but not suitable as chew toys. Experiment with throwing the squeaky toy in different directions, concealing and squeaking it, standing in different positions.

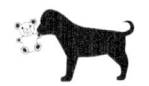

3   Frisbee toss

Frisbee throwing requires skill, coordination, and timing. Roll the Frisbee on the ground towards the dog, and most dogs will instinctually grab it. The Frisbee can then be tossed at increasingly higher levels to test the dogs' agility and acrobatic skill.

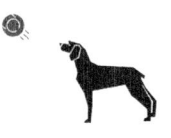

FIGURE B5 Games for dogs who like to like to fetch and carry.

6.   NAME THE TOY GAME

Dogs can also be trained to learn the name of toys, and this can be a great source of playful fun (Figure B6).

   Chaser the border collie knew the individual name of thousands of her toys, and responded to her owner John Pilley's requests to bring a toy, or place the toy somewhere specific, for example, 'Chaser bring Flipflopper. Drop Flipflopper in the bin' (Pilley, 2013). This remarkable relationship developed through playful relationships, an understanding of dogs, and time. Pilley adopted the approach of 'errorless learning'. This is a mindset that encourages trainers carefully and creatively arrange the learning environment and training plans for an animal. With the errorless learning mindset, animals experience higher levels of discretionary effort and success, which will greatly improve their welfare (Friedman, 2016, p. 8). Pilley's daughter Bianchi explains 'He would name it, show it to her, say "catch blue" and throw it to her. He'd put it in front of her and say "find blue". On the third day, when she could retrieve the ball from another room, he knew it was time to move on to another object' (Mood, 2019).

The Toy Name Game

To train a dog for this kind of activity, start by playing with the dog and one specific toy, giving it a name while you do. After some practice & praise your dog will assign that verbal name with the chosen toy. Once the dog has learned that specific toys name you can test their skills by seeing if they can pick it out among their other toys. After the dog knows the name of one toy you can move on teaching them the name of another.

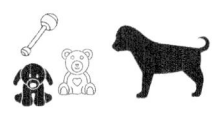

FIGURE B6 Name the Toy Game.

INDEX

Printed in Dunstable, United Kingdom